A CASEBOOK OF ETHICAL CHALLENGES IN NEUROPSYCHOLOGY

STUDIES ON NEUROPSYCHOLOGY, DEVELOPMENT, AND COGNITION

Series Editor:

Linas Bieliauskas, Ph.D.
University of Michigan, Ann Arbor, MI, USA

A CASEBOOK OF ETHICAL CHALLENGES IN NEUROPSYCHOLOGY

Edited by

Shane S. Bush

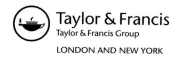

Taylor & Francis
Taylor & Francis Group

LONDON AND NEW YORK

First published 2005 by Psychology Press,
27 Church Road, Hove, East Sussex BN3 2FA

Simultaneously published in the USA and Canada
by Psychology Press
270 Madison Avenue, New York, NY 10016

Psychology Press is a part of the Taylor & Francis Group

Copyright © 2005 Psychology Press

Typeset by Charon Tec Pvt. Ltd, Chennai, India
Printed and bound in Great Britain by TJ International Ltd, Padstow, Cornwall
Cover design by Magenta Grafische Producties, Bert Haagsman and Jim Wilkie

The publisher makes no representation, express or implied, with regard to the accuracy of the information contained in this book and cannot accept any legal responsibility or liability for any errors or omissions that may be made.

This publication has been produced with paper manufactured to strict environmental standards and with pulp derived from sustainable forests.

British Library Cataloguing in Publication Data
A catalogue record for this book is available from the British Library

Library of Congress Cataloging-in-Publication Data
Applied for

ISBN 90-265-1974-5

To Dana Bush, Ph.D. and our daughters Sarah and Megan

CONTENTS

FROM THE SERIES EDITOR

Changes in the American Psychological Association's (APA's) *Ethical Principles* were published during the same year that the volume *Ethical Issues in Clinical Neuropsychology*, edited by Shane Bush and Michael Drexler, appeared in our series. This volume, *A Casebook of Ethical Challenges in Neuropsychology*, edited by Shane Bush, explores many specific applications of the new principles in the clinical neuropsychological setting. As pointed out by Richard Naugle in the forward to this text, the new principles are not always obvious in terms of appropriate application. There are changes with regard to release of test material, changes with respect to sensitivity to cultural and ethnic diversity of patients, and changes with demands of physically seeing patients vs. blindly reviewing test data as just some examples.

The authors in this volume are solid and well-known clinicians who have faced many of the situations we can imagine as clinical neuropsychologists and provide keen insight into reasonable and practical applications of the APA *Ethical Principles* in our specific practice settings. The book is organized by major settings and significant areas where ethical concerns arise, with a particularly appropriate appendix targeting one of the most nettlesome of practice arenas, forensic neuropsychology, where neuropsychologists often end up on adversarial sides in the courtroom. Guidance is provided in specific case examples along with descriptions of resolutions of ethical dilemmas. In addition to the evident utility of such a text for the practicing clinician, the mandate of APA for training in ethical issue to students at all levels makes this book and the earlier volume ideal references for teaching in programs emphasizing Clinical Neuropsychology. Dr. Bush is to be commended for his fine and readable rendering of relevant ethical issues and, again, for bringing an impressive contribution to our series. *Ethical Issues*, and *A Casebook* will undoubtedly help to improve the sophistication and humanity of the clinical services we provide.

Linas A. Bieliauskas
Ann Arbor
February, 2004

FOREWORD

In the curricula of many graduate programs, the *Ethical Principles of Psychologists and Code of Conduct* seems to receive relatively little attention. Students often learn about some aspects of the code in the context of clinical vignettes or clinical supervision, but that approach does not serve students well. A comprehensive understanding of the ethics code requires more than a piecemeal approach. Although students can readily identify the most clear-cut violations, such as initiating intimate relationships with supervisees or patients, they often lack a more detailed understanding of other aspects of the code. Even after a careful reading of its contents, I have found myself questioning the implications of this or that section in the context of some situation that presented itself in the course of my practice. Situations that seem to be black and white in the text of the code often appear in varying shades of gray in everyday practice.

For example, Section 9.02(c) states that "Psychologists use assessment methods that are appropriate to an individual's language preference and competence ..." and Section 9.06 states that, "When interpreting assessment results, including automated interpretations, psychologists take into account the purpose of the assessment as well as the various test factors, test-taking abilities, and other characteristics of the person being assessed, such as situational, personal, *linguistic, and cultural differences*, that might affect psychologists' judgments or reduce the accuracy of their interpretations. They indicate any significant limitations of their interpretations (italics added)." Certainly, to obtain valid assessment results, a patient must be able to readily understand the examiner and be equally capable of expressing his/her intended response. To test anyone in a language other than his or her primary language is to place a tremendous additional burden on the examinee. As a result, there is little defense for the neuropsychologist who, despite not speaking Spanish, examines a Hispanic patient in a region of the country where there are ample Spanish-speaking neuropsychologists. But what of the patient who speaks a less frequently encountered language or resides in a part of the country where no neuropsychologists exist who are capable of examining the patient using his/her primary language? Is it meritorious to decline to test the patient out of recognition of the threats to the validity of the results of any such examination with full understanding of the fact that the patient will then be denied service altogether? Section 3.01 state that "In their work-related activities, psychologists do not engage in unfair discrimination based on age, gender, gender identity, race, *ethnicity, culture, national origin*, religion, sexual orientation, disability, socioeconomic status, or any basis proscribed by law (italics added)." Could the denial of service even under these circumstances be regarded as unfair discrimination based on the patient's ethnicity, culture, or national origin and, consequently, constitute a violation of Section 3.01? If no one is available to examine a patient in his or her language, is it defensible to proceed with the assessment but explain the threats to validity when reporting the results of that examination? There is no clear course of action when faced with this situation; one who assumes that there is only need express that decision and brace oneself for the response from colleagues. It is advisable that, after accepting responsibility or refusing to assess a given patient, one be capable of explaining one's reasoning in the context of the ethical code.

Although the recently-released (2002) update of the ethical code was intended to answer questions that arose from the previous version published in 1992, it does not (and should not be expected to) provide answers to all possible dilemmas. For example, in the earlier version of the ethics code, psychologists were instructed in Section 2.02 to "take reasonable steps to prevent others from misusing the information [provided by assessment techniques, interventions, results and interpretations]. This includes refraining from releasing raw test results or raw data to persons, other than to patients or clients as appropriate, who are not qualified to use such information." This was typically interpreted to mean that assessment data were to be sent only to other psychologists. Practitioners whose clinical work entailed seeing patients for forensic purposes were sometimes perceived as obstructionistic when they refused to provide raw test data to attorneys on the basis that they were "not qualified to use such information." In defense of the practice of releasing raw test data to non-psychologists, it was argued by some that test protocols, test items, answers and even manuals could be readily accessed by visiting a local campus bookstore or, increasingly, surfing the internet. Attempting to limit the release of those materials by refusing to disclose them to attorneys was tantamount to closing the barn door after the cows had left. Section 9.04 of the newer version of the code states simply that, "Pursuant to a client/patient release, psychologists provide test data to the client/patient or other persons identified in the release." This broader wording suggests that test data can be provided to attorneys. Yet Section 9.11 of the same version of the code just as clearly states that psychologists continue to have a responsibility to protect the security of the test materials used by the profession in order to maintain the integrity of those materials. Releasing test data often entails distributing test stimuli, thereby ignoring the need to maintain their security. As a result, we must now ask ourselves to which portion of the code should we adhere? Which section supercedes the other? I have found that attorneys will, without hesitation, provide a decisive answer to that question but, again, it is incumbent on the psychologist to provide a

reasoned response that reflects an understanding of the ethics code.

Similarly, Section 8.06 of the 2002 code states that psychologists "avoid offering excessive or inappropriate financial or other inducements for research participation when such inducements are likely to coerce participation." For many, this principle has led to the conclusion that children should not be provided a financial or other incentive because that incentive would necessarily be paid to a parent or guardian who might in turn coerce the child's participation for their own gain. For this reason, research regarding treatment alternatives for children has sometimes lagged behind similar research with adults. To the extent that the development of potentially effective treatment interventions has slowed as a result of the effort to protect potentially vulnerable research subjects, that portion of the code will have caused harm to the very subjects it was intended to protect. Reasoning through this polemic requires a thorough understanding of the code and other documents, such as the Nuremberg Code and the Belmont Report, and the behaviors that those documents are intended to encourage or discourage. Again, it is rare that course work provides this level of understanding.

If thorough instruction regarding the code is not provided in graduate programs, then how is one to obtain that level of understanding? In my experience, that level of knowledge comes from grappling with ethical dilemmas and solving them through considerable reflection and, in some instances, consultation with peers. One need not enter clinical practice with only a superficial understanding of the ethical principles of our profession, however. This text will go a considerable distance in eliciting that reflection. By providing instances of ethical dilemmas that others have faced and the solutions they reached, the authors of the chapters of this book will dramatically advance the reader's understanding of the *Ethical Principles of Psychologists and Code of Conduct*. This book, like Dr. Bush's previous offering, *Ethical Issues in Clinical Neuropsychology*, constitutes a much needed overview of the ethical code of psychologists. It is particularly timely because it also reviews the changes from the 1992 version of the code to the newer iteration published last year. For these reasons, this text should be required reading not only for students of the profession but for all who provide neuropsychological services in order to maximize their understanding of the spirit as well as the letter of the code.

Richard I. Naugle, PhD., ABPP
November 2003

PREFACE

Ethical Issues in Clinical Neuropsychology (Bush & Drexler, 2002) was the first text devoted solely to identifying and examining ethical standards of practice in neuropsychology. As such, it offered the reader one reference for locating most of the primary ethical concerns facing clinical neuropsychologists. Such issues had previously been found in various articles and book chapters or had not been fully examined in the literature at all. Although most of the issues examined in that text transcend any single ethics code, the publication of the new Ethical Principles of Psychologists and Code of Conduct (hereinafter referred to as the Ethics Code; American Psychological Association, 2002) in the same year as the text resulted in a need for a supplement to integrate the overarching principles of ethical neuropsychological activities with the updated requirements for psychologists more generally. The current text, conceptualized as a companion to the 2002 text, is intended both to bridge that gap and to examine an expanded range of ethical challenges. This book was undertaken with two primary purposes: (1) to relate ethical issues in neuropsychology to the 2002 APA Ethics Code, and (2) to animate the ethical issues through case illustrations. Although publications are available that describe the 2002 Ethics Code in general (Fisher, 2003; Knapp & VandeCreek, 2003), this text examines in greater detail the implications for neuropsychology.

In the four-plus years since preparation for the first book began, a number of articles related to neuropsychological ethics have been published, each contributing in some way to the evolution of neuropsychological ethics. In addition to reviewing such articles, discussions of aspects of professional ethics with people who have written and lectured widely on such matters, as well as with others who are not known professionally outside of their local communities, may contribute to the further evolution of one's understanding of ethical issues in neuropsychology.

One observation stemming from my discussions with colleagues is that many of those respected as experts in neuropsychological ethics disagree on aspects of appropriate professional behavior, some quite passionately. Within this text and between this text and its predecessor, such divergence of opinions may be seen. Even authors of chapters within the same section may not agree on conceptualizations of ethical behavior or on how to approach or resolve specific ethical challenges. Similarly, I am not in complete agreement with each position held in this text, and some authors may not support statements that have been made in my introductions to the sections. Nevertheless, the authors and I have attempted to identify ethically challenging situations that are representative of those encountered by neuropsychological researchers, clinicians, and test developers and have tried to present clear and well-reasoned rationales for approaching the cases in manners consistent with ethical conduct. Research data, where it exists, has been integrated into discussions of relevant positions.

The text is comprised of thirteen sections. The first section provides a brief overview of the changes between the 1992 and 2002 Ethics Codes, with an emphasis on those areas of the Codes that may be particularly challenging in neuropsychological research and practice. Sections two through thirteen each represent a different topic area within neuropsychology. Each section is divided into two chapters, each with a different author so that the topics could be approached from more than one perspective. The exception is the Forensic Neuropsychology chapter, which was allotted five chapters in an attempt to better represent what is likely one of the most ethically challenging and controversial areas of neuropsychology.

The sections represent many of the practice settings and topic areas discussed in the first text. In addition, areas of professional activity other than clinical practice are represented, such as Neuropsychological Research (Section 12) and Test Development (Section 13). Also, new topic areas were added that seem to be areas of particular concern, such as the Neuropsychology of Pain (Section 6) and Determination of Response Validity (Section 10). In the 2002 text, Rizzo, Schultheis, and Rothbaum provided a fascinating and timely account of the ethical issues associated with virtual reality. In the current text, Browndyke and Schatz expand the discussion of ethical issues pertaining to emerging technologies to cover Information Technology and Telecommunications in neuropsychology more broadly (Section 11).

The cases in this text represent a combination of real situations, imagined situations based on actual experiences, and an integration of both real and created elements. Together, the chapters seem to reflect many of the areas of professional activity in which neuropsychologists may face ethical challenges. Given the complexity of many clinical situations and their associated ethical issues, there is considerable overlap among cases, both within and across sections. Such overlap is of value in providing multiple perspectives for understanding and negotiating ethical challenges.

The chapters within each section are simply listed in alphabetical order according to the authors' last names. The appendices include the 2002 APA Ethics Code and the *Specialty Guidelines for Forensic Psychologists* (Committee on Ethical Guidelines for Forensic Psychologists, 1991). As a result, specific quotations from the Ethics Code and the Specialty Guidelines are kept to a minimum in the text. References to the Ethics Code or the Code refer to the APA Ethics Code, although the ethics codes of different disciplines or jurisdictions may also be relevant for some readers. In addition, familiarity with the psychology ethics codes of

other jurisdictions, relevant professional publications, and the *Association of State and Provincial Psychology Boards' Code of Conduct* (ASPPB, 1990) may be of value, and knowledge of applicable jurisdictional laws is essential.

The text is intended to serve as a practical model for understanding neuropsychological ethics. The cases were developed to represent common ethical challenges encountered in various areas of practice. Although fifty-four case illustrations are presented, the text should in no way be considered exhaustive regarding the ethical challenges faced routinely by neuropsychologists. The authors in this text vary considerably in their approaches to cases. They were given both an overall format to follow and the freedom to vary within that format as needed to best convey the material and their own styles. The general format includes four sections: (a) the presentation of the vignette or scenario; (b) discussion of the relevant ethical issues; (c) discussion of how the case was resolved, given consideration of the ethical issues; and, (d) conclusions and recommendations. Where important to case analysis or resolution, changes from the 1992 Ethics Code to the 2002 Code are discussed. The sections are followed by a reference section when applicable.

As mentioned above, many colleagues influenced my work on this text, some of whom disagree with at least some aspects of what is written here, but all of whom are appreciated for their input. First, I am grateful to Linas Bieliauskas for his continued inclusion of ethics texts in this Taylor and Francis neuropsychology book series. As with the first book, Jerry Sweet's input and support have been invaluable during this process. I am fortunate to practice in the same community as Steve Honor and Mark Sandberg, both of whom have been willing to engage in frequent discussions about many of the issues and situations examined here. The Division 40 Ethics Committee, currently chaired by Michele Macartney-Filgate, and the Division 22 Social and Ethical Responsibility Committee, which I currently chair, have both been richly stimulating groups with which to work. Stephanie Hanson and Tom Kerkhoff, in our collaboration on *Health Care Ethics for Psychologists: A Casebook* (Hanson, Kerkhoff, & Bush, 2005), provided conceptualizations and discussions of numerous cases across the health care continuum. Also, the NAN Policy and Planning Committee, co-chaired at the time by Jeff Barth and Neil Pliskin, was gracious enough to allow me to draft a position paper on independent and court-ordered neuropsychological examinations (Bush et al., 2003). Glenn Larrabee and the other committee members provided input that served to clarify the many challenging ethical issues inherent in IMEs. Additional thanks goes to Michael Drexler for his thoughts and considerations. However, deepest appreciation goes to the contributing authors for their creativity, insights, and professionalism.

References

American Psychological Association (2002). Ethical principles of psychologists and code of conduct. *American Psychologist, 57*, 1060-1073.

Association of State and Provincial Psychology Boards (1990). *ASPPB Code of Conduct*. www.asppb.org/boards/code. Retrieved 8/6/02.

Bush, S.S., Barth, J.T., Pliskin, N.H., Arffa, S., Axelrod, B.N., Blackburn, L. A., Faust, D., Fisher, J.M., Harley, J.P., Heilbronner, R.L., Larrabee, G.J., Ricker, J.H., & Silver, C.H. (2003). *Independent and court-ordered forensic neuropsychological examinations: Official statement of the National Academy of Neuropsychology*. Retrieved from http://www.nanonline.org/paio/IME.shtm 1/16/04.

Committee on Ethical Guidelines for Forensic Psychologists (1991). Specialty guidelines for forensic psychologists. *Law and Human Behavior, 15*, 655-665.

Fisher, C.B. (2003). *Decoding the ethics code: A practical guide for psychologists*. Thousand Oaks, CA: Sage Publications.

Hanson, S., Kerkhoff, T., & Bush, S. (2005). *Health Care Ethics for Psychologist's: A Casebook*. Washington, DC: American Psychological Association.

Knapp, S., & VandeCreek, L. (2003). *A guide to the 2002 revision of the American Psychological Association's Ethics Code*. Sarasota, FL: Professional Resource Press.

STUDIES ON NEUROPSYCHOLOGY, DEVELOPMENT, AND COGNITION

Section 1

DIFFERENCES BETWEEN THE 1992 AND 2002 APA ETHICS CODES: A BRIEF OVERVIEW

The American Psychological Association Council (APA) of Representatives adopted the newest version of the Ethics Code on August 21, 2002 (APA, 2002), and it went into effect June 1, 2003. As with its predecessor (APA, 1992), the 2002 Ethics Code begins with an Introduction that describes its intent, organization, procedural considerations, and scope of application. The Introduction is followed by a Preamble which offers aspirational suggestions for psychological conduct. The Ethics Code then provides General Principles, which are aspirational in nature, and Ethical Standards, which are enforceable and are used to adjudicate complaints of ethical misconduct. The new code is approximately twenty percent shorter than its predecessor.

Although all of the changes to the Ethics Code have implications for neuropsychology, neuropsychologists are likely to place greatest emphasis on understanding those changes and additions that have the most relevance for their professional activities, such as Standard 9 (Assessment). Readers are referred to other resources for more general commentary on the changes to the Ethics Code (e.g., Fisher, 2003a; Knapp & VandeCreek, 2003) and to the APA Ethics Office website for redline comparisons that detail the changes (http://www.apa.org/ethics/codecompare.html, accessed December 18, 2003). Although case-based discussions of some of the changes to the Ethics Code are offered throughout the text, the following overview examines some of the changes to the Ethics Code that may be most relevant to neuropsychology.

Introduction and Applicability

The Introduction to 2002 APA Ethics Code includes the addition of a paragraph that describes the use of modifiers (e.g., reasonably, appropriate, potentially) in the Code. Modifiers (1) allow professional judgment on the part of psychologists, (2) eliminate injustice or inequality that would occur without the modifier, (3) ensure applicability across the broad range of activities conducted by psychologists, or (4) guard against a set of rigid rules that might be quickly outdated. Although some neuropsychologists may prefer that the Ethics Code provide definitive guidelines for ethical behavior that would apply in all situations, such a task is beyond the scope and purpose of an ethics code. Given the wide range of professional activities that neuropsychologists perform and the unique aspects of situations within each activity, it would be nearly impossible for any set of guidelines to state specifically how a neuropsychologist should resolve every scenario. Instead, the Ethics Code offers overarching ethical principles and a set of standards of varying degrees of specificity that provide the framework by which neuropsychologists can reason through ethical challenges. Other professional publications, such as guidelines from professional organization and peer-reviewed articles, provide further explication specific to neuropsychology, and texts such as this demonstrate how professional guidelines may be applied in actual situations.

Also in this section, a definition of the term *reasonable* is offered: "As used in the Ethics Code, the term *reasonable* means the prevailing professional judgment of psychologists engaged in similar activities in similar circumstances, given the knowledge the psychologist had or should have had at the time." Given the widely disparate views of competent neuropsychologists on a variety of topics (e.g., mild traumatic brain injury, test batteries, symptom validity testing, etc.), it seems that a well reasoned and scientifically defensible position or method of practice would be considered reasonable, whereas extreme positions or behaviors that fall well outside of the usual and customary standards of practice would not be considered reasonable.

General Principles

The revision of the General Principles incorporated widely referenced general biomedical ethical principles: autonomy, beneficence, nonmaleficence, and justice (Beauchamp and Childress, 2001). Incorporation of these commonly used biomedical ethical principles provides neuropsychologists with a useful means of conceptualizing ethical issues and a common language to use when discussing ethics with other medical professionals. In a reduction from six principles to five, the 2002 Ethics Code reflects the deletion of principles entitled Competence and Social Responsibility. Issues of Competence, based on the underlying principle of nonmaleficence, are now emphasized in the Ethical Standards (Standard 2). Content related to Social Responsibility has been incorporated into the Preamble and Introduction. General Principle D (Justice) is a new addition to the Code and emphasizes equality in access to psychological services and in the nature of the services provided. It further emphasizes the need for psychologists to ensure that potential biases and limitations of professional competence do not result in or condone unfair practices.

Ethical Standards

Changes in both the form and content of the Ethical Standards are apparent in the new Ethics Code.

Competence

In the 1992 Code, Competence was listed as a General Principle (Principle A), and was described in various standards (1.04, Boundaries of Competence; 1.05, Maintaining Expertise; 1.06, Basis for Scientific and Professional Judgments; 1.08, Human Differences; 1.22, Delegation to and Supervision of Subordinates; 7.06, Compliance with Laws and Rules). In the 2002 Code, Competence is mentioned in Principle D (Justice) but now also comprises an entire section of the Ethical Standards (Standard 2). Added are sections addressing provision of services to those who might not otherwise be served (2.01d) and provision of services during emergencies

(2.02). The increased emphasis and organization in the Standards seems to reflect the importance for psychologists to understand that professional competence is not simply something to which professionals must aspire but is an essential requirement of the successful execution of one's professional responsibilities.

Informed Consent

For the first time, the Ethics Code directly addresses issues of informed consent in assessments (Standard 9.03). Standard 9.03 outlines the consent process in considerable detail, and it describes exceptions to the need for informed consent. Because many neuropsychologists examine persons who have questionable cognitive capacity to provide informed consent, consent issues become more complicated (American Psychological Association Presidential Task Force on the Assessment of Age-Consistent Memory Decline and Dementia, 1998; Johnson-Greene et al., 1997; Johnson-Greene & National Academy of Neuropsychology, 2003). Ethical Standards 3.10(b) and 9.03(b) provide direction on how to negotiate informed consent issues when patients have or may have diminished decision-making capacity. Standard 3.10(c) is a new subsection that describes consent obligations when services are court-ordered or otherwise mandated.

Despite genuine attempts to comply with ethical standards pertaining to consent, in many situations neuropsychologists are unable provide the examinee with specific information on how test findings will be used or what the implications of the findings will be. Thus, although the consent process in such situations may not always be truly informed, neuropsychologists must nevertheless attempt to explain the potential uses and implications of the examination results to the examinee as early as possible in the examination process.

Multiple Relationships

Standards addressing multiple relationships were clarified (3.05, Multiple Relationships; 3.06,

Conflicts of Interest; 10.02, Therapy Involving Couples or Families). Neuropsychologists must refrain from taking on a professional role if it could reasonably be expected to interfere with their objectivity or otherwise negatively affect their ability to perform their duties effectively. The new Code states that multiple relationships that would not be reasonably expected to interfere with one's professional performance or result in harm would not be unethical (Standard 3.05a).

Multicultural Issues

The APA Ethics Code Task Force (ECTF) reviewed the Ethical Standards with regard to racism and other forms of disempowerment, attempting to view the code from the perspective of such groups (Knapp & VandeCreek, 2003). The results include the following.

The principle of Justice (Principle D) is new in the 2002 Ethics Code and emphasizes that all individuals are entitled to access to and benefit from psychological services of equal quality. Psychologists take steps to ensure that biases and limitations of competence do not interfere with the provision of such services. The 1992 Principle E (Concern for Others' Welfare) was incorporated into the new Principle A (Beneficence and Nonmaleficence). Both principles emphasize the need to promote the welfare of those with whom neuropsychologists interact professionally.

The 2002 Ethics Code places an increased emphasis on cultural competency in situations in which it has been determined that such competency is essential for delivery of effective services. The Code also stresses increased sensitivity to the difficulties inherent in providing psychological services when language fluency is not shared by the psychologist and the patient. New Standard 2.01(b) requires sensitivity to the impact of culture, disability, and other diversity factors on one's professional competency. Knapp and VandeCreek (2003) state, "It is not an ethical violation to provide less optimal treatment to members of … any groups; it is only

a violation if the knowledge that is lacking is essential for providing services" (p. 303).

New Standard 9.03 (Informed Consent in Assessments) has three subsections that discuss issues related to informed consent in assessments. Section (c) outlines the need for psychologists planning to use the services of an interpreter to obtain informed consent from the patient to do so. To be fully informed, the examinee should be told that the translation may result in a degree of imprecision in the test results, and the degree of imprecision will be greater the farther the interpreter and the examinee are from speaking the same dialect or regional variation of a language. Standard 9.03(c) also outlines the responsibility of psychologists to ensure that their interpreters follow requirements to maintain confidentiality of test results and maintain test security. This addition helps to emphasize the importance of psychologists clarifying with all parties involved in the provision of psychological services the need to be sensitive to the patient's rights to privacy and confidentiality, as well as to the limits of privacy and confidentiality.

Standard 9.02 (Use of Assessments), subsection (b), is new. This standard requires psychologists to use assessment instruments that have established validity and reliability for use with members of the population that the patient represents. In the absence of such validity or reliability, psychologists must describe the strengths and limitations of the test results and interpretation. Subsection (c) is also new and mandates psychologists to use measures that are appropriate given the patient's language preference and competence, unless use of an alternative language is relevant to the examination. Throughout the section on Assessment, the Code emphasizes the need to indicate the limitations of one's interpretations. Standard 9.06 (Interpreting Assessment Results) specifically states that linguistic and cultural differences must be appropriately considered when interpreting assessment results. Also, psychologists are expected to indicate any significant limitations of their interpretations.

Release of Test Data and Materials

During the revision process and following finalization of the 2002 Code, Standard 9.04 (Release of Test Data) received the greatest attention (Fisher, 2003b; Knapp & VandeCreek, 2003). The 2002 Ethics Code distinguishes between *test data* and *test materials*. *Test data* (Standard 9.04a) refers to "raw and scaled scores, client/patient responses to test questions or stimuli, and psychologists' notes and recordings concerning client/patient statements and behavior during an examination." With a release from the client/patient, psychologists are to provide such data to the client/patient or to other persons identified by the client/patient. However, psychologists "may refrain" from releasing such data in order to protect the client/patient or others from substantial harm or in order to avoid misuse or misrepresentation of the data. Without a release from the client/patient, psychologists are to provide others with test data only as required by law or court order. Under the 1992 Code, psychologists were required to refrain from releasing raw data to anyone (other than the patient under certain circumstances) not qualified to interpret or appropriately use the data. Under current guidelines, with a client/patient release, psychologists must provide test data to the patient/client or to anyone identified in the release, unless the psychologist believes that "substantial harm, misuse, or misrepresentation" may result.

In Standard 9.11 (Maintaining Test Security), *test materials* are defined as "manuals, instruments, protocols, and test questions." In contrast to *test data*, psychologists are required to "make reasonable efforts to maintain the integrity and security of test materials ..." Because the test data are often written on the test materials, determining how to release test data without releasing test materials becomes problematic. The ability to comply with the requirements of both standards appears further limited when one considers that for some tests, the *data* and the *materials* are inseparable (Bush & Macciocchi, 2003). For example, with measures of verbal memory, the stimuli provided by the neuropsychologist and the data produced by the examinee are one and the same. A similar situation is found with graphomotor reproduction tests. Thus, in such situations, it is impossible to meet the APA mandate to release test data but not test materials.

Standard 9.04(a) attempts to provide further guidance in reference to this matter where it states, "Those portions of test materials that include client/patient responses are included in the definition of *test data*." That is, the test materials "convert" to test data (Behnke, 2003). Thus, according to the 2002 Ethics Code, test materials, such as protocols, should be safeguarded when they have no answers written on them but no longer need to be safeguarded after answers have been written on them. It appears that this position requires further clarification.

Additionally, Standard 9.04 requires neuropsychologists to refrain from releasing data when the potential for misuse or misrepresentation of the data exists. However, it appears likely that if the item responses are provided without the context of the questions and other stimuli that are present on the protocols, there would be a high potential for misuse or misrepresentation of the data. Misuse and misrepresentation have the potential to result in harm to the examinee.

The ability, or responsibility, to release test data may be seen as still more ambiguous in situations in which the examinee is not the neuropsychologist's client. For example, in the context of an independent examination, the neuropsychologist has been retained by an attorney, insurance company, or other entity rather than the examinee, rendering the retaining party the "client". In such situations, the question arises as to whether or not it would be consistent with ethical practice, according to the APA Ethics Code, for the neuropsychologist to release completed test forms to the client (e.g., an attorney) and to others specified by the client (e.g., opposing counsel).

In situations such as this in which either course of action may be supported by the Ethics Code, neuropsychologists must decide for themselves whether they want to do what is simply acceptable according to the Code (release the data) or what may be seen as a higher standard of ethical practice (provide access to test materials and data to those qualified to interpret them). These two possible courses of action pit ethical principles against each other. Providing data to the client is consistent with respecting the right of the client to self-determination (Principle E, Respect for People's Rights and Dignity). That is, the client has the right to choose what is done with the product of the work for which they paid. In contrast, providing data to an individual that is not qualified to interpret it and is not bound by the same ethical requirement to safeguard it may result in harm to the examinee (Principle A, Beneficence and Nonmaleficence) and may result in invalidation of future examinations of others (Principle D, Justice). In dilemmas such as this, the greater harm must be determined. Disservice to many would likely outweigh the restricted service to one. Although it has been suggested that when provided with a patient release it is probably now ethical to release neuropsychological data even to those not qualified to interpret or appropriately use it (Adams, 2003), further consideration of the contradictory requirements of the new code do not seem to support such conclusions.

The ethics of releasing neuropsychological records has been extensively debated in the neuropsychology literature (Barth, 2000; Lees-Haley & Courtney, 2000a; Lees-Haley & Courtney, 2000b; Shapiro, 2000; Tranel, 2000), without the emergence of a general consensus on how to handle requests for records. Given the wide variability of professional contexts in which neuropsychologists work, it may be that the general nature of the standards provided by APA cannot be applied with equal success in all contexts. It may be that discussions of the risks and benefits of releasing test data and materials must be context specific.

Additional Assessment Issues

The 2002 Code includes a section on record reviews and consultations conducted in which an individual examination is not needed for the opinion (Standard 9.01c). In such situations, psychologists explain the reasons why an examination was unnecessary and detail the information upon which their decisions were based. This new standard gives general authorization to procedures which previously were exceptions to the requirement to perform a face-to-face examination when offering diagnostic or evaluative statements or recommendations, particularly in forensic contexts (1992 Standards 2.01 and 7.02b,c; Knapp & VandeCreek, 2003).

Professional Subspecialties

Unlike the 1992 Code with the section on Forensic Psychology (Standard 7), the decision was made for the 2002 Code not to address specialty areas within psychology, such as forensic psychology, health psychology, etc. The 2002 Ethics Code was written with the intention of providing global guidelines that would apply to all psychologists, leaving subspecialties to develop their own relevant standards of practice. As a result, Standard 7 from the 1992 Code was deleted, with much of its content disbursed throughout the 2002 Code. For example, the admonition to not make false or deceptive statements in legal proceedings can be found in Standard 5.01 (Avoidance of False or Deceptive Statements). Although some mention is given to forensic contexts or testimony in the 2002 Code, forensic neuropsychologists should continue to refer to the *Specialty Guidelines for Forensic Psychologists* (Committee on Ethical Guidelines for Forensic Psychologists, 1991; currently under revision), as well as relevant articles, chapters, and case illustrations (e.g., Sweet, Grote, & van Gorp, 2002).

Conclusions

Neuropsychologists may face a number of ethical challenges in the execution of their professional responsibilities. Staying abreast of changes to the ethics codes that govern one's professional activities is as vital to success as staying informed of advances in neuropsychological research and practice. To avoid ethical misconduct, neuropsychologists must understand the recent changes to the APA Ethics Code and integrate the Code's Principles and Standards with other relevant professional resources. Such resources include other relevant ethics codes (e.g., Canadian Code of Ethics for Psychologists; Canadian Psychological Association, 2000), the Standards for Education and Psychological Testing (American Educational Research Association, APA, National Council on Measurement in Education, 1999), other relevant professional publications (e.g., American Academy of Clinical Neuropsychology, 2000, 2003; Committee on Ethical Guidelines for Forensic Psychologists, 1991; National Academy of Neuropsychology Policy and Planning Committee, 2000a,b,c & 2003), and jurisdictional laws. The most ethically challenging situations do not have "black or white" solutions. As a result, neuropsychologists who seek the opinions of ethics committees and other colleagues experienced in such matters, possibly including those who hold opinions different from their own, may be in the best position to pursue a successful course of action.

References

Adams, K.M. (2003). It's a whole new world: Or is it? Reflections on the new APA Ethics Code. *Newsletter 40, 21 (1)*, 5-6 & 18.

American Academy of Clinical Neuropsychology (2000). Statement on the presence of third party observers in neuropsychological assessments. *The Clinical Neuropsychologist, 15*, 433-439.

American Academy of Clinical Neuropsychology (2004). Official position of the American Academy of Clinical Neuropsychology on ethical complaints made against clinical neuropsychologists during adversarial proceedings. *The Clinical Neuropsychologist, 17*, 443-445.

American Educational Research Association, American Psychological Association, National Council on Measurement in Education (1999). *Standards for educational and psychological testing.* Washington, D.C.: American Educational Research Association.

American Psychological Association (1992). Ethical principles of psychologists and code of conduct. *American Psychologist, 47*, 1597-1611.

American Psychological Association (2002). Ethical principles of psychologists and code of conduct. *American Psychologist, 57*, 1060-1073.

American Psychological Association, Committee on Psychological Tests and Assessment (n.d). *Statement on disclosure of test data.* American Psychological Association, Science Directorate, 750 First Street, NE, Washington, DC 20002-4242. http://www.apa.org/science.

American Psychological Association Presidential Task Force on the Assessment of Age-Consistent Memory Decline and Dementia (1998). *Guidelines for the evaluation of dementia and age-related cognitive decline.* American Psychological Association, Practice Directorate, 750 First Street, NE, Washington, DC 20002-4242. http://www.apa.org/practice.

Barth, J.T. (2000). Commentary on "Disclosure of tests and raw test data to the courts" by Paul Lees-Haley and John Courtney. *Neuropsychology Review, 10*, 179-180.

Beauchamp, T.L., & Childress, J.F. (2001). *Principles of biomedical ethics* (5th ed.). New York: Oxford University Press.

Behnke, S. (2003). Release of test data and APA's new Ethics Code. *Monitor on Psychology, 34 (7)*, 70-72.

Binder, L.M., & Thompson, L.L. (1995). The ethics code and neuropsychological assessment practices. *Archives of Clinical Neuropsychology, 10 (1)*, 27-46.

Bush, S.S., & Drexler, M.L. (Eds.) (2002). *Ethical issues in clinical neuropsychology.* Lisse, NL: Swets & Zeitlinger Publishers.

Bush, S., & Macciocchi, S.N. (2003). The 2002 APA Ethics Code: Select changes relevant to neuropsychology. *Bulletin of the National Academy of Neuropsychology, 18 (2)*, 1-2 & 7-8.

Canadian Psychological Association (2000). *Canadian code of ethics for psychologists – third edition*. Attawa, ON: Author.

Committee on Ethical Guidelines for Forensic Psychologists (1991). Specialty guidelines for forensic psychologists. *Law and Human Behavior, 15*, 655-665.

Fisher, C.B. (2003a). *Decoding the ethics code: A practical guide for psychologists*. Thousand Oaks, CA: Sage Publications.

Fisher, C.B. (2003b). Test data standard most notable change in new APA ethics code. *The National Psychologist*, Jan/Feb, 12-13.

Johnson-Greene, D., Hardy-Morais, C., Adams, K., Hardy, C., & Bergloff, P. (1997). Informed consent and neuropsychological assessment: Ethical considerations and proposed guidelines. *The Clinical Neuropsychologist, 11*, 454-460.

Johnson-Greene, D., & National Academy of Neuropsychology Policy and Planning Committee (2003). *Informed consent: Official statement of the National Academy of Neuropsychology*. Retrieved from http://www.nanonline.org/paio/informed_consent.shtm 1/16/04.

Knapp, S., & VandeCreek, L. (2003). An overview of the major changes in the 2002 Ethics Code. *Professional Psychology: Research and Practice, 34*, 301-308.

Lees-Haley, P.R., & Courtney, J. C. (2000a). Disclosure of tests and raw test data to the courts: A need for reform. *Neuropsychology Review, 10*, 169-174.

Lees-Haley, P.R., & Courtney, J. C. (2000b). Reply to the commentary on "Disclosure of tests and raw test data to the courts". *Neuropsychology Review, 10*, 181-182.

Macciocchi, S.N. (2001). Informed consent and neuropsychological assessment. *Newsletter 40*, Winter/Spring, 34-36.

National Academy of Neuropsychology Policy and Planning Committee (2000a). Test security: Official position statement of the National Academy of Neuropsychology. *Archives of Clinical Neuropsychology, 15*, 383-386.

National Academy of Neuropsychology Policy and Planning Committee (2000b). Presence of third party observers during neuropsychological testing: Official position statement of the National Academy of Neuropsychology. *Archives of Clinical Neuropsychology, 15*, 379-380.

National Academy of Neuropsychology Policy and Planning Committee (2000c). The use of neuropsychology test technicians: Official position statement of the National Academy of Neuropsychology. *Archives of Clinical Neuropsychology, 15*, 381-382.

National Academy of Neuropsychology Policy and Planning Committee (2003). *Test Security: An update. Official statement of the National Academy of Neuropsychology*. Retrieved 2/17/2004 from http://nanonline.org/paio/security_update.shtm

Shapiro, D.L. (2000). Commentary: Disclosure of tests and raw test data to the courts. *Neuropsychology Review, 10*, 175-176.

Sweet, J.J., Grote, C., & van Gorp, W.G. (2002). Ethical issues in forensic neuropsychology. In S. Bush & M. Drexler (Eds.), *Ethical issues in clinical neuropsychology*, 103-133. Lisse, NL: Swets & Zeitlinger Publishers.

Tranel, D. (2000). Commentary on Lees-Haley and Courtney: There is a need for reform. *Neuropsychology Review, 10*, 177-178.

Section 2

ETHICAL CHALLENGES IN FORENSIC NEUROPSYCHOLOGY

Introduction

For the purposes of this text, the term "forensic neuropsychology" is used broadly to refer to all adversarial administrative and judicial neuropsychological activities (Sweet, 1999; Sweet, Grote, & van Gorp, 2002). This broad definition extends beyond the contexts of civil and criminal litigation to include administrative determinations such as disability determination, worker's compensation, competency, civil commitment, fitness for duty, educational due process, and other adversarial cases.

Many clinical neuropsychologists intentionally or inadvertently become involved in forensic matters. Understanding one's role in forensic contexts is a critical first step in avoiding ethical misconduct. The roles of neuropsychologists, as with other medical fields, have commonly been defined as either "Treating Doctor" or "Forensic Expert"[1] (Fisher, Johnson-Greene, & Barth, 2002; Macartney-Filgate & Snow, 2000). However, it seems that this distinction could benefit from re-examination and further elaboration and clarification. In addition, the role of "Trial Consultant" is included as an area of professional neuropsychological activity. Although understanding the distinctions between roles and avoiding engaging in multiple roles with one client is important for maintaining ethical conduct, it is also necessary to attend to intrarole conflicts that may interfere with objective presentation of neuropsychological evidence to the trier-of-fact. The following four roles are described: forensic

---

[1]The distinction between *fact witness* and *expert witness*, although common in psychological writings, is not found in the *Federal Rules of Evidence* (Committee on the Judiciary, House of Representatives, 2002). The F.R.E. (Article VII, Opinions and Expert Testimony) distinguishes only between expert and lay witnessess. The determination is made by the court based on the potential for the knowledge, skill, experience, training, or education of the witness to assist the trier of fact. The term "fact witness" is not found in the Federal Rules of Evidence.

examiner, trial consultant, clinical examiner, and treating doctor.

Forensic Examiner

In the traditional Forensic Examiner role, the neuro-psychologist is retained by plaintiff or defense counsel, although at times retention is directly by the court. As should be the case in all evaluations, the neuropsychologist collects and reviews information and administers measures sufficient to answer the referral question. Compared to some clinical situations, the forensic examiner may have more time and resources, including financial resources, to obtain extensive background information through record review and, when allowed and appropriate, interviews of all relevant collateral sources of information. Patient report may be relied upon less than in the clinical context. The forensic examiner may conduct extensive evaluation of response validity and consider all possible explanations for impaired test results and other findings. Based on the extensiveness of the evaluation, the neuropsychologist is in a position to offer opinions with a relatively high degree of confidence.

In the performance of such an evaluation, the forensic examiner aspires to be objective and free from bias, thereby allowing the conclusions reached and the diagnostic and/or causality opinions to be credible. However, it has been suggested elsewhere (e.g., Martelli, Bush, & Zasler, 2003) and is again noted here that one is not free from bias simply by performing a forensic evaluation. The nature of forensic work is inherently fraught with multiple and competing demands (Lees-Haley & Cohen, 1999; Shuman & Greenberg, 2003). Neuropsychologists performing forensic services are subject to "competing tensions" when attempting to integrate the various demands. "All experts, however competent and well intentioned, are human, meaning that they are subject to limitations, bias and error" (Lees-Haley & Cohen, 1999; p. 446). As a result, neuropsychologists, regardless of which side of the adversarial forensic process has retained them, must be proactive in addressing their own potential for bias (e.g, Brodsky, 1991). The use of self-examination questions may help to reduce the potential for bias (Sweet & Moulthrop, 1999). It appears that a lower potential for bias would come only from the examiner being retained by a party that has no financial or emotional stake in the outcome of the case (e.g., the court).

The independent neuropsychological examination represents a common forensic practice, one in which a traditional doctor-patient relationship does not exist. Although neuropsychologists do not have the same obligations to examinees in independent forensic examinations that they do in clinical contexts, certain professional responsibilities exist whenever a neuropsychologist conducts an examination (Bush et al., 2003). Despite the uniqueness of this type of examination, and consistent with all other areas of practice, neuropsychologists are responsible for maintaining appropriate ethical standards of practice.

Trial Consultant

The trial consultant assists one side of a forensic neuropsychological case in determining the strengths and weaknesses of the neuropsychological case presented by the other side. The trial consultant does not testify, and his or her identity may be unknown to the opposing side.

Treating Doctor

Traditionally, the term "Treating Doctor" has been applied to any neuropsychological services (evaluation or treatment) performed in a clinical context. In the traditional treating doctor role, as in the forensic examiner role, the neuropsychologist has a responsibility to collect information and administer measures sufficient to answer the referral question and initiate treatment. However, in the interest of expediency, the neuropsychologist may proceed from evaluation to diagnosis and treatment recommendations without reviewing extensive, if any, objective archival records or interviewing collateral sources of information.

The neuropsychologist may then follow the patient for treatment, becoming more sympathetic to the patient's perspective, which may be less consistent with the degree of objectivity required for offering forensic opinions.

Some authors have described the treating doctor as an advocate, using the terms synonymously (e.g., Fisher, Johnson-Greene, & Barth, 2002; Iverson, 2000). Webster's Dictionary defines an advocate as "one that pleads the cause of another" (Merriam-Webster, 1988). Although advocacy may be an important component of treatment in some situations (see Chapter 3 by Honor below), advocacy does not seem to be an integral component of most psychotherapeutic approaches (Corsini, 1984). Thus, the term "advocate" applies to the treating doctor role only in specific and relatively infrequent situations.

The neuropsychologist treating doctor is invested in the patient's clinical progress and overall well-being. As such, the objectivity required for critical examination of data and alternative hypotheses may be reduced (Strasburger, Gutheil, & Brodsky, 1997). Such partisanship may be acceptable in the treatment context, although if conflicting information emerges that puts the patient's treatment plan in question, the treating doctor must consider the new information and adjust or discontinue treatment or seek consultation from an independent colleague as indicated. Even with subsequent collection of extensive objective background information, the therapeutic alliance would limit the neuropsychologist from changing roles and attempting to offer a new, forensic report or offering a forensic opinion. Performing a forensic evaluation of a patient with whom one a preexisting therapeutic relationship would constitute a dual role and is considered unethical (Barsky & Gould, 2002; Lees-Haley & Cohen, 1999; Melton, Petrila, Poythress, & Slobogin, 1997).

Clinical Examiner

The clinical examiner is distinguished from the treating doctor. Survey results indicate that neuropsychologists devote a substantially greater amount of practice time to assessment than to treatment (Sweet, Peck, Abramowitz, & Etzweiler, 2002). The purpose of the clinical evaluation is typically to determine if deficits exist and, if so, why, and to facilitate treatment if needed. In this role, the neuropsychologist performs the same evaluation as does the forensic examiner, but, in the interest of expediency, may not gather and review equivalent objective background information and may not interview all relevant collateral sources of information about the examinee. Some authors argue that such reliance on patient self-report represents bias in favor of the patient on the part of the examiner. However, the neuropsychologist performing a clinical evaluation attempts to maintain objectivity, to the same degree as the forensic examiner, in all aspects of the evaluation, including review of the available information and test data. The neuropsychologist uses measures sufficient to answer the referral question, including measures of response validity, and considers explanations other than what the patient reports, thus demonstrating critical acceptance of the information provided by the patient.

In addition to the manner in which "advocacy" was used above, other authors have used the term "advocacy" to describe support for a certain philosophical position or belief system about an issue (Barsky & Gould, 2002), such as postconcussion syndrome, rather than for an individual, such as one's patient. Such advocacy, if based on objective facts or research, may be quite valuable in public policy matters. However, the neuropsychologist who consistently provides the same type of diagnosis or prognosis regardless of the unique features of each case, thus arguing for only one point of view, would be engaging in unethical advocacy. As can be seen, the term "advocacy" has been used in forensic psychology writings to describe quite different situations. If used in forensic contexts, the meaning of the term should be clearly defined.

The ethical neuropsychologist performing a clinical evaluation is an advocate for neither the examinee nor a particular clinical condition. Contrary to what some have proposed, performing a clinical evaluation does not give one license to subordinate objectivity regarding test data interpretation, nor does it automatically make one's impressions biased. The neuropsychologist in possession of limited background information, depending on the context, discusses limitations of the conclusions drawn.

Some authors consider diagnosis and causality the sole purview of the forensic examiner. However, such a position represents an oversimplification of the many situations that clinical neuropsychologists face. Context must be considered. Clinical neuropsychologists routinely provide diagnoses on a variety neuropathological and psychological conditions, and they offer opinions about causation of the disorders. In the case of severe brain injury, a neuropsychological evaluation is typically not needed to make a diagnosis. However, a neuropsychological evaluation may be needed to help plan cognitive rehabilitation and to address emotional/behavioral issues. Although occurring in a clinical context, a diagnosis of such brain injury can be made by the neuropsychologist with a reasonable degree of certainty. In addition, there may occasionally be clinical situations in which patients with more ambiguous symptoms present for clinical evaluation, with instruction from the examiner, with objective background records. With such information, the neuropsychologist can place increased confidence, where previously less certain, in conclusions regarding causality.

The clinical examiner may testify to any aspect of the evaluation, including diagnostic and causal impressions, determined within the scope of clinical practice. However, the neuropsychologist who does not address causality in the clinical report but then later, when provided with additional documents by the patient's attorney, adds statements reflecting such opinions, has entered into a dual role. In contrast, transitioning from the clinical examiner role to the treating doctor role following completion of the evaluation is appropriate.

Conclusions

It is acknowledged that the descriptions of neuro-psychologist roles provided here will not be met with universal acceptance. It is likely that those who believe that they can first be a treating doctor and then transition into, or simultaneously serve as, the patient's forensic examiner will disagree. Similarly, those who maintain that only the forensic examiner is an objective nonadvocate will also disagree. Nevertheless, it is hoped that the clarification of terms will facilitate more meaningful exchanges on the subject of neuropsychologist roles and that practitioners willing to consider more moderate positions will find the descriptions beneficial in their understanding of forensic neuropsychology.

Through both administrative and litigated cases, the authors of this chapter present scenarios that reflect each of the roles described above. Within the cases and their analyses, the authors guide the reader through some of the most common ethical hurdles and offer guidance on how to negotiate such challenges.

References

Barsky, A.E., & Gould, J.W. (2002). *Clinicians in court: A guide to subpoenas, depositions, testifying, and everythings else you need to know.* New York: The Guilford Press.

Brodsky, S.L. (1991). *Testifying in court: Guidelines and maxims for the expert witness.* Washington, D.C.: American Psychological Association.

Bush, S.S., Barth, J.T., Pliskin, N.H., Arffa, S., Axelrod, B.N., Blackburn, L.A., Faust, D., Fisher, J.M., Harley, J.P., Heilbronner, R.L., Larrabee, G.J., Ricker, J.H., & Silver, C.H. (2003). *Independent and court-ordered forensic neuropsychological examinations: Official statement of the National Academy of Neuropsychology.* Retrieved from http://www.nanonline.org/paio/IME.shtm 1/16/04.

Corsini, R.J. (1984). *Current psychotherapies, third edition.* Itasca, IL: F.E. Peacock Publishers.

Fisher, J., Johnson-Greene, D., & Barth, J. (2002). Evaluation, diagnosis, and interventions in clinical neuropsychology in general and with special populations: An overview. In S. Bush & M.L. Drexler (Eds.), *Ethical issues in clinical neuropsychology,* (pp. 322). Lisse, NL: Swets & Zeitlinger Publishers.

Iverson, G.L. (2000). Dual relationships in psycholegal evaluations: Treating psychologists serving as expert witnesses. *American Journal of Forensic Psychology, 18 (2),* 79-87.

Lees-Haley, P.R., & Cohen, L.J. (1999). The neuropsychologist as expert witness: Toward credible science in the courtroom. In J.J. Sweet (Ed.), *Forensic neuropsychology: Fundamentals and practice,* (pp. 443-468). Lisse, NL: Swets & Zeitlinger Publishers.

Macartney-Filgate, M., & Snow, G. (2000). Forensic assessments and professional relations. *Newsletter 40, 18,* 28-31.

Martelli, M.F., Bush, S.S., & Zasler, N.D. (2003). Identifying, avoiding, and addressing ethical misconduct in neuropsychological medicolegal practice. *International Journal of Forensic Psychology 1 (1),* 26-44. http://ijfp.psyc. uow. edu.au/

Melton, G.B., Petrila, J., Poythress, N.G., & Slobogin, C. (1997). Psychological evaluations for the courts, second edition. New York: The Guilford Press.

Merriam-Webster (1988). *Webster's ninth collegiate dictionary.* Springfield, MA: Merriam-Webster Inc.

Shuman, D.W., & Greenberg, S.A. (2003). The expert witness, the adversary system, and voice of reason: Reconciling impartiality and advocacy. *Professional Psychology: Research and Practice, 34 (3),* 219-224.

Strasburger, H., Gutheil, T., & Brodsky, B. (1997). On wearing two hats: Role conflict in serving as both psychotherapist and expert witness. *American Journal of Psychiatry, 154,* 448-456.

Sweet, J.J. (1999). *Forensic neuropsychology: Fundamentals and practice.* Lisse, NL: Swets & Zeitlinger Publishers.

Sweet, J.J., Grote, C., & van Gorp, W.G. (2002). Ethical issues in forensic neuropsychology. In S.S. Bush & M.L. Drexler (Eds.), *Ethical issues in clinical neuropsychology*, (pp. 103-133). Lisse, NL: Swets & Zeitlinger Publishers.

Sweet, J.J., & Moulthrop, M. (1999). Self-examination questions as a means of identifying bias in adversarial assessments. *Journal of Forensic Neuropsychology, 1*, 73-88.

Sweet, J.J., Peck, E.A., Abramowitz, C., & Etzweiler, S. (2002). National Academy of Neuropsychology/ Division 40 of the American Psychological Association practice survey of clinical neuropsychology in the United States, part I: Practitioner and practice characteristics, professional activities, and time requirements. *The Clinical Neuropsychologist, 16 (2)*, 109-127.

Chapter 1[1]

ETHICAL CHALLENGES IN FORENSIC NEUROPSYCHOLOGY, PART I

Robert L. Denney

Scenario 1

A neuropsychologist in private practice receives a telephone call from the District Attorney's office in his local district in Texas requesting that he perform a neuropsychological evaluation of a man charged with a capital offense. The man has been charged with murder arising from his participation in an armed robbery of a grocery store. While not suspected of killing the clerk, the defendant's participation in the robbery makes him eligible for the death penalty under Texas Law. The prosecutor tells the neuropsychologist he is concerned the defense attorney thinks the defendant is not competent to proceed to trial because he is a "little slow" and has a long history of illicit drug abuse, including inhalants. The neuropsychologist is to address competency to stand trial. The neuropsychologist agreed to perform the evaluation, as he had done many such evaluations in the past and understands the legal issues related to competency to stand trial. He subsequently receives a court order to evaluate the defendant's

mental status, with a focus on competency to stand trial.

The neuropsychologist meets with the defendant at the county jail, introduces himself, and explains he is there to evaluate the man's competency to proceed. Initially, the defendant is hesitant and unwilling to participate in the evaluation, but the neuropsychologist makes it clear he is evaluating competency to proceed, will prepare a report on the matter, and possibly testify if called to do so. The defendant ultimately indicates he understands the reason for the evaluation and agrees to proceed with it.

The neuropsychologist performs his standard clinical interview, interviews the defendant specifically about competency-related issues, and administers a neuropsychological test battery (including standard checks of test result validity). During the interviews, the defendant describes his history and his recollection of the events in question. The neuropsychologist writes a report to the judge indicating his opinion that the defendant is slightly below average in intellect but has no significant neuropsychological impairments. He considers the man to have antisocial personality disorder and to be competent to proceed.

The neuropsychologist testifies in court that the defendant is competent to proceed, and the

[1]Opinions expressed in this chapter are those of the author and do not necessarily represent the position of the Federal Bureau of Prisons are the U.S. Department of Justice.

judge finds the man competent. He is convicted. In Texas capital cases, there is a "bifurcated trial", meaning that the jury first decides the issue of guilt or innocence (guilt phase) and then decides whether or not to invoke the death penalty (sentencing phase) based on three criteria. One of these criteria is "whether there is a probability that the defendant would commit criminal acts of violence that would constitute a continuing threat to society." The neuropsychologist receives another call from prosecuting attorney requesting that he come testify before the jury during the sentencing phase regarding the nature of the man's personality disorder and his propensity for dangerousness as a result.

Relevant Ethical Issues

The practice of neuropsychology in the forensic arena is fraught with potential ethical dilemmas. Because of the uniqueness of the forensic environment, and the fact that the American Psychological Association's (APA) Ethics Code did not cover important issues in forensic psychology (particularly criminal forensics), the Specialty Guidelines for Forensic Psychologists were jointly developed and adopted by Division 41 of the APA (American Psychology-Law Society) and the American Academy of Forensic Psychology (members of the forensic board affiliated with the American Board of Forensic Psychology) in 1991. The Guidelines were intended to be consistent with the 1990 APA's Ethical Principles of Psychologists, but they also provide more specific guidance for psychologists providing forensic services. The 1992 Ethics Code included a section on forensic activities. This section was eliminated and its contents subsumed under various sections in 2002 Ethics Code. While the Specialty Guidelines are aspirational in nature, they outline appropriate professional conduct when providing psychological expertise to the judicial system. In this regard, it is important for neuropsychologists who present themselves

as experts to attorneys and courts to be familiar with these guidelines as well as the current Ethics Code.

The Specialty Guidelines define forensic psychology as "all forms of professional psychological conduct when acting, with definable foreknowledge, as a psychological expert on explicitly psycholegal issues, in direct assistance to courts, parties to legal proceedings, correctional and forensic mental health facilities, and administrative, judicial, and legislative agencies acting in an adjudicative capacity." The Specialty Guidelines were not written to apply to psychologists asked to provide professional psychological services when the psychologist was not aware at the time of the service that it would become forensic in nature. For these individuals, however, the Specialty Guidelines may be helpful in preparing to communicate professional opinions in the forensic arena. The vignettes in this section are discussed in light of the Specialty Guidelines as well as the 2002 Ethics Code.

There are several relevant ethical issues at play in this vignette. Keeping one's work within areas of expertise, avoiding harm, providing for informed consent, and basing opinions on an adequate data base are all ethical concerns within this vignette. While not a major focus in this vignette, the need to consider implications of working on capital cases is a personal issue which must be resolved prior to engaging in such work.

Competence

The neuropsychologist performed a type of evaluation for which he had appropriate training and experience. Competency to stand trial (or competency to proceed) is a legal question that has specific legal criteria. Rather than the common notion of competency or incompetency to perform a task well, it refers to the ability to understand, both factually and rationally, the nature and consequences of the charges/proceedings and the ability to assist properly in a defense. The absence of competency must be due to a mental illness or defect. This neuropsychologist is in good stead in this regard because the vignette indicated he understood the legal issues involved and had experience completing such evaluations. Ethical standards clearly indicate that neuropsychologists are to practice within their areas of competence.

Avoiding Harm in Forensic Assessments

General Principle A (Beneficence and Non-maleficence), General Principle E (Respect for People's Rights and Dignity), Ethical Standard 3.04 (Avoiding Harm), and Specialty Guideline IV.E.2 all address the need to avoid causing harm to those with whom neuropsychologists interact professionally. It could seem to many that providing an opinion that a man is competent, or more directly here – dangerous, in a legal proceeding where the man faces a potential death penalty sentence might be unethical because it could pave the way for a future execution, but such is not the case. It is easy to become confused as to who is the client in this case. When working in the forensic arena, particularly under court order, the judicial system is the client. Neuropsychologists are to provide expert opinion on matters from within the sphere of scientific knowledge. In this regard, neuropsychologists simply provide the judge and jury unique information about mental illness and behavior. It is up to the triers of fact to make legal decisions (i.e., *findings*). Allowing for violation of constitutional rights is allowing harm, but providing a reasoned and thoughtful opinion based on sufficient and appropriate information sources is not. Appreciating who the client is and accepting the fact that our opinions may not always "help" the defendant are issues the neuropsychologist must resolve before engaging in forensic work, particularly in capital cases (Denney & Wynkoop, 2000).

Neuropsychologists need to resolve in their own minds their opinion regarding the death penalty and assess their own ability to provide

objective service prior to engaging in such service. As forensic examiners, neuropsychologists are not advocates for a social cause one way or the other. Strong personal beliefs on the issue could potentially, and unknowingly, cloud judgment and make objective assessment difficult. It is imperative that evaluators consider these issues and decide what aspect of a capital case they are willing to participate in prior to accepting the work (Melton et al., 1997).

Informed Consent

This evaluation was done under court order, which sets into place unique circumstances regarding informed consent (Standards 3.10c, 9.03a & b). Normally, neuropsychologists need consent from the person being evaluated, but under a court order such consent is not needed. In this case it is best to acquire informed *assent* (Standard 3.10b) if at all possible. Here the neuropsychologist explained the purpose for the evaluation and acquired appropriate assent, even though it was initially hesitant. The man's hesitancy will be addressed, but it was actually the *informed* aspect of assent where his major ethical dilemmas arise. He informed the man the evaluation was dealing with competency to proceed, not potential future dangerousness. In addition, evaluating future potential dangerousness is a significantly different evaluation which generally requires a different data base.

This aspect of the vignette is based, loosely, on a real case addressed by the U.S. Supreme Court in 1981, called *Estelle v. Smith*. In this case, James Grigson, a psychiatrist, received an informal request from the judge to perform a competency evaluation of defendant Smith. He evaluated Smith regarding competency to proceed and testified during a competency evaluation. During a later sentencing hearing, Dr. Grigson provided testimony on the man's potential dangerousness without having informed him he would be doing so and without competently evaluating the issue. The U.S. Supreme Court ruled that defendant Smith's 6th Amendment right to counsel and

5th Amendment right to be free of self-incrimination were both violated. He should have had counsel (he had no counsel at the time of the evaluation) who was aware of the evaluation prior to performing that evaluation, and he should have been informed that information provided by him could be used to address future potential for dangerousness during a later sentencing phase of his trial. These are certainly issues relevant for neuropsychologists performing evaluations in the criminal forensic arena.

The neuropsychologist provided informed consent in that he explained the nature and purpose of the evaluation and who requested it. In this scenario, the defendant was initially hesitant. The hesitancy apparently resolved after thorough explanation in this case, but significance hesitancy and unwillingness to proceed dictates a course of action for the evaluator. Here is where the Specialty Guidelines provide more direct guidance than the Ethics Code (Specialty Guidelines IV.E, E.1, & E.2). The evaluator is to stop the evaluation until the defendant has opportunity to interact with his attorney. Many times defendants have very good reasons for not wanting to participate in evaluations, but many times concerns can resolve easily with a quick phone call to the attorney. As this evaluation was presumably based on court order, the defendant's consent is not required; however, it is always appropriate to help resolve the concern by allowing contact with counsel. The issue becomes more problematic in the absence of a court order. Because the evaluation is for competency to proceed, the evaluator must not assume the defendant is making a competent decision. When defense attorneys request the evaluation, it is possible they will want the evaluation to continue and seek a court order to have it done. As a result, it is important to make the defense counsel aware of the situation and seek direction. In addition, prosecuting and defense attorneys as well as judges have the freedom to raise the issue of competency to proceed over the objection of the defendant him or herself. In such cases, a court

order is the only reasonable course of action. Judges have the moral and legal mandate to not allow an incompetent defendant to progress through the legal process. Ethical neuropsychologists should have a similar viewpoint.

In this scenario, the neuropsychologist informed the defendant that he was being evaluated for competency to proceed with his legal case. Implied in the Informed Consent sections of the Ethics Code is a mandate to only use that information for the purpose described. Coming back and testifying about future dangerousness without proper informed consent is exactly what Dr. Grigson did in the *Estelle v. Smith*. He used information provided to him from defendant Smith for competency to arrive at a conclusion regarding his dangerousness. Smith's consent was not "informed." In essence, defendant Smith's 5th Amendment right to avoid self-incrimination was violated as described by the U.S. Supreme Court. The Specialty Guidelines address this issue specifically in III.D., "Forensic psychologists have an obligation to understand the civil rights of parties in legal proceedings in which they participate, and manage their professional conduct in a manner that does not diminish or threaten those rights." Similarly, IV.E.3 reveals, "After a psychologist has advised the subject of a clinical forensic evaluation of the intended uses of the evaluation and its work product, the psychologist may not use the evaluation work product for other purposes without explicit waiver to do so by the client or the client's legal representative." This information clearly reveals it would be inappropriate for the neuropsychologist to testify regarding issues other than that on which he was initially consulted. Informed consent is such a serious concern, particularly with death penalty cases, that it behooves the clinician to provide very thorough informed consent by discussing all foreseeable future uses of the work product. Consequently, it is good practice to explain that one could be required to testify about information gathered in the evaluation at a later sentencing hearing as well as an obvious competency hearing or trial. Many forensic practitioners use a written informed consent form. By disclosing all foreseeable potential uses, the evaluator likely resolves the issue of informed consent, but it does not resolve the potential pitfall of providing opinions beyond the scope of the initial evaluation.

Bases for Assessments

The second issue regarding this neuropsychologist testifying to the defendant's future dangerousness was the fact the neuropsychologist did not evaluate the defendant on that issue. More often than not, the specific referral question dictates the nature of the evaluation, including what collaborative sources and what tests will be used. The knowledge domain relevant to assessment of future risk of violence is not the same as that of competency to proceed and certainly includes corroborative information about past history of violence as well as other issues. The neuropsychologist did not establish an adequate data base, as is required by Ethical Standards 2.04 (Bases of Scientific and Professional Judgments) and 9.01 (Bases for Assessments). In this scenario, the neuropsychologist may have stayed within the scope of his evaluation at the time of the sentencing phase if he kept his opinion solely to whether or not the defendant had a mental illness or neurocognitive defect and how this might affect his behavior. The corroborative information was not acquired to provide an expert opinion that the man was, or was not, dangerous.

Case Resolution

When contacted to testify to future potential dangerousness during the sentencing phase, this neuropsychologist decided the appropriate thing to do, given the limited nature of his informed consent and scope of his evaluation, was to explain his ethical dilemma and encourage the referral source to have the defendant evaluated

again on that specific issue. He explained he had not provided informed consent regarding this possibility prior to the evaluation, and testifying to future dangerousness could potentially be considered a violation of the defendant's 5th *Amendment* right to be free of self-incrimination under *Estelle*. In addition, he could not provide an opinion on the man's future dangerousness because he did not evaluate that issue. Specialty Guidelines IV.G reveals this appropriate behavior when pressed to move beyond our ethical boundaries:

> When conflicts arise between the forensic psychologist's professional standards and the requirement of legal standards, a particular court, or a directive by an officer to the court or legal authorities, the forensic psychologist has an obligation to make those legal authorities aware of the source of the conflict and to take reasonable steps to resolve it. Such steps may include, but are not limited to, obtaining the consultation of fellow forensic professional, obtaining the advice of independent counsel, and conferring directly with the legal representatives involved.

If he was still called to testify after his objections, he would instruct the attorney he would have to limit his testimony to only those issues he evaluated, namely presence and nature of any mental illness.

Conclusions and Recommendations

1. *Understand your personal views about suspected and convicted criminals and about the death penalty.* Such consideration must occur before engaging is such practice, because extreme views on this matter can cloud judgment.
2. *Elicit informed consent/assent.* It is best to presume you could be called to testify during any phase of the criminal judicial process.

Consequently, such a possibility needs to be communicated to the defendant so he/she can decide what information to provide. Many evaluators provide written explanation and seek written consent/assent from defendants. While not always necessary, it would be prudent in most situations but particularly in capital cases.

3. *Develop and maintain competency*. Develop competency in criminal forensic practice, and maintain that competency through continued educational activities.
4. *Practice only within your competencies*. Seek supervision, decline, or refer out those cases where you do not have competence regarding unique populations and particular referral questions.
5. *Limit opinions to the referral question and provide opinions only based on sufficient data sources*. Mental health professionals cause numerous difficulties in the judicial system when they do not limit their opinions to the referral questions. Make sure opinions are based on appropriate and adequate, empirically derived, information sources.

Scenario 2

A clinical neuropsychologist provides routine neuropsychological evaluation and treatment services at a state funded head injury rehabilitation hospital in a large metropolitan community. She also maintains a part-time private practice where she focuses on civil and criminal forensic issues. At the rehabilitation hospital, she worked with a young man who survived a severe TBI from a MVA for about three months before he transitioned home and to the day treatment program. As part of her work in the inpatient unit, she completed a routine neuropsychological evaluation and performed much of the face-to-face cognitive rehabilitation. She continued to work with this man in a treatment capacity within the day treatment program. One day, he did not

arrive for day treatment, and she learned he was arrested the evening before and charged with bank robbery. Two weeks later she received a telephone call from the young man's defense attorney asking her if she would complete a neuropsychological evaluation to determine the defendant's competency to stand trial. The attorney said he particularly wanted her to do the examination because she already knows the man quite well, and he was familiar with her previous good work in criminal competency evaluations.

Relevant Ethical Issues

Relevant ethical issues certainly include competency to perform an evaluation on competency to stand trial, but it was apparent from the attorney's familiarity with her previous work (in her private practice) that she had experience performing such evaluations. The major ethical concern here is her recent relationship with the defendant. She was a treating clinician prior to the request for what amounts to an independent forensic examination. A treating clinician, under most circumstances, cannot adequately provide an objective, independent expert opinion about competency to proceed after maintaining a treatment relationship. This change in role is significant enough to constitute a potential dual role under the general issue of multiple relationships.

Multiple Relationships
Ethical Standard 3.05(a) states in part, "A psychologist refrains from entering into a multiple relationship if the multiple relationship could reasonably be expected to impair the psychologist's objectivity, competence or effectiveness in performing his or her functions as a psychologist ..." Additionally, Specialty Guideline IV.D states in part, "(1) Forensic psychologists avoid providing professional services to parties in a legal proceeding with whom they have personal or professional relationships that are inconsistent with the anticipated relationship. (2) When

it is necessary to provide both evaluation and treatment services to a party in a legal proceeding (as may be the case in small forensic hospital settings or small communities), the forensic psychologist takes reasonable steps to minimize the potential negative effects of these circumstances on the rights of the party, confidentiality, and the process of treatment and evaluation."

At first glance, the situation described does not appear to be a multiple relationship based on the description of multiple relationships in the Ethics Code (Standard 3.05) and the Specialty Guidelines (IV.D). At the time of the attorney request, the defendant was no longer in the rehabilitation program. Such a distinction is rather artificial in this instance because the neuropsychologist still remains the treatment provider in the eyes of the defendant; more significantly, the defendant remains a patient in the eyes of the neuropsychologist. When a neuropsychologist is hired to provide an expert opinion, she is expected to provide an independent and objective assessment of the person's condition and apply that information to the forensic question. Ethical Standard 3.05 does not make this situation clear. It is difficult for a neuropsychologist to provide an objective assessment after having been in a treatment relationship with a patient. Forensic Guideline IV.D was written for just such an instance. The guideline recommends avoiding these dual roles except under rare circumstances, such as in small communities or small forensic hospitals where there is simply no other professional available to provide the much needed service. In these instances, it is incumbent on the neuropsychologist to minimize potential conflict, possibly through peer review or consultation.

To better understand this scenario, the reader must realize the difference between a fact witness and an expert witness, and the fact that there can be different roles for expert witnesses (Melton et al., 1997). Fact witnesses provide testimony regarding what they experienced with their own senses; they cannot provide opinion beyond obvious opinions that everyday laymen could conclude from the circumstances, nor can they rely on third party information (called hearsay evidence). Expert witnesses can testify to factual events just as a fact witness, but they can also form opinions regarding the situation based on their specialized education, knowledge, training, and experience. In addition, they can rely on hearsay evidence if it is what other professionals in their field customarily rely upon, such as X-ray technologists, radiologists, psychometricians, et cetera. There would be no concern for the neuropsychologist to testify as a fact witness on the nature of the defendant's head injury, diagnosis, treatment, and such. It is also possible for her to testify as an expert witness, but here is where it becomes complicated. She could testify as an expert regarding the nature of his brain injury, neurocognitive functioning, general mental health, diagnoses, treatment, and prognosis without addressing the *ultimate issue*. The ultimate issue in this scenario is his competency to stand trial; that is the question the "trier of fact" (judge in this instance) must answer. In order to perform in this role as expert, she would not need to evaluate him further as she had her previous evaluation and ongoing treatment interactions to draw from. In this capacity, she could provide insights derived from her knowledge of the patient and her expert knowledge and experience as a neuropsychologist. Providing professional services in the area of criminal forensics is rather complex and requires specialized knowledge, which is exactly why the Specialty Guidelines were developed.

Case Resolution

Given this neuropsychologist's understanding of the need to avoid potential conflict inherent in multiple relationships, she made it very clear to the referring attorney what her role could, and could not, be given her professional ethics and the Specialty Guidelines. She indicated she would be willing to provide expert testimony regarding the nature of the defendant's brain injury, treatment program, response to treatment, and prognosis, but she could not provide an expert opinion regarding the ultimate issue of his competency to stand trial. She recommended the attorney use her as the treatment specialist to describe the serious impact of the defendant's past head injury, but that the attorney hire another forensic expert to evaluate the man and address his competency to stand trial. She then provided her recommendations for competent and ethical forensic providers in the community.

Conclusions and Recommendations

1. *Be aware of the Specialty Guidelines for Forensic Psychologists.* The Ethical Principles and Code of Conduct do not adequately address the complexities inherent in practicing forensic psychology, particularly in the criminal forensic arena.
2. *Keep abreast of other competent and ethical practitioners in the community.* It is tremendously helpful to have at your fingertips a list of competent clinicians, particularly those who have criminal forensic experience, not only to provide to those requesting services, but also to have as colleagues in arms and consultants to rely upon for guidance in ethically complex forensic situations.
3. *Anticipate attempts by attorneys to ignore neuropsychologists' role clarifications while on the stand.* Although the neuropsychologist may have explained the limits of her opinions as a treating neuropsychologist, it is possible the attorney calling her as a witness could ignore her request and press on to ultimate opinion questions while she was on the witness stand. In such instances, it may be wise to first allow the opposing attorney time to object before beginning to answer (Behnke, Perlin, & Bernstein, 2003). If no objection is

forthcoming, it is incumbent of the neuropsychologist to simply indicate she does not have an opinion regarding the man's competency. The attorney may even ask questions which set the stage for her to come to a "professional opinion" based on the facts of the case or "hypotheticals." Nevertheless, she should not provide such an ultimate issue opinion unless she has actually evaluated that issue (asked the defendant questions about specific competency related issues in this case). There might be times, when the expert does have an opinion about that issue even though she did not evaluate the specific issues. In this instance, such opinions are based on personal impression and incomplete information rather than sound evaluation techniques. As a general rule, experts should refrain from providing opinions that are not based on "reasonable scientific or professional certainty." In fact, we are ethically bound to withhold them by simply indicating we do not have an expert opinion on that issue.

References

Behnke, S.H., Perlin, M.L., & Bernstein, M. (2003). *The essentials of New York Mental Health Law: A straightforward guide for clinicians of all disciplines.* New York: W.W. Norton & Company.

Committee on Ethical Guidelines for Forensic Psychologists (1991). Specialty Guidelines for Forensic Psychologists. *Law and Human Behavior 15 (6)*, 655-665. Available at http://www.abfp.com/downloadable/foren.pdf

Denney, R.L., & Wynkoop, T.F. (2000). Clinical neuropsychology in the criminal forensic setting. *Journal of Head Injury Rehabilitation 15*, 804–828.

Estelle v. Smith 451 U.S. 454 (U.S. Supreme Court, 1981).

Melton, G.B., Petrila, J. Poythress, N.G., & Slobogin, C. (1997). *Psychological Evaluations for the Courts.* (2nd ed.). New York: Guilford.

Chapter 2

ETHICAL CHALLENGES IN FORENSIC NEUROPSYCHOLOGY, PART II

Christopher L. Grote

Scenario 1

An attorney was injured in a motor vehicle accident and claimed cognitive deficits as a result of a mild head injury incurred at the time. He then claimed that he was unable to practice law and applied for benefits through his disability carrier. He was referred for an independent neuropsychological evaluation. During the interview, some of his responses raised questions about whether he was still licensed, or license-eligible, to practice law. He appeared evasive when asked if he still has his law license and whether any complaints had been filed against him with the state agency that disciplines attorneys. His medical records did not refer to these issues. Neuropsychological testing resulted in many impaired scores on tests of cognitive ability, but the patient also failed two "tests of effort". A subsequent "Google" internet search indicated that an attorney, with the same name and state of residence as the patient, had an upcoming disbarment hearing because of allegations of embezzlement of a large sum of money.

Relevant Ethical Issues

Dilemma: Should a neuropsychologist play the role of "private detective"?

This case was generated in the context of a "forensic neuropsychology" setting. The patient was referred by his disability carrier for an "independent medical evaluation". Therefore, it was made clear to the patient, prior to any interview or testing, that: (a) there was no traditional treating or "doctor-patient" relationship; (b) there were limits of confidentiality and anything from the interview or testing that was deemed relevant to the evaluation would be reported to the disability carrier; and (c) the patient or "client" would not receive any feedback directly from the psychologist unless there was authorization to do so from the disability carrier.

Do the Ethical Principles of the American Psychological Association (APA) (2002) speak to the appropriateness of accessing publicly-available information without the patient's knowledge, or consent, and if so, do these principles differentiate between "treating" and "forensic" cases? In short, the answer appears to be "no" to both of these questions. Reference to the 2002 Ethics Code indicates that Standard 3.10 (Informed Consent) has a number of potentially relevant provisions. These include that the psychologist "obtain the informed consent of the individual", although the breadth or extent of detail to be provided is not specified. Standard 3.10 also states that when the evaluation is court ordered or otherwise mandated, psychologists tell the patient of the "anticipated services, including whether the services are court ordered or mandated and any limits of confidentiality, before proceeding". Finally, Standard 3.10 states that "psychologists appropriately document written or oral consent, permission, and assent".

Consider for a moment that the Google search did not turn up an attorney with the patient's name. Would it be appropriate, in that case, for the neuropsychologist to call the registrars of the schools from which the patient claimed to have graduated in order to confirm attendance and graduation? Johnson-Greene et al. (1995, 1997) have reported that patients' self-report of their educational attainment is often inaccurate, and that confirmation of claims of school attendance or graduation can easily be confirmed by simply phoning a school's registrar. However, Standard 4.06 (Consultations) states that psychologists "do not disclose confidential information that reasonably could lead to the identification of a client/patient ...". This implies that it would be unethical to have called the registrar if the patient's status (as a patient) and the reason for the request were revealed.

Finally, Standard 9 (Assessment) also has a few potentially relevant subsections. These include 9.01 (Bases for Assessments), which states that psychologists base their opinions on "information and techniques sufficient to substantiate their findings". This indicates that psychologists need sufficient information on which to base their judgments and interpretations. In many situations, it is vital to determine the patient's level of education so that test results can be properly interpreted. Standard 9.03 (Informed Consent in Assessment) dictates that psychologists usually obtain informed consent for assessments, and that such consent includes an explanation of the nature and purpose of assessment. This standard seems to largely say the same thing as the earlier-reviewed Standard 3.10, the problem again being that there is no guidance on how much or how little information should be provided in obtaining informed

consent. Finally, Standard 9.06 (Interpreting Assessment Results) states that psychologists need to account for things that might affect their interpretation of the results, including "various test factors, test-taking abilities, and other characteristics of the person being assessed ...". This seems reminiscent of Standard 9.01 in reminding psychologists that they need to understand the context in which their data is being collected.

Case Resolution

In the above case, one could not be absolutely sure that the person identified in the Google search was the same person being evaluated. The issue was resolved by asking the disability carrier to determine if they could obtain information from the state's Attorney Registration and Disciplinary Committee as to whether the patient was licensed to practice law. The carrier later forwarded a document which showed that the patient indeed was scheduled for a hearing to determine whether he should be disbarred because of allegations of embezzlement. This information was extremely relevant to questions being asked of the psychologist regarding the patient's ability to work as an attorney. The patient was disbarred several months after the psychological evaluation.

Conclusions and Recommendations

Neither the 1992 nor the 2002 Code appears to offer any specific guidance as to whether accessing public information during the course of an evaluation is even an ethical issue. The notion that this might be an ethical or problematic issue arose only after a colleague questioned whether certain activities, such as confirming that a patient attended a certain school, would be better described as "detective work" rather than that of psychological evaluation. A question was raised as to whether the patient had adequate knowledge of what might happen during the evaluation, and whether "snooping" would violate informed consent requirements or the right to privacy and dignity (Principle E, Respect for People's Rights and Dignity).

Inquiries were then made of other colleagues as to what they thought of such practices. Most responded that such activities were not only ethical but incumbent upon psychologists who wish to offer fully-informed opinions that would be of maximal utility both to the patient and the referent. Some pointed out that psychologists have the same right as other members of the public in accessing publicly-available information, and that there was no reason for evaluating psychologists to deny themselves such information. However, one colleague commented that although this practice may not be precluded by the Ethical Principles, he would not do it for fear of alienating the patient. Another colleague commented that such activities might change the "playing field" to one that is "not level" as the psychologist is accessing certain information without the patient's knowledge. Yet another colleague suggested that patients be approached to sign a "release of information" to gather such information so that both the psychologist and the patient understand what information will be gathered and that the patient's refusal to sign such a document might in itself provide diagnostic information. Another colleague replied that a patient who would use this opportunity to deny release would then put the psychologist in the position of having less information available to him or her than an ordinary citizen.

In conclusion, one might argue that these may be "non-issues" since even a broad reading of the 1992 and 2002 Ethical Principles does not indicate any reason to think that accessing publicly-available information is prohibited. Indeed, in recent years there have several accounts of public figures, including politicians, celebrities and coaches, who have admitted to falsifying accounts of their military or educational records. One recent article cited the findings of an executive recruiter who found evidence of misrepresentation of

education reports among some 11 to 23% of job seekers (Parker, 2002).

Resolution of this type of case may depend on how one interprets, and weighs, the relative obligations of "Informed Consent" versus "Bases for Assessment". The Ethics Code only gives general outlines of what is meant by each term, and it is unclear as to how much or how little detail should be provided to obtain informed consent. It may be a matter of opinion as to how much information is needed for a clinician to have a sufficient basis to make a clinical decision. For example, should pre-evaluation informed consent include a warning that the patient's "effort" will be measured with a "malingering" test, or that the MMPI-2 includes validity scales to determine the over- or under-reporting of symptoms of psychopathology? To this end, some authors (Youngjohn, Lees-Haley, & Binder, 1999) suggested that "warning malingerers" only produced more sophisticated attempts to malinger but did not change the problem.

In terms of Bases for Assessment, one could argue that it is or is not vital to confirm the details of a patient's self-report. While the importance of these details will vary on a case-by-case basis, in general it should be remembered that psychological testing typically is meant to predict some specific "real world" behavior, such as ability to work. As such, more times than not it will be crucial for the psychologist to obtain records that reflect other aspects of the patients functioning outside the neuropsychology laboratory.

The 1992 and 2002 Ethics Codes do not preclude a psychologist from accessing publicly-available information to confirm aspects of patients' self-reports. However, information gathered from these methods should be used very cautiously, as misidentifications may occur. For example, a patient may have attended a school under a different name, or a school may simply be in error when it reports that there are no records for a particular person. Additionally, one should not be surprised if a patient were to become angry at learning that somebody "checked up" on them. Despite these potential problems, psychologists should not be dissuaded from checking publicly-available records as a means of increasing the utility and accuracy of their evaluation reports.

Scenario 2

A stock broker had been in treatment for depression when he applied for disability benefits, and was then referred for a neuropsychological evaluation. The insurer forwards relevant records, including the broker's resume. The resume indicates a number of job changes and some periods of unemployment in the years pre-dating the issuance of his disability insurance. During the interview with the broker, he clearly states his anger at the disability carrier, and feels that the neuropsychological evaluation is an attempt for the carrier to go on a "fishing expedition" to find some reason not to pay his claim. He states that he will answer only those interview questions that he feels are relevant. It is explained that his feelings are understood, but that such feelings will not preclude his being asked about topics deemed relevant by the neuropsychologist. In subsequent interview, the broker does reply to initial questions about his background, but becomes agitated when he is asked about his vocational history. He repeatedly tells the neuropsychologist to "move on" to questions about his current symptoms, and is firm in his refusal to answer any additional questions about his background.

Relevant Ethical Issues

Dilemma: What information is needed to complete a neuropsychological evaluation, and who should determine this?

It is not unusual for litigants and insurance claimants to voice their displeasure at being evaluated by a neuropsychologist retained by an insurance company or a defense attorney. Some have gone so far as to specifically voice their concern that the evaluator is a "hired gun" whose goal is to disprove their claim. Attempts to build some rapport with such patients may be difficult if not impossible, and an evaluator's self-perception of being objective and their attempts to communicate this to the client may be answered with scornful looks or derisive comments from the patient. At times, evaluators may feel that they're on the "on the defensive" and subsequently feel a need to demonstrate their sympathy with the client, or may even be tempted to accede to the patient's preferences for not being asked certain questions or completing certain tests.

How does an evaluating psychologist balance a client's desire for non-disclosure against the responsibility to offer fully-informed neuropsychological opinions? This issue does not seem to have been discussed in previous publications on ethics in psychological assessment, and is not specifically mentioned in the 1992 or 2002 editions of the Ethics Code. However, several principles and standards in the 2002 version may offer some guidance. Principle E (Respect for People's Rights and Dignity) is among several aspirational and non-enforceable goals aimed at guiding psychologists "towards the highest ideals of psychology". Principle E states that psychologists respect "the rights of individuals to privacy, confidentiality and self-determination".

An enforceable standard that is related to Principle E is Standard 4.04 (Minimizing Intrusions on Privacy), which states, in part, that "Psychologists include in written and oral reports and consultations, only information germane to the purpose for which the communication is made". This obviously raises the question of how to determine what is or is not relevant, and it is likely that a psychologist's interpretation of this issue may differ from that of the client/patient. It is possible, for example, that even questions about a patient's religious affiliations and beliefs, political leanings or sexual orientation may be useful in framing a context from which neuropsychological interpretations are made. However, in such cases, the psychologist should be ready to detail how the information is potentially relevant to the diagnosis and treatment of the patient.

Additional concerns or limits on the collection and distribution of patient information may arise from provisions contained in the Health Insurance Portability and Accountability Act (HIPAA) which took effect in April 2003. Originally designed to simplify and protect the confidentiality of electronic billing and transmission of health information, this legislation has evolved into a complex series of administrative rules that impact both the clinical and research activities of neuropsychologists. For example, it has been reported that one provision of HIPAA is that only the "minimum necessary" information be collected from patients, placed in their charts and then transmitted to others. Of course, what constitutes minimum necessary is debatable. Consultation with a hospital HIPAA officer indicates that this would be determined by the "clinician's judgment" and would ordinarily not be second-guessed as long as other clinicians agreed that such information was necessary to complete an evaluation.

In addition to increased privacy rights, HIPAA provides for increased patient access to their medical records, and for the rights of patients to amend their medical records to clarify errors. However, of particular relevance to this chapter is the caveat that because forensic services are designed to serve a legal purpose, they do not constitute health services (Connell & Koocher, 2003). As a result, information compiled in anticipation of use in *civil, criminal, and administrative* proceedings is not subject to the same right of review and amendment as is health care information in general [§164.524(a)(1)(ii)] (U.S. Department of Health and Human Services, 2003). That is, according to Connell and Koocher (2003), HIPAA and the privacy rules included therein do not apply to forensic assessment. Finally, when considering applicable laws, state laws must be considered, and the more stringent of the state and federal laws will apply.

The need to limit invasions on a patient's privacy has to be balanced against the obligation to have sufficient information available to interpret test data and to offer suitably-informed opinions. As earlier reviewed, Standard 9.01 (Bases for Assessments) states that "Psychologists base the opinions contained in their recommendations, reports, and diagnostic or evaluative statements, including forensic testimony, on information and techniques sufficient to substantiate their findings". This would seem to suggest that it is necessary in some cases to ask, or to even insist upon obtaining, information relevant to a patient/client's previous and current functioning. This information might include academic transcripts, medical and military records, or the patient's self-report of vocational, family, health and psychiatric history, to cite just some examples. Failure to obtain and incorporate this information into a clinical evaluation could cause a psychologist to lack sufficient bases for their judgments and interpretations.

Finally, it should be noted that Standard 3.06 (Conflict of Interest) states that "Psychologists refrain from taking on a professional role when personal, scientific, professional, legal, financial or other interests or relationships could reasonably be expected to (1) impair their objectivity, competency or effectiveness in performing their functions as psychologists …". The most obvious implication of this standard is that psychologists indeed cannot serve as a "hired gun", and that their opinions and judgments should not be influenced by whom has retained them or will pay their fee. Checklists on how one can maintain their objectivity can be found in other publications (Sweet & Moulthrop, 1999; van Gorp & McMullen, 1997).

Case Resolution

Again, the APA Ethics Code does not appear to offer specific guidance on ways to resolve potential conflicts between a patient's desire for non-disclosure and the psychologist's need to have appropriate bases for their judgment and interpretation. Resolution in at least some cases may depend on whose conviction is stronger: the psychologist's "need to know" versus the patient's feeling that self-disclosure is irrelevant and/or may hurt their claim.

In the vignette, the patient was referred to determine whether he was competent to work in his usual occupation and if possible/applicable to determine at what point in time he had lost the ability to work at that job. Given that the patient was unwilling to answer any additional questions about his background after a certain point in interview, it was decided that the evaluation should be terminated. A subsequent call was made to the referring defense attorney to explain the situation, including that neuropsychological test data could later be collected but would be of limited value if the neuropsychologist could not understand the patient's perception of why he couldn't work and when this problem started. The attorney understood the neuropsychologist's concerns and stated that her opinion that the patient was required to answer the questions that had been attempted in the interview. It was later reported to the neuropsychologist by another attorney, at the same defense firm, that the patient's claim had been dismissed in court although they did not know if it was related to the patient's refusal to answer all interview questions during the neuropsychological evaluation, or some other reason.

Conclusion and Recommendations

Neuropsychologists are obligated to offer objective opinions, whether the client/patient was referred by a treating physician, attorney or insurance company. What makes an opinion objective? At a minimum, it includes appropriate and relevant information gathered from interview, review of records, and a dispassionate interpretation of neuropsychological and psychological test data. Lack of data from any of these three areas could pose a problem for interpretation.

Some cases of insufficient data may not preclude one from answering the questions-at-hand, and the neuropsychologist may not even need to comment on the issue. At the other end of the spectrum, neuropsychologists should be prepared to withdraw from a case, or to at least not write a report, if they feel they have been denied access to records or if a patient has not answered all questions asked of them.

Unfortunately, it may be inevitable that an evaluator will be "at loggerheads" with the occasional patient during an interview for a forensic neuropsychological evaluation. It is recommended, based in part on the 2002 Ethics Code, that the neuropsychologist keeps in mind what information is deemed necessary to complete the evaluation. If the requested information has the potential of being critical in obtaining an understanding of the patient's history and functioning, then it is recommended that the neuropsychologist politely persist in trying to get the information in interview. Of course, the patient may not agree that the information is a relevant topic for the interview, so the neuropsychologist should be prepared to offer a polite and reasonable explanation of why such information is necessary. If the patient persists in refusing to answer certain questions, the neuropsychologist should respect this position and not necessarily try to trick or brow-beat an answer out of the patient. Instead, the neuropsychologist should inform the patient of reasonably foreseeable consequences of their not answering the questions. These outcomes might include termination of the evaluation, or that the neuropsychologist will not be able to do what was asked of them that day, and subsequent visits with the patient might be requested. The neuropsychologist should not make any predictions about the effect of the patient's refusal-to-answer in terms of pending litigation or claims, obviously enough, as such information is probably not known. Instead, the neuropsychologist should attempt to remain calm and polite, but firm, in requesting information that is deemed important to the evaluation. In general, there seems to be little to no risk of running afoul of the Ethics Code by trying to obtain relevant information from a patient. In contrast, it seems possible that violations of the Code might take place when a neuropsychologist fails to obtain critical information or fails to acknowledge that missing information places limits on the ability to offer fully-informed opinions.

References

American Psychological Association, (1992). Ethical principles of psychologists and code of conduct. *American Psychologist, 47*, 1597-1611.

American Psychological Association, (2002). Ethical principles of psychologists and code of conduct. *American Psychologist, 57*, 1060-1073.

Connell, M., & Koocher, G. (2003). HIPAA & forensic practice. *American Psychology Law Society News, 23 (2)*, 16-19.

Johnson-Greene, D., & Binder, L. (1995). Evaluation of an efficient method for verifying higher educational credentials. *Archives of Clinical Neuropsychology, 10*, 251-253.

Johnson-Greene, D., Dehring, M., Adams, K., Miller, D., Arora, S., Beylin, S., & Brandon, R. (1997). Accuracy of self-reported educational attainment among diverse patient populations: A preliminary investigation. *Archives of Clinical Neuropsychology, 12,* 635-643.

Parker, I. (2002, November 4). Dept. of padding dishonorable degrees. *The New Yorker, 78 (33)*, 46-47.

Sweet, J., & Moulthrop, M. (1999). Self-examination questions as a means of identifying bias in adversarial assessments. *Journal of Forensic Neuropsychology, 1*, 73-88.

U.S. Department of Health and Human Services (2003). Public Law 104-191: Health Insurance Portability and Accountability Act of 1996. Retrieved November 24, 2003 from http://www.hhs.gov/ocr/hipaa/

van Gorp, W., & McMullen, W. (1997). Potential sources of bias in forensic neuropsychological evaluations. *The Clinical Neuropsychologist, 11*, 180-187.

Youngjohn, J., Lees-Haley, P., & Binder, L. (1999). Comment: Warning malingerers produces more sophisticated malingering. *Archives of Clinical Neuropsychology, 14*, 511-515.

Chapter 3

ETHICAL CHALLENGES IN FORENSIC NEUROPSYCHOLOGY, PART III

Stephen Honor

Scenario 1

The patient is a fifty-five year old man referred by his neurologist for neuropsychological examination and treatment following head and physical injuries sustained in a motor vehicle accident (MVA). The patient experienced posttraumatic amnesia with no recall of the accident. The neurological examination report indicated that following the accident the patient had "very little active cognitive functioning." The patient presented with a number of neurocognitive and neurobehavioral symptoms that reportedly did not exist prior to the MVA. Because the referral was less than two months post MVA, rather than conducting a comprehensive neuropsychological examination, a shorter neurobehavioral screening examination was administered. The results of the screening indicated moderate to severe impairments in memory, attention, language functions and visuoconstructional ability. On a nonverbal test of intelligence, the patient, a college graduate, obtained a score of 81, which was below the average range of intelligence.

Following the neurobehavioral screening assessment, the treatment plan was to monitor the patient's (hoped for) recovery, to provide neuropsychological counseling services to the patient and his wife in order to help them to understand what had happened to the patient

apparently as a result of the accident, and to help the patient cope and adapt to his deficits and inability to function adequately as a result of the head injury. Referral to a cognitive rehabilitation program was also to be considered. A more comprehensive neuropsychological examination was deferred for several months and would be performed if the patient's cognitive deficits did not begin to remit.

The patient's past medical history was significant for psychiatric disability due to depression, for which he continued to receive psychotherapy and antidepressant medication. This information was reported in the initial Neurobehavioral Screening Examination Report. Notwithstanding this premorbid condition, the patient, and his wife, reported that he had not previously exhibited the significant cognitive and neurobehavioral symptoms that reportedly developed after the MVA. In obtaining copies of medical records pertaining to the accident, two of the patient's health care professionals reported that they had provided services to the patient for physical problems prior to the MVA. Both practitioners were clear that prior to the MVA, they were not aware of any (overt) cognitive problems; both independently reported that they observed significant changes in the patient's cognitive functioning post MVA.

Following three months of neuropsychological services, the patient was notified by his no-fault insurer that, as a result of the findings of a neuropsychological IME, payment for further treatment and evaluation services was being denied. The insurance company denial stated that the IME examiner had "determined the subjective information relating to cognitive impairment has origins predating the motor vehicle accident … and are not causally related to that accident."

Since this opinion was not consistent with the information provided by the patient, his spouse, and two long-term health care practitioners, the treating neuropsychologist questioned the basis on which the IME neuropsychologist had made his determination.

A copy of the IME neuropsychological evaluation report was obtained. The report correctly described the history of the accident, including the PTA, and the patient's physical and cognitive complaints. Also of note, the IME neuropsychologist stated that "no medical records were made available" at the time of the IME.

The IME examiner reported that, in addition to interview information, a screening examination was conducted (in fact, the same screening test that was utilized by the treating neuropsychologist in initially assessing the patient's reported cognitive problems was used); the findings indicated several areas of prominent cognitive deficit. The IME examiner further reported that the patient acknowledged that he was experiencing some level of depression and anxiety, as well as reporting a prior history of psychiatric treatment (although there was little specificity as to medications or type and duration of psychotherapy).

In the Diagnostic section, the IME neuropsychologist suggested a "working diagnosis" of unresolved adjustment disorder with possible exacerbation of a pre-existing psychiatric history. At that time the IME examiner did not recommend denial of payment for further services. However, an Addendum report was filed with the insurer within two months, which suggested that the insurer had requested copies of post-MVA

medical records and had provided them to the IME neuropsychologist. In the Addendum report, the examiner specified all of the documents that were supplied and reviewed; the examiner then stated that the post-MVA records made it "more apparent" that the patient presented with "longstanding depression" which predated the MVA, and that the cognitive impairment also predated the MVA and was therefore not causally related. Based upon that Addendum report, the no-fault insurer denied payment for further neuropsychological services. What was problematic about the IME examiner's opinion was that the treating neuropsychologist was in possession of all of the post-MVA medical records that the IME examiner had reviewed, and there was no indication whatsoever that the patient had reported to anyone that he was experiencing cognitive difficulty prior to the car accident. The treating neuropsychologist responded to the IME examiner's Addendum report by questioning the basis of the modified conclusion that the cognitive problems were of a premorbid nature. It was suggested that the IME examiner, in the absence of any confirming data, had made a speculative assumption that was inappropriate and unsubstantiated.

What ensued was a series of communications, with the IME examiner maintaining the same position without actually responding to the question of the basis of the specified conclusions. At a point, the IME examiner requested that the insurer obtain a copy of all premorbid psychiatric records to assess whether or not there was an indication of premorbid cognitive deficit. The treating neuropsychologist supported this recommendation, making the request that the insurer reinstate the patient's neuropsychological benefits until such time that the records confirmed the IME examiner's opinion. The reasoning was that since there was no information provided to demonstrate the accuracy of the examiner's conclusions regarding premorbid cognitive deficits, the results of the IME were therefore inconclusive, and the patient should not be further penalized due to an inconclusive IME. The no-fault insurer refused, suggesting that not only should their examiner review the premorbid medical records, but that the same examiner should also conduct further testing to assess whether or not the patient was malingering or suffering from psychological/psychiatric problems that could affect cognitive functioning. In fact, the patient received notification specifying a date for a second neuropsychological IME with the same examiner. The reasoning of this recommendation was vigorously challenged by the treating neuropsychologist and the patient's attorney. Not only had their examiner not suggested a consideration of malingering in the reports already provided to the insurance carrier, but it was acknowledged that the patient was certainly suffering from psychological problems which in all likelihood had been exacerbated not only by the effects of the MVA, but by the manner in which the insurer was handling his case, notably the denial of payment for services that were deemed essential. Additionally, confirmation of significant psychological distress and cognitive deficit obtained by further testing would in no way answer the question as to whether or not the cognitive deficits were of a premorbid nature. It is of note that during the several months that this situation was unfolding, the patient became significantly depressed, at one point potentially suicidal.

A request was made of the carrier that, based upon the written authorization of the patient, the treating neuropsychologist be provided with a copy of all of the IME neuropsychologists records, including all raw data. After a period of "haggling" with the insurer and IME examiner, and with the assistance of the patient's attorney, those records were supplied. Careful review of the records, which included copies of the raw data from the IME examiner's "examination," as well as history forms completed by the patient and the IME examiner's notes, made it clear that while the IME examiner's tests confirmed significant cognitive deficits, neither the examiner's notes

nor any of the history forms suggested that the patient experienced cognitive difficulties before his accident. There was nothing in any of these records that supported the IME examiner's opinion that the patient had exhibited premorbid cognitive deficit.

While the insurer was requesting the fourteen years of premorbid psychiatric records, the treating neuropsychologist also independently obtained the same records; in addition, the treating neuropsychologist spoke on the telephone with the patient's prior therapist (who had been the same individual throughout the entire fourteen years of treatment). Both the therapist's verbal information and a very careful review of the premorbid medical records confirmed the information provided by the patient; notwithstanding the acknowledged psychological problems, neither the therapist nor the medical records indicated any cognitive deficits. Based upon this additional information, the insurer was contacted again by the treating neuropsychologist and the patient's attorney to insist that they reinstate the patient's neuropsychological benefits. While the request for reinstated benefits included a request to the IME examiner to issue an additional Addendum report modifying the opinion that the cognitive deficits were of a premorbid nature, not only did the examiner never issue such an Addendum or directly deal with the question as to the basis of the opinion of premorbid cognitive functioning, but the insurer continued to refuse to rescind their denial of payment for neuropsychological services.

Relevant Ethical Issues

The issues involved in this case represent questions concerning the professionalism and objectivity of the initial IME neuropsychologist. The examiner's unsupported, speculative opinion (Standard 2.04, Bases for Scientific and Professional Judgments; Standard 9.01, Bases for Assessments; and Standard 9.02, Use of

Assessments) not only interrupted the necessary examination and treatment services, but did harm to the patient as well (Principle A, Beneficence and Nonmaleficence; Standard 3.04, Avoiding Harm). Although the IME examiner was protected from a malpractice claim because of what are recognized as the restrictive rules that govern "independent medical evaluations," which states (among other things) that there is no "doctor/patient relationship," does this release such individuals from professional and ethical responsibilities to individuals undergoing such IMEs?

In fact, there is an American Medical Association (AMA) position paper that states that a "limited" doctor-patient relationship does exist even in such circumstances (AMA, Council on Ethical and Judicial Affairs, 1999), and a recent position paper by the National Academy of Neuropsychology (Bush et al., 2003) details the professional and ethical responsibilities of the independent forensic neuropsychological examiner. There are patients who are hurt, or whose problems become exacerbated, due to the results of questionable IMEs at the hands of biased health care practitioners, such as this IME neuropsychologist. Neuropsychologists have a responsibility to monitor their own potential biases and to avoid allowing those biases to impact on those whom they examine and treat (Principle B, Fidelity and Responsibility; Principle C, Integrity; Standard 3.06, Conflict of Interest).

In this case, the nature of the professional and ethical concerns was made known to the IME neuropsychologist who did not respond in a professional manner to those issues. Although there may be occasional cases in which health care practitioners who are not treating professionals are held accountable for the effect(s) of their opinions on the examinees, at this time, the ability to enforce ethical mandates in such situations remains insufficient. Thus, the question remains, what redress does an individual, such as the patient depicted in this case, have against non-treating professionals whose opinions are the basis of denial of services deemed necessary by the patient and his treating health care professionals?

In contrast to the potential threats to the ethical standards and principles discussed above in relation to the IME neuropsychologist, the treating neuropsychologist seemed to employ the principle of Beneficence. By taking a strong advocacy role and fighting for the patient's rights in a system with which the patient was unfamiliar and unable to engage, the treating neuropsychologist was able to secure additional benefits for the patient, thus helping him during a very difficult period.

Case Resolution

During the several months that this issue was unfolding, a formal complaint was made to the State Insurance Department; this agency did contact the insurer in support of the request to clarify the basis of their decision to deny payment for the patient's services, given the results of an equivocal and non-definitive IME. Once again, the insurer refused to reinstate the patient's benefits. However, at no time during the several month period of time did the no-fault insurer, or the IME neuropsychologist, address the treating neuropsychologist's challenge that the IME examiner's conclusions were speculative assumptions not based on any existing data. While this was seen as the main issue, it was not ever addressed. After being continuously challenged, and with the pressure of the state insurance department, the no-fault insurer "spontaneously" issued a cancellation of the second IME with the neuropsychologist in question, indicating that they would arrange for the proposed second IME with a different neuropsychologist. Approximately two months later the patient was notified that he had been scheduled for a neuropsychological IME with a practitioner a great distance from the patient's residence. However, since the treating neuropsychologist was aware of the reputation of this second examiner as being an objective and "honest" practitioner (based upon prior IMEs conducted by this neuropsychologist), in spite of the great inconvenience to the patient, that IME was conducted.

Of additional interest is the fact that the no-fault insurer did not supply the treating neuropsychologist, the patient, or his attorney with a copy of the results of this second neuropsychological IME. It was necessary to write several letters, renew the complaint with the state insurance department, and finally to make a personal call to the claim representative to obtain a copy of the IME report. The results of the second IME indicated that the patient exhibited significant cognitive and emotional deficits, and that there was no evidence that the cognitive problems were of a premorbid nature. Appropriate examination and treatment were recommended (the patient to date had never undergone comprehensive examination to assess his status), effectively "overturning" the opinion of the first IME.

Conclusions and Recommendations

There exist a variety of professional roles that a neuropsychologist can assume in a personal injury forensic case. Although provided against a backdrop of litigation, the neuropsychologist seen for treatment upon referral from another healthcare professional or upon self-referral occupies the position of treating doctor, one who may advocate for the neuropsychological rights of the patient when such action is indicated. Consistent with the Ethics Code's aspirational General Principles, there may be occasions when treating neuropsychologists *should* advocate for the neuropsychological rights of patients who have limited ability to advocate for themselves.

Scenario 2

The patient is a man of Portuguese birth who was involved in an MVA at 37 years of age,

which was several years ago. The patient was a pedestrian who was hit by a car while crossing the street. He brought a law suit against the driver of the car, and in the course of his care he was examined by two qualified neuropsychologists. The plaintiff was referred to the first neuropsychologist by his physician. The second neuropsychologist was retained by the plaintiff's attorney. Another neuropsychologist was retained by the attorneys for the defense insurance company to review the medical records and neuropsychological examination reports and to offer an opinion as to the accuracy of the findings and the processes used by the previous two neuropsychologists in evaluating the plaintiff. The neuropsychologist for the defense did not meet or directly examine the plaintiff. The retaining defense attorneys were advised that in the absence of conducting a formal examination or directly evaluating the plaintiff, opinions offered by the neuropsychologist would be restricted to assessing the work of the treating and plaintiff neuropsychologists, and that no opinion regarding the status of the plaintiff could be offered.

The patient emigrated to the United States approximately nine years prior to the car accident and was non-English speaking. Therefore, in order for the plaintiff neuropsychologist to conduct the examination, a interpreter provided by the plaintiff's attorneys was used for all meetings and examination sessions.

The information provided pertaining to the MVA included the following: the patient was seen in the ER and was discharged with head injury instructions; in addition to diagnoses of the patient's physical injuries, a diagnosis of traumatic brain injury with postconcussive headaches was made by the treating physiatrist; the treating neuropsychological examination was conducted approximately two months after the MVA (although no report was written specifying the findings of that examination, diagnoses of concussion, dementia due to head injury, and posttraumatic stress disorder were attributed to the first neuropsychologist); the second (plaintiff) examination was conducted approximately two years post MVA; referral was by the plaintiff attorneys; the basis of referral of the plaintiff was to "determine the nature of his residual cognitive and affective impairments secondary to a traumatic brain injury"; the plaintiff reportedly suffered a "possible head trauma" with "a brief period of loss of consciousness"; the plaintiff's ability to report his own background information was compromised, and there was a vagueness to the information that was provided; there was no history of prior head injury or psychological/psychiatric difficulty; chronic pain and sleep/wake cycle disturbance were reported; and two months subsequent to the MVA, the plaintiff had a fall in which he again injured his head with reports of dizziness and poor balance.

Personal background information provided by the plaintiff included (in part): 8th grade education completed in Portugal; employment in construction prior to the MVA; and he was married and had one child.

The plaintiff neuropsychologist conducted the examination in two extended sessions with translations provided by the plaintiff attorney's interpreter. Because of the language problems, the neuropsychologist indicated that "select verbal tasks" and motoric and visually mediated tasks were used. The neuropsychologist reported the opinion that because of the "ease of translation" and the patient's cooperation, the test scores were an "accurate reflection of the patient's maximal abilities."

Based upon performance on the examination, the plaintiff neuropsychologist came to the following conclusions: pre-accident intellectual abilities were estimated to have been in the average to low average range; test performance was considered to be significantly below the "projected pre morbid average to low average I.Q. level" and his "prior educational achievements"; the neuropsychologist indicated that the plaintiff met DSM-IV criteria for major depression and posttraumatic stress disorder; the deficits noted in testing were considered to be reflective of a

"TBI" with significant deficits in attention, information processing, memory and executive functioning; and, no evidence of malingering was noted.

Recommendations included (in part): psychiatric referral for evaluation of medication needs; neurological evaluation with EEG to rule out potential petit mal seizures; cognitive remediation (ideally provided by a therapist able to speak Portuguese); and, psychotherapy (also by a therapist speaking the patient's language).

Relevant Ethical Issues

There are a number of professional and ethical concerns that arise with respect to the manner in which the second neuropsychologist evaluated and managed this case. Given that the reviewing neuropsychologist was retained by defense counsel, the specific nature of the professional "concerns" was provided to them for use in their litigation of the case. The following represents the major problems which, after the outcome of the case, would be addressed.

Third-Party Presence

All examination sessions were conducted with a third party, the interpreter, in the room. There was no consideration by the examiner of the possible effects of the presence of that third party on the plaintiff's performance on the examination, a factor which has been explored by a number of researchers and writers (Hamsher, Lee & Baron, 2001; McCaffrey, Williams, Fisher, & Laing, 1997; National Academy of Neuropsychology, 2000). The interpreter was provided by plaintiff's counsel. The neuropsychologist did not appear to take into consideration the effect of translation itself on the test results and thusly on the validity of the test data (e.g., the neuropsychologist had no idea as to how accurately the interpreter translated the instructions for the tests) nor any consideration of the possibility that plaintiff attorney's interpreter may have provided "helpful" information to the plaintiff during the course of translation. Thus, the neuropsychologist appeared to have violated Standard 2.01 (Boundaries of Competence) and Standard 9.06 (Interpreting Assessment Results).

Test Adaptation

The neuropsychologist adapted some of the test material to meet the demands of a non-English speaking individual. The problem is essentially one of validity, both in terms of using tests that were standardized on an English-speaking population for a non-English speaking examinee as well as deviating from the standardized instructions by administering only selected parts of those tests (Standard 9.02, Use of Assessments).

Forensic Examination

The neuropsychologist was retained by plaintiff's attorney. Thus, this was obviously a forensic referral and the neuropsychologist had a "duty" to conduct a forensic examination. The neuropsychologist's statement that "No evidence of malingering is noted within formal testing" is a gratuitous statement in light of the fact that no formal measures of effort/honesty were included in the test battery. The neuropsychologist had no educational data and no measure of premorbid academic or intellectual functioning, yet the statement was made that premorbid intelligence was considered to be low average to average in the absence of this information in an individual who had completed only the 8th grade in another country. There appeared to have been no attempt on the part of the neuropsychologist to obtain premorbid medical or educational data. Although the plaintiff had emigrated from another country, in a forensic case one must at least make the attempt to obtain such information in order to better understand the results of neuropsychological testing. The neuropsychologist specified many symptoms reported by the plaintiff, including physical pain, sleep disruption and significant emotional distress yet, in confirming and diagnosing "TBI",

the neuropsychologist did not appear to take into consideration the possible effects of these variables on cognitive functioning, hence the diagnosis of traumatic brain injury. Also, there appeared to be no consideration of alternative hypotheses to explain the plaintiff's symptoms, which is required of an objective, impartial forensic neuropsychological evaluation. In fact, this plaintiff suffered a second head injury in a fall that occurred approximately two months post-MVA, the omission of which from the neuropsychologist's report suggested that the possible effects of that second head injury were not factored into the neuropsychologist's opinion regarding the etiology of the "TBI". Thus, the neuropsychologist failed to satisfy the ethical requirement to establish appropriate bases for his conclusions (Standard 2.04, Bases for Scientific and Professional Judgments; Standard 9.01, Bases for Assessments).

Consistent with the role as the defense neuropsychologist, this information was shared with the defense attorneys. The legal suit that had been filed on behalf of the plaintiff was asking for an award in the seven figures. The defense counsel was advised by the reviewing neuropsychologist that the plaintiff may very well have suffered a TBI in the car accident, but because of the many errors that had been committed by the plaintiff's neuropsychologist, it was not appropriate to conclude that the plaintiff had actually suffered a TBI, or that if he actually did exhibit cognitive deficits that they were due to the MVA-based head injury. The neuropsychologist had simply not taken into account the above-specified variables that can affect cognitive functioning, and in many ways had not met the burden of conducting a comprehensive forensic neuropsychological evaluation. Although knowing from the outset that he was being retained as a forensic neuropsychological expert, the plaintiff neuropsychologist did not obtain the necessary information nor consider the other possible explanations for the plaintiff's difficulties. As a results, there appeared to be a breach of Principle A (Beneficence and Nonmaleficence) and Principle B (Fidelity and Responsibility).

In this case, it is believed that the plaintiff neuropsychologist was not aware of the probable ethical infractions. Unfortunately, this does not absolve the neuropsychologist from responsibility for the actions described in this vignette.

Case Resolution

This case did go to trial and the plaintiff neuropsychologist was cross-examined based upon the information provided by the reviewing neuropsychologist. Sadly for the plaintiff, since that individual may well have sustained the cognitive and neurobehavioral injuries attributed to the accident, the neuropsychologist was not able to adequately defend the conclusions specified in the report under cross-examination. The jury returned a verdict on behalf of the plaintiff for physical injuries but not the diagnosed TBI; the award was a fraction of that which had been sought.

Conclusions and Recommendations

What was the responsibility of the plaintiff neuropsychologist towards the injured individual? Certainly, since the plaintiff neuropsychologist took on a forensic role, it would be reasonable for the reader to conclude that he should have been knowledgeable about the process and procedures of conducting more than a clinical examination. Having not met that burden, the neuropsychologist may well have been responsible for the outcome of the jury verdict that, for all intents and purposes, did not lead to a reasonable financial award if the man did in fact suffer a TBI in the accident. While the restrictive rules of service that operated in the first case are also operative here, did the neuropsychologist's

errors, and their effect on the plaintiff, actually rise to the level of malpractice? Was the "performance" of the neuropsychologist detrimental to the plaintiff?

Based upon the higher standards for forensic assessment, the neuropsychologist did not conduct a "proper" evaluation. Thus, under cross-examination, this professional was unable to defend the diagnosis that had been specified. In that context, the plaintiff was harmed by the work of the neuropsychologist. One may question the competence of the plaintiff neuropsychologist in this forensic situation, questioning as well the manner in which the professional and scientific responsibility that our ethics suggest in providing our services was managed. The neuropsychologist did not appear to be aware of many of the errors that were committed during the evaluation, and therefore may have gone beyond the boundaries of that individual's experience and competence. This author has noted similar types of errors committed by other otherwise competent clinical neuropsychologists who become involved in forensic assessment but who appear not to be trained or truly knowledgeable about the differences between forensic and clinical assessment. One of the tenets of our ethical principles is also to avoid harm. It seems reasonable to suggest that the type of harm experienced by this plaintiff was foreseeable.

Related issues in this kind of case include concerns about the effects of the neuropsychologist's work on the outcome of the plaintiff's litigation. Since the reviewing neuropsychologist believed that the plaintiff may have sustained a TBI in the MVA, and ultimately the plaintiff neuropsychologist's testimony did not stand up under cross-examination, what is our responsibility in such circumstances? In forensic situations, it is our obligation to advocate not for the plaintiff whom we may have examined, but for our opinions. But when the level of work does not allow us to effectively advocate in this manner in a court of law, in effect we cause harm to the plaintiff's case in a manner that can have long term and potentially devastating repercussions. As specified, this presents both ethical and professional challenges that if, as neuropsychologists, we are to remain a viable force in the personal injury litigation of head injury, we simply have to be able to function at the highest level of our profession, consistent with the general as well as forensic ethical and practice guidelines for psychologists.

This section has explored the professional and ethical use of neuropsychological assessments under two conditions: (1) the no-fault system, designed to allow parties injured in MVAs to obtain necessary and appropriate medical services regardless of "fault"/responsibility for the accident, and (2) defense assessment in personal injury litigation. Neuropsychologists working with known or potential forensic cases must try to anticipate potential ethical and professional challenges and be prepared to confront them in a competent, objective, and ethical manner. Those neuropsychologists evaluating and/or treating patients with accident-related neuropsychological deficits who are not prepared to negotiate the forensic arena should seek appropriate training/supervision in order to best serve their patients and protect themselves. Nevertheless, even with appropriate preparation, neuropsychologists practicing in forensic contexts are likely to face ethical dilemmas and should be prepared to seek consultation with experienced and ethically-knowledgeable colleagues when such challenges arise.

References

American Medical Association, Council on Ethical and Judicial Affairs (1999). *Code of Medical Ethics: Current Opinions with Annotations. 100. Patient-Physician Relationships in the Context of Work-Related and Independent Medical Examinations*. Washington, D.C.: Author.

American Psychological Association, (2002). Ethical principles of psychologists and code of conduct. *American Psychologist, 57*, 1060-1073.

Bush, S.S., Barth, J.T., Pliskin, N.H., Arffa, S., Axelrod, B.N., Blackburn, L.A., Faust, D., Fisher, J.M., Harley, J.P., Heilbronner, R.L., Larrabee, G.J., Ricker, J.H., & Silver, C.H. (2003). *Independent and court-ordered forensic neuropsychological examinations: Official statement of the National Academy of Neuropsychology*. Retrieved from http://www.nanonline.org/paio/IME.shtm 1/16/04.

Hamsher, K., de S., Lee, G.P., & Baron, I.S. (2001). Policy statement on the presence of third party observers in neuropsychological assessments. *The Clinical Neuropsychologist, 15*, 433-439.

McCaffrey, R.M., Williams, A.D., Fisher, J.M., & Laing, L.C. (1997). *The practice of forensic neuropsychology: Meeting challenges in the courtroom*. New York: Plenum Press.

National Academy of Neuropsychology Policy and Planning Committee (2000). Presence of third party observers during neuropsychological testing: Official statement of the National Academy of Neuropsychology. *Archives of Clinical Neuropsychology, 15*, 379-380.

Chapter 4

ETHICAL CHALLENGES IN FORENSIC NEUROPSYCHOLOGY, PART IV

Brad L. Roper

Scenario 1

A neuropsychologist received a call from the Director of Human Resources at a mid-sized manufacturer of top-secret military widgets. "Doctor," began the director, "We are having some problems with one of our security guards, and I was wondering whether you might check him out to make sure he can do his job and he isn't a danger to other employees." Fitness-for-duty (FFD) evaluations had never been part of the neuropsychologist's practice, which consisted largely of seeing acute rehab patients at the local hospital where he had trained students for decades. However, the director went on to say that the security guard, who had been with the company for two years, had possibly suffered a head injury while off-duty three months ago. The neuropsychologist felt comfortable enough with head injury to accept the case. The director emphasized that the neuropsychologist should not provide the examinee with any feedback or recommendations.

The examinee, a soft-spoken African-American man, arrived early and was seated in the waiting room, jiggling his right leg fiercely. He rose quickly and greeted the neuropsychologist with a firm handshake and averted eyes.

Once in the testing room, the neuropsychologist told the examinee that he was conducting an independent examination and presented his standard informed consent form and a release form authorizing results to be sent to the director. The examinee appeared dubious as he read the forms. He signed them, but wrote on each form, "I am doing this under duress!" The neuropsychologist eyed the additions curiously but, unfazed, proceeded with the interview. The examinee said that he has always been an exemplary employee and all of his recent problems stem from conflicts with his new supervisor. He admitted that he did have an accident one early morning as he hit a patch of ice and slid off the road, adding that he hit his head and was a little dazed. The wreck also strained his neck, which kept him out of work for three weeks. When he returned to work, he had been moved to the day shift and assigned to a supervisor newly transferred from a plant in a different part of the country. He repeatedly denied any ongoing problems from the accident.

The neuropsychologist had not thought to ask the director more about the examinee's job duties, but he imagined that the examinee should be able to describe them. When the examinee mentioned that he wears a handgun as part of his job, the neuropsychologist became a little nervous, wondering if there were any particular questions he should ask armed officers. Suddenly remembering something the director had said about assessing dangerousness, the neuropsychologist asked about homicidal ideation or intent, which the examinee, of course, denied.

When testing began, the examinee's nervousness shot through the roof. He was sweating profusely and, despite encouragement, he catastrophized his performance, saying that he would surely lose his job. The neuropsychologist tried to put him at ease, but the examinee's nervousness continued, as he quickly responded to the WAIS-III (Wechsler, 1997) Vocabulary subtest like it was a timed quiz on a game show. During the Block Design subtest, the examinee became so excited that he stood up to see the designs directly from above, but his hands were shaking so much that he had difficulty positioning the blocks. The neuropsychologist tried to get as much testing done as possible, but eventually he decided that he had given enough tests to write a passable report. He felt sorry for putting the examinee through such an obviously uncomfortable ordeal. On the way out, the examinee apologized for performing poorly and implored the neuropsychologist to help him keep his job. As a neuropsychologist, he was uncharacteristically moved with compassion. He winked at the examinee, who, after all, was a nice man, and replied, "Don't worry, I'll do all I can to take care of you."

After the evaluation, the neuropsychologist called the examinee's new supervisor. The supervisor was polite on the phone, but said he did not have much time to chat. "I'll tell you one thing," commented the supervisor, "Although I have nothing against the boy's heritage, he could never be the kind of 'All-American' employee that you're looking for, if you know what I mean." The neuropsychologist was shocked at the supervisor's apparently prejudiced remarks. In order to correct the situation, he called the examinee and advised him to file an EEO complaint against the supervisor.

Feeling relieved, the neuropsychologist sat down to write the report, following his typical clinical outline. Then he paused and thought, "You know, I'm feeling a little over my head here. I believe I should consult with someone who has experience with these types of evaluations." His rolodex directed him to a colleague who was a former trainee and who now did FFD evaluations. He gave her a call, thinking it would be nice to chat a little as well.

Relevant Ethical Issues

The neuropsychologist presents to us as quite a dunderhead, his actions fraught with ethical violations. What's worse, although he has blundered into all sorts of trouble, he seems mostly oblivious to it. Given his many years of experience as a neuropsychologist, one may wonder how he could have committed such a range of ethical violations.

In accepting the case, the neuropsychologist has ignored Standard 2.01 (Boundaries of Competence) of the Ethics Code (APA, 2002), and evidence of his incompetence is sprinkled throughout the scenario. Because the referral pertains to head injury, he assumed that he was qualified, ignoring his inexperience in performing FFD evaluations. Among specific knowledge and skills needed for FFD evaluations, examiners should be familiar with the job duties of the referred employee (Allen, Hibler, & Presant, 2000), minimally via obtaining a detailed job description from the employer. Furthermore, examiners should have general familiarity with high-risk occupations, such as those that require training and provision of a sidearm, before conducting evaluations of individuals in such professions (Borum, Super, & Rand, 2002).

Another example of knowledge needed is familiarity with the Americans with Disabilities Act of 1990 (ADA, 1991), including the rights provided to the employee as well as the implications regarding any recommendations that might be made by the examiner. In his apparent lack of familiarity with relevant law, the neuropsychologist violated Standard 2.01, Section (f), which states, "When assuming forensic roles, psychologists are or become reasonably familiar with the judicial or administrative rules governing their roles." In addition to the request to assess ability to perform job duties, the director requested assessment of the examinee's potential for workplace violence. The neuropsychologist interpreted the request as merely reflecting a need to assess homicidality, a standard part of a mental status exam. However, assessing the risk of workplace violence is a much more involved activity (Kausch & Resnick, 2001) requiring familiarity with relevant literature and assessment methods. As such, the neuropsychologist violated Section (a) of Standard 9.01 (Bases for Assessments).

The neuropsychologist also ran into several problems in the process of defining his role, explaining the evaluation to the examinee, and obtaining appropriate documentation of consent and release. The neuropsychologist appropriately informed the examinee that he was conducting an independent exam, but it is unclear how this was explicated in terms of the neuropsychologist's role and the limits of confidentiality. Moreover, the neuropsychologist used a generic informed consent form from his clinical practice, which would not appropriately explain the limits of confidentiality, the absence of a doctor-patient relationship, and the involvement of a third party as the neuropsychologist's client. Furthermore, he dismissed as inconsequential the examinee's addition to the forms that he was entering the evaluation "under duress." Although the examinee's predicament may not reflect a legal definition of "duress," the statement suggests that he was not entering into the evaluation willingly. Instead of accepting the examinee's amendment to the forms, the neuropsychologist should have sought to insure that the examinee was entering into the evaluation willingly and that he was willing to have the report sent to the employer. Sections of the Ethics Code relevant to role clarification and informed consent include the clarification of professional roles and obligations in Principle B (Fidelity and Responsibility) and Standards 3.10 (Informed Consent), 9.03 (Informed Consent in Assessments), 3.07 (Third-Party Requests for Services), and 4.02 (Discussing the Limits of Confidentiality).

During testing, the examinee's performance was clearly affected by his anxiety level. The neuropsychologist showed some awareness of this, but in light of the severity of the examinee's anxiety, his decision that he had obtained valid testing is at best very questionable. Relevant standards include Section (b) of Standard 9.01 (Bases for Assessments) and Standard 9.06 (Interpreting Assessment Results).

The neuropsychologist's parting comment that he would "take care" of the examinee served to further confuse his role, inconsistent with the commitment he made to the employer as his client (Standard 3.07). Although the comment might have temporarily reduced the examinee's anxiety, if the neuropsychologist was merely trying to be nice, he was essentially being disingenuous to the examinee (Principle C, Integrity). If he was indeed promising to write the examinee a favorable report, he would still run into problems with Standard 3.07 and Principle C, and he would be left with conflicting roles (Standard 3.05, Multiple Relationships).

Although the neuropsychologist was justifiably concerned when confronted with the supervisor's racially prejudiced remarks, contacting the examinee and advising him to file an EEO complaint was misguided, again violating Standards 3.07 and 4.02. At another level, communication of such remarks could provoke unpredictable actions from the employee, and might further strain the relationship between the employee and the supervisor (Standard 3.04, Avoiding Harm). With the employer as the client, information obtained from other employees should not have been shared with the examinee (Standard 4.01, Maintaining Confidentiality). Instead of telling the examinee, the neuropsychologist should have conveyed the comments of the supervisor to the director, as such comments may have had a direct relationship to the examinee's difficulties on the job. In any case, given that the conversation with the supervisor was very brief, the neuropsychologist should have arranged to gain more information from him or others who work with the examinee (Standard 9.01).

Finally, the neuropsychologist was wise to seek advice from a colleague prior to writing a report following his "typical format." In general, reports to employers should focus on functional abilities related to employment, as inclusion of the information in a typical clinical report could result in undue harm to the employee. Relevant sections of the Ethics Code include Standards 3.04 (Avoiding Harm) and 4.04 (Minimizing Intrusions on Privacy).

Case Resolution

In discussing the case with the colleague, the neuropsychologist began to think he might have made a few mistakes in the evaluation. The colleague suggested that the neuropsychologist write a brief letter to the director, explaining that the evaluation was not valid and providing the names of nearby neuropsychologists who had experience in FFD evaluations. The thought occurred to the colleague that the examinee might be more willing to speak explicitly to an African-American neuropsychologist regarding possible racial discrimination. Unfortunately, there were no African-American neuropsychologists within a 300-mile radius of the examinee's home. Although not suggested by the colleague, with the letter the neuropsychologist included a bill for his time.

While speaking with the neuropsychologist, the colleague noticed that her former mentor could not avoid mentioning the name of the company as well as the names of all the employees involved in the evaluation, despite gentle reminders to keep the information anonymous,

which violated Standard 4.01 (Maintaining Confidentiality) and, more specifically, Standard 4.06 (Consultations). After further discussion with the neuropsychologist, she decided that he may not be capable of satisfying Standard 2.06 (Personal Problems and Conflicts) and, consistent with Standard 1.04 (Informal Resolution of Ethical Violations), she decided that some action was needed on her part. With the assistance of the neuropsychologist's family, the colleague arranged for him to be evaluated in the memory disorders clinic at a nearby university. With the neuropsychologist's help, the colleague developed a list of all the tests with which he was familiar, which was sent to the university neuropsychologist before the evaluation. The neuropsychologist was subsequently found to have the early stages of a frontal dementia.

With the neuropsychologist's permission, the colleague then endeavored to act on his behalf. She notified the director that paying the neuropsychologist's bill was not necessary. The neuropsychologist agreed to retire from active practice, but he had never made plans for closing down his practice (Standard 3.12. Interruption of Psychological Services). The colleague assisted him in doing so, attending to his records consistent with Standards 6.01 (Documentation of Professional and Scientific Work and Maintenance of Records) and 6.02 (Maintenance, Dissemination, and Disposal of Confidential Records of Professional and Scientific Work). She offered to pay the neuropsychologist for his test materials (Standard 9.11, Maintaining Test Security), but he insisted that she take them as a token of his gratitude for her help.

The neuropsychologist now lives with his daughter and her family. He has no worries and he loves watching his grandsons play Little League.

Conclusions and Recommendations

Before conducting FFD evaluations, neuropsychologists should obtain the necessary knowledge and skills to perform such assessments and consult with colleagues as needed when uncertainties arise. Although FFD evaluations are broadly considered "forensic" (Sweet, Grote, & van Gorp, 2002), they are unique in several respects. Typically, employees are justifiably concerned that they may lose their job and, thereby, their security and means of livelihood. Under such a threat, employees may present as very anxious, upset, angry, or hostile, and such emotions and behaviors may themselves interfere with the valid assessment of abilities. Accordingly, it is incumbent on the neuropsychologist to attempt to ease such emotions and consider the impact of emotions on performance. Furthermore, at least some defensiveness is expected, and extreme defensiveness is not uncommon, with employees potentially withholding important information about their history and current difficulties. As such, neuropsychologists must carefully assess for under-reporting, comparing examinees' reports to available records and the results of collateral interviews.

Whereas individuals in other forensic settings may be accustomed to personal questions, perceived invasions of privacy, and the process of providing informed consent, employees may have little exposure to these and may easily be taken aback by activities that we consider routine. Employers often provide employees with scant information about the nature of the evaluation, and employees may begin evaluations feeling both uninformed and suspicious. As such, neuropsychologists should insure that employees understand the nature of the evaluation and its possible outcomes. Employees should be given the opportunity to ask questions and contact their employer for more information. Although employees are typically informed by employers that they must take part in the evaluation or lose their job, it is important from the neuropsychologist's perspective to establish that the employee is entering into the evaluation willingly. Employees should be informed that they may wish to consult with an attorney before proceeding with the evaluation.

Regarding documentation, findings shared with employers should typically be limited to those which are directly relevant to the employee's work-related abilities. Inclusion of diagnostic labels may be interpreted inappropriately by the employer, potentially resulting in undue harm to the employee. Likewise, communicating even seemingly benign information to employers regarding psychosocial or medical history could potentially harm employees. Finally, despite the need to limit the scope of feedback to employers, neuropsychologists should maintain professional records of the evaluation that are adequate to justify the work-related opinions provided.

Scenario 2

A neuropsychologist received a referral from a private physician serving as an Aviation Medicine Examiner designated by the Federal Aviation Administration (FAA), to perform a neuropsychological evaluation on a former commercial airline pilot who had obtained a DUI conviction and was subsequently grounded from flying. He had entered a recovery program and was diagnosed with Alcohol Abuse. He had remained abstinent for six months, and neuropsychological evaluation was requested to assess possible neurocognitive impairments from prior alcohol use. Although the neuropsychologist was experienced in aviation psychology, she had not previously received a referral from this physician. The physician did not have the pilot's contact information handy, but he said that the pilot should be calling to schedule an appointment in a couple of days. It was two months before a man with the pilot's name called, stating that he needed a psychological evaluation for "special issuance" as a commercial airline pilot.

While reviewing informed consent, the neuropsychologist told the examinee that she was an independent examiner working on behalf of the physician and the FAA, appropriately detailing her role and specifying that she could provide no immediate feedback to him but would send the report and test scores to the physician, who would make them available to the FAA. She also told the examinee that he could have a copy of the report, if desired, once it was completed. The neuropsychologist mentioned that the examinee would be billed directly for the evaluation, explaining that most health insurance companies would not reimburse for the evaluation because it is not considered medically necessary. The examinee expressed irritation at having to pay for the evaluation and insisted that he would seek reimbursement through his healthcare insurance anyway. The examinee signed the informed consent form but seemed unaware of the referring physician and said, "I remember talking to a doctor but I don't know his name." The neuropsychologist explained that the evaluation may or may not be favorable to his return to work as a commercial airline pilot. The examinee angrily retorted, "It better be favorable if I'm paying for it." The neuropsychologist endeavored to elaborate her role, but the examinee remained miffed.

During testing, the examinee was initially mildly anxious. Although his anxiety did not appreciably impact performance, he continued to openly express his frustration, at times showing hostility toward the neuropsychologist, requiring limit-setting and role clarification. After lunch, the examinee returned and behaved like a changed man. He was extremely polite with the neuropsychologist, expressed his appreciation for being treated fairly, and began asking many questions about the tests being used. The neuropsychologist answered some general questions, but repeatedly told the examinee that she could not give feedback or reveal the answers to test items.

The neuropsychologist's pager went off, and she stepped away to another room to respond. The call proved to be a complex problem that took over fifteen minutes to resolve. Upon returning, she noticed that the examinee's performance on the WAIS-III Information subtest was flawless. Later in the afternoon, she noticed that the examinee performed extremely well on a verbal learning test, recalling 14 of 16 words on the first trial and acing the rest of the test. The examinee performed closer to expectations on CogScreen Aeromedical Edition (Kay, 1999), a computerized test commonly used with commercial airline pilots.

At the completion of testing, the neuropsychologist reviewed her paperwork to make sure it was complete. She could not find the informed consent form. The examinee admitted that he had taken the form while the neuropsychologist was out of the room, adding that he did not want results sent to the physician. He explained that he did not have a problem paying for the evaluation, so long as the neuropsychologist would spend more time with him reviewing the tests and his performance. The neuropsychologist repeated that she was an independent examiner and that she could not give feedback but that her agreement with the physician did allow for the examinee to also receive a copy of the report. She told the examinee that the consent form is her property and that he must return it, but he refused. She added that she has an obligation to the physician and the FAA as an independent examiner. The examinee replied, "If that's true, then why isn't the physician paying you?" The neuropsychologist was momentarily at a loss for words, and the examinee continued, "Listen, what if I hired you as a consultant to help me prepare for doing the evaluation with someone else later? I'll even pay you $500 extra." The neuropsychologist, marshalling control of her rising anger, replied that such an arrangement was not possible.

By that time, it was late in the day and the receptionist had gone home. Feeling exhausted and angry, the neuropsychologist escorted the examinee to the waiting room and immediately took a restroom break. She returned to the testing room, looking forward to unwinding at home with her husband and daughter. She was glad that she kept clinical reports, as well as computerized tests such as CogScreen and the MMPI-2 (Butcher, Dahlstrom, Tellegen, Graham, & Kaemmer, 1989), on a hot-pluggable external hard drive, making it easy for her to work from home. Hastening to gather her things, she stopped short and stared in shock at the empty space on her desk. Her WAIS-III manual and her hard drive were gone.

Relevant Ethical Issues

Whereas the neuropsychologist's bumbling actions in the first scenario may sound to us like a tragicomedy, the neuropsychologist's situation in this scenario hits closer to home. Reflecting on her predicament, we may empathize with her and wonder how vulnerable we might be to such misdeeds. Admittedly, the situation described is very rare, perhaps representing to some readers a "nightmare scenario" that nevertheless may be instructive in tackling ethical issues. Of course, the scenario also includes legal aspects, such as those of reporting a crime and limiting legal liability, but the focus below is on the ethical issues involved.

Beginning with the referral and initial contact with the pilot, the scenario contains vagaries regarding the connection between the physician and the examinee. One might assume that the pilot to which the physician referred was the same pilot that came for the evaluation. However, the neuropsychologist had never obtained contact information from the physician and obtained no identification other than the man's self-report. Clarification that the referred individual was the same pilot would fall under Standard 3.07 (Third-Party Requests for Services).

Of note, the neuropsychologist acted appropriately in obtaining informed consent and repeatedly clarifying her role with the examinee. The examinee's hostility aside, he held the commonsensical view that the one paying for a service should be considered the client of those services, and his sense of justice was apparently offended by the disjunction. However, later in the day, it became more apparent that the examinee's ostensible conflation of the roles was a

thinly veiled attempt at manipulation. From the standpoint of the Ethics Code, the particular person or entity paying for an evaluation has no bearing on determining who is the client. Although the Code addresses potential pitfalls of fees and fee arrangements when a client is also the payor or partial payor (Standard 6.04, Fees and Financial Arrangements; Standard 6.05, Barter with Clients/Patients), there is, of course, no inherent connection between client and payor. To the contrary, the Code makes specific reference to our obligations to payors distinct from clients (e.g., Standard 6.06, Accuracy in Reports to Payors and Funding Sources). The linchpin of establishing the relationships of client and payor is the process of informed consent. The neuropsychologist appropriately followed the standards relevant to these issues, which are the same as those in the first scenario and include Standards 3.10, 9.03, 3.07, 4.02, and 4.05. However, she could have avoided some misunderstanding by an earlier explication of the fee arrangement, as in an appointment letter, which would have better addressed Standard 6.04 (Fees and Financial Arrangements).

The neuropsychologist's need to manage an emergent situation regarding a prior evaluation is not uncommon in neuropsychology practice, when an examinee may be left alone in a room with easy access to tests. Unfortunately for the neuropsychologist, her actions led to a breech of test security (Standard 9.11, Maintaining Test Security), which resulted in some test performance that was much higher than expected. In situations such as FFD evaluations in which there are strong external incentives for examinees to appear cognitively intact, extra care should be taken in meeting Standard 9.11. Additionally, any indications that performance overestimates ability should be considered in test interpretation (Standard 9.06 Interpreting Assessment Results).

In a surprising move, the examinee swiped the consent form in the neuropsychologist's absence. It is important to decouple the two aspects of this action, which include the theft and the withdrawal of consent. Although there is no specific requirement in the code that informed consent for assessments be documented, such activity is routinely performed for liability reasons and in attending to Standard 6.01 (Documentation of Professional and Scientific Work and Maintenance of Records). By not taking the examinee's file with her when she left the room, the neuropsychologist opened herself up to problems with the maintenance of her records. Even so, the examinee's theft is certainly unexpected and perhaps difficult to completely guard against, and the form's absence clearly does not negate the fact that informed consent was originally obtained. In the more likely scenario in which consent is withdrawn and the form is not pilfered, complete documentation of consent-related events can be obtained by having the examinee write "I withdraw consent" on the original form, including the date and time with his or her signature. Since the examinee refused to return the form, the neuropsychologist should document this fact, as well as the withdrawal of consent.

What are the neuropsychologist's obligations in response to the examinee's withdrawal of consent? In her exasperation over the purloined form, the neuropsychologist seemed uncertain about what she should do. Although the Ethics Code speaks to the need to inform research participants of their right to withdraw and its consequences (Standard 8.02 Informed Consent to Research), no such provision is explicitly given in standards for Standard 3.10 (Informed Consent) or Standard 9.03 (Informed Consent for Assessments). Notably, the latter standard makes an exception to the need for informed consent when "testing is mandated by law or governmental regulations." Although psychological testing had been requested by the FAA, a governmental organization, the mandate for testing was contingent upon the examinee's interest in pursuing medical certification to return to work as a pilot. As such, governmental regulations do not strictly mandate the assessment.

Despite her anger at the examinee, the neuropsychologist clearly felt an ethical requirement to honor his demand that no information be sent to the physician or the FAA. She also felt that she had a competing obligation to her clients (Standard 3.07) to report results of the evaluation, but she wondered if that would get her into legal trouble. At the same time, she felt that she had been duped into releasing the content of the tests. Did she have an obligation to protect the flying public, consistent with Principle A (Beneficence and Nonmaleficence)? In her indignation over the examinee having studied test materials while she was out of the room – further aggravated by the subsequent burglary – the neuropsychologist felt that he should suffer consequences for his actions. Otherwise, couldn't he continue the pattern until he had the tests memorized?

The examinee's next attempt was to alter the nature of the evaluation by redefining himself as the client, which the neuropsychologist appropriately countered. Although some uncertainties exist in the vignette regarding whether the physician referred the examinee, clearly the intended client is not the examinee himself. The neuropsychologist obviously has an obligation to the physician and the FAA as the identified clients (Standard 3.07), as had been detailed in the informed consent process. The examinee's withdrawal of consent might limit the neuropsychologist's ability to report findings to her clients, but it does not allow her to provide immediate feedback to the examinee. Although the examinee may, if he wishes, obtain a copy of the report when it is completed, it would not seem appropriate to send him a copy and withhold the information from the third-party clients.

Let us assume for a moment an alternative scenario, in which another commercial airline pilot initiates a self-paid consultation with the neuropsychologist in the absence of an outside referral. If this second pilot is interested in learning more about the tests or doing a "dry-run" assessment, this would not be permissible for the neuropsychologist to perform, as it would constitute a violation of test security (Standard 9.06). Furthermore, engaging in an underhanded disclosure of tests, even by their mere administration, to a commercial airline pilot would run afoul of "safeguard[ing] the welfare and rights of those with whom they interact professionally and other affected persons" in Principle A (Beneficence and Nonmaleficence); psychologists' "professional and scientific responsibilities to society" in Principle B (Fidelity and Responsibility); and the statement that psychologists do not "steal, cheat, or engage in fraud, subterfuge, or intentional misrepresentation of fact" in Principle C (Integrity). In this case, neuropsychologists have a duty to protect the flying public and must refuse such overtures. If the consultation the second pilot seeks involves cognitive remediation, the neuropsychologist may ethically engage in such, but she should make efforts to preserve test security in the context of any assessment or remediation performed.

Finally, we encounter the issue of the stolen test materials and hard drive. In escorting the examinee back to the waiting room and not outside of a locked door before using the restroom, the neuropsychologist was unreflective about her actions and their possible implications regarding Standards 4.01 (Maintaining Confidentiality), 6.02 (Maintenance, Dissemination, and Disposal of Confidential Records of Professional and Scientific Work), and 9.11 (Maintaining Test Security), particularly in light of the examinee's prior actions. Despite her exhaustion and nature's call, the neuropsychologist should have kept an eye on the examinee at all times prior to his leaving, and in failing to do so she risked much more than the items she later found missing.

Case Resolution

After searching her briefcase and the testing room, the neuropsychologist decided that the examinee must have taken the items. She then looked out the window and saw that his car was gone. She called the police and reported the theft, providing the examinee's address, phone number, and a physical description. As she was reporting the theft, she cursed herself for not placing security and encryption measures on her hard drive. She then left a message for the receptionist to check for any missing files or other items and instruct others in the group practice to check as well. She sent an email to all staff to apologize for her lapse, offering to organize a meeting to discuss office security issues. The neuropsychologist then rescheduled the next day's appointment and returned home to a fitful night's sleep.

The next day, the neuropsychologist called her liability insurance carrier to ask about the implications of the stolen hard drive. A claims manager told her that he appreciated her reporting the theft, but he advised her that the company would not need to formally respond unless someone filed a suit against her. He suggested she call the police and her property insurance carrier. The neuropsychologist then contacted an attorney who she thought had experience in liability and risk management, and told him about the withdrawal of consent. He advised her that, in order to protect her best interests, she should not respond to the physician with any feedback from the evaluation, although he supposed that it was okay to report the circumstances of the theft, because theft was behavior that was not privileged and had already been made public via the police report. The neuropsychologist then consulted with the ethics officer of her state psychological association. He advised her to identify the individuals who were on the hard drive and try to notify them of the theft. He said he needed to "noodle" over the issue of withdrawn consent and would call her back later. In reviewing files, the neuropsychologist determined that the hard drive contained reports and test scores from 23 examinees. "Whew," she said to herself, "It could have been worse." She sent letters to the examinees and to third-party clients, stating that records that contain personal and potentially sensitive information were stolen from her office.

She urged them not to become alarmed, and she invited them to contact her if they wished to discuss the issue further. The neuropsychologist then called the physician's office and, without mentioning the previous day's appointment, confirmed that the examinee was indeed the pilot whom the physician had referred.

The same day, the police visited the examinee, who claimed that he had taken the materials "mistakenly" and agreed to return them. Of course, the neuropsychologist believed that the theft was purposeful. Irritated at the examinee's dishonesty, she decided to press charges. The neuropsychologist presumed that the examinee easily could have copied the materials before returning them. She had yet to hear back from the ethics officer about withdrawing consent. Seeking further consultation, she called several colleagues. The first responded, "If consent is withdrawn, that's the only thing you can tell the referring doctor. Including any interpretive information could get you into trouble." The next colleague said, "After testing is over, he can't withdraw consent any more than he could withdraw consent for sex. It's done, and you have an obligation to the doctor to send your report. Of course, don't mention anything about the theft." "But," responded the neuropsychologist, "that's the exact opposite of what the lawyer told me!" Another colleague exclaimed, "You may not think this is personal medical information under HIPAA, but your state licensure board doesn't care what you think. Don't even tell the doctor that you saw him!"

"AAAGH!" All the conflicting advice caused the neuropsychologist's head to spin, and she swiftly supinated onto a soft sofa. For no clear reason, she thought about an old psychotherapy supervisor from graduate school, an odd man whom she suspected must be some sort of mystic. Feeling silly, she did what he had taught her, and took a few slow, deep breaths. Instead of concentrating on all of the externals and opinions, she closed her eyes and looked inward. To her surprise, a measure of insight dawned.

She realized that she could not respond to the physician with a clinical report. First of all, her anger at the examinee, although quite justified, was so strong as to compromise her objectivity in formulating clinical impressions (Standard 2.06, Personal Problems and Conflicts). Furthermore, her decision to press charges also precluded her ability to serve as an independent examiner (3.05, Multiple Relationships). Finally, she felt that, on balance, the withdrawal of consent should probably be honored.

The following day, the neuropsychologist returned to the office and dictated a letter to the physician, stating that the examinee had withdrawn consent to have any results released. She also stated that a theft of test materials had occurred when the examinee was the only other person in the office, and she added that the examinee's exposure to the tests would compromise the validity of future evaluations. The receptionist typed the letter as the neuropsychologist donned her coat. The receptionist asked, "Should we send an invoice to the examinee?" "Oh, yes," smiled the neuropsychologist, "Bill him for every minute."

Conclusions and Recommendations

First of all, although words have been put into an attorney's mouth in this scenario, please note that the fictional attorney could indeed be incompetent, and no legal advice is intended in any part of this tale. Secondly, although I chose a commercial airline pilot as the story's antagonist, pilots as a group have been among the most respectful and appropriate individuals whom I have assessed, and no aspersions on them are intended. Rather, the scenario is meant to highlight that FFD-referred examinees are under unique motivational contingencies, which may lead to behaviors that compromise test security, confidentiality, agreements with third-part entities, and the welfare of the public. In such contexts, the potentially competing demands of various aspects of the Ethics Code, as well as the need to limit liability, can combine to form thorny dilemmas indeed.

Laptop computers and removable computer peripherals are often used to store both patient information and computerized psychological tests. Their use should be carefully monitored, especially in situations where examinees might benefit from knowledge of computerized tests. Neuropsychologists should insure that information is carefully password-protected to protect test security and patient records. In the scenario, the neuropsychologist's allowing the examinee access to her easily stowable, non-encrypted hard drive is analogous to leaving other patients' files in his presence.

The bulk of forensic referrals in neuropsychological practice are those in which examinees have contingencies to malinger or "fake bad." Recent interest in the area has led to a flurry of useful research on effort measures, and perhaps our profession has some past sins for which to atone in this regard. However, relatively little attention has been paid to forensic assessments in which the contingency is to "fake good." Although faking good is usually considered impossible on performance-based tests, this is only true of the *test-naïve* examinee.

Threats of job loss or efforts to enter or re-enter a high-risk occupation may serve as powerful motivators for individuals to seek a "leg up" in neuropsychological evaluations. Accordingly, neuropsychologists should be particularly mindful of protecting test security in FFD and pre-employment evaluations. Additionally, neuropsychology as a profession should closely monitor any violations of test security that might take place on the internet or via other media.

Self-referrals for neuropsychological evaluation from individuals in high-risk occupations are always suspect and may represent an attempt at a "dry run." Gifted individuals may glean much from prior evaluations (Rapport, Brines, Axelrod, & Theisen, 1997). In general, such referrals should not be accepted, and an appropriate referral source and referral question should be obtained before conducting the evaluation.

Although opinions vary widely regarding the specific actions to take after an FFD examinee withdraws consent, it is probably best to honor such demands from the standpoint of the Ethics Code. The neuropsychologist would then inform the third-party client that consent had been withdrawn and no impressions could be released. However, in cases where the third-party client is paying for the evaluation, the client may interpret failure to release information as reneging on an agreement. When individuals in high-risk occupations withdraw consent, inclusion of feedback to third-party clients that the validity of future evaluations may have been compromised serves to protect the public good.

In the rare event that an examinee steals materials from a neuropsychologist's office, the neuropsychologist, of course, may report the theft and press charges. However, such actions may impact the neuropsychologist's ability to fulfill his or her obligation to third-party clients. Even if the theft were not reported, the neuropsychologist would need to reflect upon whether the personal nature of the theft would bias his or her opinions. Furthermore, failure to report a theft could itself have legal and liability ramifications. Whether or not the third party should be informed of the theft remains debatable.

References

American Psychological Association (2002). Ethical principles of psychologists and code of conduct. *American Psychologist, 57,* 1060-1073.

Americans with Disabilities Act of 1990, 42 U.S.C.A. 12101 *et seq.*

Allen, M.G., Hibler, N.S., & Presant, N.L. (2000). Psychiatric evaluations: By the Federal Occupational Health Procedures. *The Forensic Examiner, 9,* 13-18.

Borum, R., Super, J., & Rand, M. (2002). Forensic assessment for high-risk populations. In

A.M. Goldstein (Ed.), *Handbook of Psychology Volume 11: Forensic Psychology,* 133-147. Hoboken, New Jersey: John Wiley & Sons.

Butcher, J.N., Dahlstrom, W.G., Graham, J.R., Tellegen, A., & Kaemmer, B. (1989). *Minnesota Multiphasic Personality Inventory-2 (MMPI-2): Manual for Administration and Scoring.* Minneapolis: University of Minnesota Press.

Kausch, O., & Resnick, P.J. (2001). Assessment of employees for workplace violence. *Journal of Forensic Psychology Practice, 1*, 1-22.

Kay, G.G. (1999). *CogScreen Aeromedical Edition: Professional Manual*, Washington, DC: CogScreen LLC.

Rapport, L.J., Brines, D.B., Axelrod, B.N., & Theisen, M.E. (1997). Full Scale IQ as mediator of practice effects: The rich get richer. *Clinical Neuropsychologist, 11*, 375-380.

Sweet, J.S., Grote, C., & van Gorp, W.G. (2002). Ethical issues in forensic neuropsychology. In S. Bush & M.L. Drexler (Eds.) *Ethical Issues in Clinical Neuropsychology*, 103-133. Lisse, Netherlands: Swets & Zeitlinger.

Wechsler, D. (1997). *Manual for the Wechsler Adult Intelligence Scale – Third Edition*. San Antonio, Texas: The Psychological Corporation.

Chapter 5

ETHICAL CHALLENGES IN FORENSIC NEUROPSYCHOLOGY, PART V

Jerry J. Sweet

Scenario 1

A middle-aged individual was involved in a multiple vehicle car accident. Stopped in a line of traffic, waiting for the roadway ahead to be cleared, the plaintiff was the driver of one of a number of cars that in domino fashion was struck in the rear bumper and then in turn struck the bumper of the car in front. The defendant was the driver who had failed to notice that the cars in line were in fact not moving, and thereby triggered the chain reaction of bumper-to-bumper accidents. Immediately after the accident, witnesses noted the plaintiff to be acting normally as all the drivers awaited the police. The witnesses described very little visible damage to the plaintiff's car. At the scene, no medical care was provided to the plaintiff, who drove to work as planned following completion of police paper work. Eventual medical evaluation of neck pain and general feeling of ill health resulted only in prescription of muscle relaxants and a neck brace.

Nearly ten years later, the plaintiff was still involved in the litigation process related to the multiple vehicle accident. Within a year of one another, but again almost ten years after the accident, both the plaintiff's and the defendant's attorneys retained expert neuropsychologists to render opinions. As one might expect, many intervening events had taken place in the years subsequent

to the accident and numerous records were available for review by both experts. In the intervening years, a seizure disorder had been diagnosed and continuously treated. Some records suggested the possibility of pseudoseizures and at least one neurologist opined that a seizure disorder was not present. The plaintiff had a long list of problems attributed to the accident, but it was uncontested that the plaintiff opened and operated successful businesses in the ten years following the accident.

The neuropsychology experts disagreed on a number of points. The expert retained by the plaintiff's attorney concluded that the initial injury, subsequent complaints and medical findings, as well as the plaintiff's pattern of performances on neuropsychological testing were all highly consistent with persistent effects of traumatic brain injury. The expert retained by the defense, viewing the same information, plus data from the second neuropsychological evaluation, expressed the opposite opinion. The test results obtained by the two neuropsychologists were substantially different in a number of ways, the details of which are unimportant in this particular instance in terms of consideration of possible ethical issues. Even the specific points of disagreement between the experts are unimportant for our discussion of ethical issues. In fact, *disagreement between expert witnesses is common and rarely cause for concern from an ethical perspective.*

One of the two neuropsychology experts rendered a series of opinions, first within the formal report of the plaintiff and then during subsequent discovery deposition, which are pertinent in that they involve professional behaviors that frequently seem to cause concern regarding ethical standards. The numbered items that follow constitute the relevant opinions rendered by the neuropsychologist. (1) The neuropsychologist noted in formal written opinion that two of the specific test scores proved there was a seizure focus in one area of the brain and a mirror focus in another area of the brain, both of which could only be attributable to the accident ten years earlier. (2) The neuropsychologist claimed special training and expertise as a neuropsychologist that allowed diagnosis of seizures, which was acknowledged as otherwise within the practice domain of neurology. (3) The neuropsychologist claimed special expertise in making neuropsychological diagnoses and asserted that this special expertise had been recognized by another state's court system and documented in a ruling that barred other neuropsychologists from rendering certain opinions that he/she was permitted to make. (4) The neuropsychologist claimed that any neuropsychologist who did not use neuropsychological test battery A, which was alleged to be the only scientifically validated battery, could not render valid opinions and, related, opinions based upon tests other than battery A had been determined not to be admissible under Daubert standards. (5) In one of numerous claims of special and unique expertise, the neuropsychologist claimed that a credential that was obtained through purchase and which had not been associated with a peer review process also was proof of his/her special expertise. (6) A major foundation of the neuropsychologist's opinion was discovered upon examination of the raw test protocols to be due to a scoring error.

In this particular instance, there was no disagreement between plaintiff's and defendant's attorneys regarding *liability*. That is, attorneys for both parties agreed that the defendant was liable for the accident. The only disagreement was the question of *damages*, which made the opinions of the neuropsychologists quite salient in determining the ultimate outcome of the case.

Relevant Ethical Issues

To understand what did or did not happen related to the initial ethical concerns, it is best to consider each individually.

Bases for Scientific and Professional Judgments

The first issue pertained to whether a neuropsychologist should claim that the result of any particular formal neuropsychological test, in isolation, "proved" the presence of a seizure disorder. While many clinical research studies of deficits associated with groups of individuals suffering from seizure disorders could be cited to justify the general relevance and usage of neuropsychological test procedures, there is no research indicating that a specific test finding can be used to validate the presence or absence of a seizure disorder in an individual patient. Although a concern could be expressed relevant to Ethical Standard 2.04 (Bases for Scientific and Professional Judgments), simply holding and espousing a belief is, in and of itself, not truly unethical. Moreover, when an erroneous or unsupportable belief is made within a forensic context, the lack of foundation for such an opinion can be demonstrated and the opinion effectively negated. Making this statement was not deemed unethical.

Avoidance of False or Deceptive Statements

Neuropsychologists are specialists in understanding behavior that may be associated with brain dysfunction. As such, neuropsychologists often work closely with physicians to determine whether the source of a behavioral anomaly is best understood as brain dysfunction versus a psychological problem. In this instance, the neuropsychologist's statement of being able to diagnose seizures appeared idiosyncratic and self-serving, in that it strongly suggested engaging in a medical practice that by statute falls within the domain of a physician. Within the broader context of this case, some physicians had deemed the behavior to be due to seizures, whereas others had not. The neuropsychologist's position was clearly stated; it was not that the special skill that he/she claimed was allowing agreement with some of the physicians, but instead that because of his/her particular training an independent diagnosis could be made, without *any* involvement or consideration of opinions of physicians. It was merely coincidental in the expert's mind that any physician had offered a similar opinion. Moreover, the expert indicated in no uncertain terms that *no other* neuropsychologist was able to render this same opinion; only he/she possessed the requisite medical training. This ethical concern is perhaps best understood in the context of the next *three* items of concern, which are elaborated below.

(1) The neuropsychologist claimed that his/her unique skill in neuropsychological assessment had been noted within a particular state jurisdiction that allowed no other psychologist to render opinions on certain topics. The details of the specific ruling were not provided.

(2) The neuropsychologist claimed that the particular constellation of tests he/she had used was proven in scientific research to be the only reliable and valid battery available, and further that court rulings had upheld that it was the only constellation of tests that met the Daubert evidentiary standards. In reality, the particular battery espoused was not exactly the battery that had been used by the neuropsychologist, and there were numerous

points of overlap between the tests used by both neuropsychologists. Nevertheless, the position taken was that the "other" neuropsychologist's work was not acceptable scientifically and should be discounted wholly as not valid.

(3) One of the credentials held by the neuropsychologist was obtained by purchase from a company that had become well known in legal circles (see Hansen, 2000) for selling sham credentials. The neuropsychologist nevertheless defended the credential and insisted that not only had the honor been difficult to attain, but also few were worthy to possess it.

Considering the above points together, it seems obvious that the neuropsychologist in question felt special and unique and was trying to convince the attorneys, and ultimately the "triers of fact", involved in the case that any disagreement with his/her opinions meant the other person was wrong. Whether this behavior is associated with his/her own psychopathology *or* is situation specific is a moot point. Regardless, both the 1992 (Standards 3.03, Avoidance of False or Deceptive Statements, and 7.04, Truthfulness and Candor) and 2002 (Standard 5.01, Avoidance of False or Deceptive Statements) versions of ethical standards make it clear that psychologists are not to make false, deceptive, or fraudulent statements regarding, among other items, their training, experience, competence, or credentials. Clearly, at least some of the neuropsychologist's claims to unique and special expertise likely were known by the neuropsychologist to be completely without support. In litigation scenarios, extreme and unsupportable opinions generally are easily exposed for what they are. However, even though such statements in a forensic context frequently will be discounted in the course of attorneys "proving up" a case, it is not the probable, eventual benign impact that determines whether they are ethical or not. The neuropsychologist likely knows that some of the statements are false. Therefore, an independent review by peers would likely conclude that these statements indicate unethical behavior.

Test Results

The neuropsychologist had based a significant portion of his/her opinion on a test result that turned out upon inspection of raw data by the second neuropsychologist to be a very significant scoring error. True mistakes by a professional catch the attention of forensic experts and attorneys and are likely to elicit pointed questions regarding the possibility of additional invalidity in the remaining data. However, such mistakes would not routinely raise concern regarding ethical violations and were not deemed unethical in this instance.

Case Resolution

Deposition testimony and numerous authoritative peer reviewed publications entered into evidence seriously undercut the opinion of the self-aggrandizing neuropsychologist and rendered it fairly impotent. In that sense, the system worked; the case was settled just as trial began for a relatively trivial amount, which had been offered for many months before the trial. Apparently, the retaining attorneys ultimately had so little faith in the ten-year-long case, which fundamentally had rested largely upon the extreme claims of only one of their experts, that they elected not to even allow the judge and jury to hear the details of the case.

At the conclusion of such a case (i.e., when the forensic outcome is complete), questions of an ethical nature can be addressed. To do so any earlier would normally be inappropriate, as the mere involvement in an adversarial matter can and should place contemporaneous ethical complaints in a self-serving light or as deliberate obfuscation of more substantive matters. Once the case is over, and with no other agenda in

mind, a clearer and less emotional conclusion regarding possible unethical behavior seems possible. However, even this seemingly conservative position may not be clear-cut if, for example, because of practice geography or referral patterns the two neuropsychologists are likely to be retained by opposite sides in adversarial proceedings in the future. In such a circumstance, the onus of appearing or actually having a hidden agenda cannot be removed even when the case at hand is complete and no further action would be appropriate. This latter scenario was determined to be the situation in this instance and therefore, even though significant ethical concerns remained at the conclusion of the case, anonymous discussions with other forensic expert colleagues determined that no further action was deemed appropriate.

Conclusions and Recommendations

The most recent changes in the *Ethical Principles of Psychologists and Code of Conduct* (cf. American Psychological Association, 1992; 2002) had the general effect of dispersing a number of specific issues formerly contained within a section titled "Forensic Activities" into more general sections. It remains clear, and is so stated in the introduction to the latest revision, that the ethical standards continue to apply to psychologists who are involved in forensic activities. Very few primary ethical standards have been changed substantively, as applies to forensic neuropsychology. Among the few exceptions, changes have (1) removed the implication that psychologists always try to personally evaluate forensic referrals, rather than perform only records review, when they offer opinions, (2) revised the definition of the information referred to as "test data" that should be released upon court order, while retaining security of "test materials", and (3) noted the exception to reporting an ethical violation if discovered while being retained to review the work of another psychologist whose professional conduct is in question. To be clear regarding the latter point, this instance could occur when a licensing board has retained a forensic neuropsychologist to review the work of another forensic neuropsychologist against whom a professional complaint has been lodged. Mere retention to render a professional opinion that may or may not differ with another neuropsychologist's expert opinion would not be included within this latter point.

If ethical concerns that arise *within* a forensic context remain salient *after* the case has concluded, then it is appropriate to consider whether any action is necessary. In general, the guidelines for specialty practice in forensic psychology (Committee on Ethical Guidelines for Forensic Psychologists, 1991) are informative and helpful in making this determination. The specific issues that arise for neuropsychologists involved in forensic activities can be somewhat unique and challenging. In this regard, the writings for neuropsychologists in particular by Binder and Thompson (1995), Grote, Lewin, Sweet, and van Gorp (2000), Guilmette and Hagan (1997), and Sweet, Grote, and van Gorp (2002) are relevant to these considerations. Consonant with virtually all ethical situations involving psychologists, when appropriate, the first step is to attempt an informal resolution by bringing the concerns to the attention of the psychologist. Failing resolution in this fashion, if appropriate, the matter can be referred to state or national ethics committees, licensing boards, or institutional authorities.

Scenario 2

The second case for consideration involved an automobile accident between two cars. The first automobile, driven by the plaintiff, was struck by the defendant's automobile in the rear. The force of the collision was great enough to cause airbag deployment; the plaintiff was also in a seatbelt harness. At the scene, witnesses and paramedics reported normal behavior and no signs of brain injury. All at the scene denied that loss of consciousness had occurred. In the emergency room, memory for all events was intact, but the plaintiff changed her report to include the possibility of a brief loss of consciousness. In subsequent reports to physicians, the plaintiff's description involved increasing numbers and severity of symptoms suggestive of brain injury. However, not until years later when an attorney referred the plaintiff for neuropsychological and psychiatric evaluations by two experts who share office space was the plaintiff advised that a brain injury had taken place. The relevant details of the plaintiff's background are significant and numerous. To be brief, the plaintiff had stopped working years before the accident because of "chemical sensitivity" and had a social history that included serious childhood abuse and a chaotic adulthood, during which ineffectual social and vocational functioning was evident. The history and symptoms provided by the plaintiff to various health care professionals and ultimately to expert witnesses were at times *very* discrepant.

Within a general clinical practice, a generalist clinical psychologist who provided testing for all manner of forensic cases also provided neuropsychological assessment. In the particular case under consideration, the psychologist used a first year practicum student as an assistant in evaluating a personal injury litigant. Most of the relatively few neuropsychological tests used in the case were administered, scored, and initially interpreted by the practicum student. It was later revealed that this case was one of the first to be seen by the practicum student, and there were so few neuropsychological referrals to this general practice that the student's practicum experience was discontinued and completed elsewhere. Interestingly, the practicum student had a career in mental health prior to beginning the retooling educational process required to become a doctoral level clinical psychologist. In this prior career the practicum student would have qualified as an expert and been able to render independent opinions regarding psychopathology and psychiatric diagnoses.

Of greatest interest, the majority of this information documented by the practicum student strongly supported hypotheses *other* than traumatic brain injury as a cause for the plaintiff's presentation. The student's documentation included recording different elements of history that were revealed during testing and were at odds with the information contained within the formal report subsequently rendered by the psychologist. The supervising psychologist acknowledged having deliberately kept out of the report all of the observations and history documented by the practicum student, which was only discovered when the separate records kept by the student were subpoenaed. It turned out that history discrepancies of the plaintiff's psychologist and psychiatrist (who worked in the same office) had been brought to the attention of both by the student, and both the psychologist and the psychiatrist had excluded the information from consideration. The first neuropsychological evaluation by the generalist clinical psychologist failed to report any history or test observations that did not support the plaintiff attorney's theory of brain injury and even failed to disclose that a specific test finding had occurred. The undisclosed test result was one that knowledgeable neuropsychologists would have construed as strong evidence of insufficient effort. In fact, it turned out that the practicum student had reported all the test observations and test findings independently to a university professor, who was also a neuropsychologist. This "curbside" consult was motivated solely by the practicum student's desire to learn. The professor told the student that the plaintiff's presentation and test results were not credible. In an effort to reconcile the professor's viewpoint with that of her clinical supervisor, the student conveyed the opinion of the professor to the psychologist, who ignored all of it. Finally, despite the fact that the psychologist was being retained as an expert to render a forensic opinion, no effort tests were administered during the first evaluation. In the final report issued by the psychologist, all results and history information were interpreted as supporting diagnoses of mild traumatic brain injury and post-traumatic stress disorder (PTSD).

A neuropsychologist was retained to provide an independent opinion. The plaintiff failed numerous effort measures and validity indicators in the second neuropsychological evaluation. Numerous non-neurological and extremely unrealistic and inconsistent findings were documented. Additionally, during the second evaluation, the plaintiff provided very different history information (e.g., not having *ever* suffered some of the prominent PTSD symptoms listed in the prior neuropsychological evaluation report; having been an average student in a vocational track, rather than a valedictorian in high school) compared to that contained within prior records. The conclusions of the neuropsychologist were that malingering and personality disorder were both prominent in the plaintiff.

Relevant Ethical Issues

Integrity

Principle C (Integrity) appears directly relevant to the appearance that the generalist psychologist deliberately covered up and failed to note the presence of information that cast a very negative light on the hypotheses and conclusions favored by the plaintiff. The discrepant test result was not reported in the formal report and was only evident in the student's separate file. The observations of the test examiner are normally important to the opinion of a psychologist who was not present to make his or her own observations. Even though the observations came from a student, which in some instances legitimately might lead to being discounted, this student had a former career in which expertise of judging human behavior and clinical phenomena was well established.

Along the same line of concern, Ethical Standard 6.01 (Documentation of Professional and Scientific Work and Maintenance of Records) appears relevant, in that records under the control of the psychologist should not have been altered, withheld, or disposed of. Stated differently, within a forensic context of litigation, all expert witnesses have an obligation to maintain and, when appropriately requested to do so, fully disclose all records received and created during the course of a case. Even outside a forensic context, the ethics code of psychologists requires that we be honest and complete in recording and maintaining information upon which we base our opinions.

Similarly, Ethical Standard 9.01a (Bases for Assessment) requires that psychologists base their opinions, "including forensic testimony, on information and techniques sufficient to substantiate their findings." In this instance, the formal opinion should have at least acknowledged the existence of addressed disagreements with the observations of the test examiner. Instead, the presence of the observations and information from the test examiner were kept secret and not revealed in the standard disclosures that are inherent in litigation proceedings. Related, Ethical Standard 2.04 (Bases for Scientific and Professional Judgments) appears also to suggest that bases for opinions be consistent with scientific and professional knowledge; it is common and accepted practice to rely upon the test observations of trained examiners.

At the very least, even if not a violation of one or more Ethical Standards, the appearance of actions by an expert witness that represent bias are a serious matter, which in almost all forensic contexts can and should lead to a significant discounting of an expert's opinions. The reader is referred to discussions pertaining to possible bias and inappropriate advocacy versus rendering of objective neuropsychologist expert opinions (cf. Sweet & Moulthrop, 1999; Lees-Haley & Cohen, 1999). One would not ever expect in routine clinical work that suppressing or distorting of information could be consistent with rendering an objective differential diagnosis. Within a forensic context, such behavior is likely to represent serious bias.

Delegation of Work

A different concern could be raised regarding Ethical Standards 2.05 (Delegation of Work to Others) and 9.07 (Assessment by Unqualified Persons). If a psychologist allows an important part of a clinical or forensic service to be performed by an individual whose observations are later viewed as so unreliable as to be wholly excluded from the light of day, one wonders if the psychologist breached ethical obligations in allowing an unqualified individual to practice under his or her auspices. In this instance, the context of a training environment for the practicum student appears to represent a mitigating circumstance. Though likely this ethical concern would not be deemed a true violation if subject to peer review, within a forensic context it is unquestionably a poor judgment by an expert witness, one that serves to undercut the expert's credibility and opinions.

Professional Competence

A final area of ethical concern is the possibility that the generalist is practicing outside his or her areas of competency, which falls under Ethical Standard 2.01 (Boundaries of Competence). In this particular instance, concern regarding competence pertains to: (1) having rendered a forensic opinion on a far less than comprehensive evaluation that did not include assessing some of the more important domains relevant to possible brain injury, (2) having so few relevant neuropsychological testing cases in past or present practice experience that it seems likely even minimal criteria associated with demonstrating expertise in neuropsychology would not be satisfied (i.e., he/she would not be deemed an expert in neuropsychology by peers or by evidentiary standards used by courts), and (3) because of glaring knowledge deficiencies, an apparent unwillingness to consider important relevant information, even that which could effectively rule out brain injury and posttraumatic stress disorder. Importantly, with regard to the broad issue of competency, the generalist had been practicing many years and had never attended neuropsychology conferences, pursued continuing education in neuropsychology, subscribed to journals on neuropsychology or related areas (i.e., brain injury), and acknowledged not performing neuropsychological evaluations with any regularity. In instances such as this, a competing hypothesis in terms of ethical concerns regarding extreme bias is lack of competence, which is sometimes a difficult distinction.

Case Resolution

As with Case 1, the deposition and trial proceedings allowed full disclosure of all the unusual omissions and commissions associated with the opinions of the generalist clinical psychologist. At trial, the opinion of the psychologist had been so seriously undermined that he/she was not called to testify at trial. Moreover, the defense attorney easily demonstrated the impressive inconsistency and unrealistic presentation of the plaintiff across time.

With the trial completed, an attempt at informal resolution of ethical concerns was attempted. A straightforward and non-threatening letter was sent to the psychologist (i.e., complainee) by the neuropsychologist (i.e., complainant). In the letter, a non-judgmental educational tone was taken. The complainee called the complainant on the telephone and discussed the issues that had been contained within the complainant's letter. During the conversation, the complainee acknowledged discomfort and regret about several aspects of his/her work on the case. Given that the complainee appeared as a result of the letter and subsequent discussion to appreciate a broader understanding of his/her prior actions within an ethical context, the complainant considered the matter closed, and no further action was taken.

Conclusions and Recommendations

The distinction between bias versus lack of competence, when the question arises within the conduct of forensic cases, can be difficult.

It should be noted that both bias and lack of competence can lead to unsupportable opinions that lack objectivity and, of course, both can influence a forensic case in a direction that is misleading to the "triers of fact". Is it possible for incompetence, or even ignorance, to in fact be a conscious bias that is therefore relevant to ethical concerns? Yes. If an expert in a series of forensic case experiences fails to modify his/her lack of knowledge even after multiple salient learning trials (e.g., aggressive cross-examinations during which the expert's opinions are shredded by presentation of large literatures to the contrary), but continues to render uninformed and unenlightened opinions in which the previously exposed literatures are denied, then conscious bias is likely to be the cause. After all, how does one explain that a psychologist, who earlier in life having demonstrated learning ability that allowed the granting of a doctoral level degree, has (without onset of brain dysfunction) suddenly lost the ability to learn and benefit from experience? In such an instance, Principle C (Integrity) and Ethical Standard 5.01 (Avoidance of False or Deceptive Statements) apply.

Weissman and DeBow (2003) have presented a relevant discussion of ethical principles and professional competencies within a text for forensic psychologists. These authors have captured an important insight and perspective in the following quote, which also applies to forensic neuropsychologists:

> Ethical behavior in the individual, although subserved by personal motivations and characterological features, nonetheless can be understood as a set of learnable functional skills. When properly implemented (e.g., in the formulation of assessment methodologies that address psycholegal issues and protect rights and privileges of all the parties to a legal action), these ethical skills constitute an essential component of competent forensic practice (p. 52).

Overall Conclusions

Examination of relevant studies of professional practice (e.g., Sweet, Peck, Abramowitz, & Etzweiler, 2003) reveals that involvement in forensic activities is now common and in fact a prominent part of professional life for clinical neuropsychologists. Yet, examination of publication content in the forensic neuropsychology literature across a decade of marked growth in this practice area showed relatively few publications concerning ethics (Sweet, King, Malina, Bergman, & Simmons, 2002). Professional ethics are generally deemed to be "principles of conduct governing an individual or a group" (Merriam-Webster, 2002). Although sometimes ethical considerations are viewed as "aspirational", rather than mandatory (cf. *Black's Law Dictionary*; Garner, 1999), psychologists have generally viewed the standards promulgated by the American Psychological Association as a necessary context for acceptable clinical practice. As difficult to understand and apply as ethical standards can be in the increasingly complex reimbursement, regulatory, legal, and societal "real world" of clinical practice, ethical standards within a context of forensic practice can be even more enigmatic.

As noted earlier, there are some relatively unique situations that can arise in the course of rendering an opinion in a forensic case. Examples include (a) being asked by a plaintiff's attorney to delete mention of unsavory history information that was revealed in the interview of the plaintiff, (b) finding that the "other" neuropsychology expert is not a neuropsychologist at all and has relied entirely upon a hired psychology intern's work in rendering a forensic opinion, and (c) discovering that the "other" neuropsychologist's assessment consists of a brief interview and a few idiosyncratic, unnormed "tests" that have not undergone any peer-reviewed research trials. Whereas these brief descriptions are reason for ethical concern, an actual determination of ethical misconduct requires much more detail and context.

The two cases above were presented in similar fashion to the approach used by Nagy (2000), who constructed numerous fictional, but lifelike, vignettes to illustrate a vernacular interpretation of ethical standards. Different than Nagy, the experiences described above were based on numerous actual practice experiences, amalgamated to maximize their heuristic value into two cases. For the purposes of these case illustrations, the emphasis has been on potential ethical considerations related to professional behavior of neuropsychologist expert witnesses, rather than the nuances of the litigated cases themselves. Readers may notice that when the specific ethical concerns were discussed, mention of the particular neuropsychologist's position within the litigated case (i.e., whether retained as expert by the defense or retained as expert by the plaintiff) was not mentioned. Even though the reader may have construed the side of retention from the details of the case, it was not overtly mentioned because ethical concerns can be raised in forensic situations on both sides. Stated differently, being retained by one or the other side of a litigated case is, across experts, not systematically associated with being either less or more ethical. Rather, ethical problems occur in response to specific case situations and may for an individual expert recur across his or her cases. Thus, with regard to consideration of ethical standards as applied to neuropsychological activities within forensic proceedings, *Axiom 1* is that no one can claim a more ethical position simply by virtue of the fact that he or she is retained more by the plaintiff or more by the defense in adversarial proceedings.

Although questions regarding ethical behavior are raised more frequently within forensic proceedings than with the provision of routine clinical services, the number of actual ethical violations is not necessarily higher. It appears that because of the adversarial nature of forensic activities associated with its unique context (i.e., different roles, goals, and expectations), the application of ethical standards that were intended primarily for routine clinical activities is even less clear with forensic activities. Due to this lack of clarity and the need to address a host of issues typically not found within routine clinical service, it is only natural that as practitioners seek to understand situation-specific behaviors of their peers, questions regarding the possibility of ethical violations arise. However, importantly, one cannot help but observe in frequent conversations with other neuropsychologists who engage in forensic activities that concerns regarding ethical standards, even though regularly entertained in the minds of neuropsychologists who are functioning as expert witnesses, are much less often made explicit within the forensic proceeding. Frequently, this is due to the fact that initial concerns devolve to a subsequent less emotional conclusion that a standard has not been violated. As we have considered for educational purposes some common issues that frequently trigger concerns, readers should note that most often, at least within a forensic context, it is ultimately concluded by one neuropsychologist that the "other" neuropsychologist has not committed an ethical violation.

Thus, with regard to consideration of ethical standards as applied to neuropsychological activities within forensic proceedings, *Axiom 2* is that the rate of actual ethical violations is not proportionate to the increased number of ethical concerns raised during forensic proceedings. Moreover, if set aside until the end of a forensic proceeding, very few initial ethical concerns will be deemed necessary to pursue. This fact explains why licensing boards and ethics committees routinely adopt a policy of not accepting complaints for investigation if the situation involves civil (e.g., personal injury, malpractice), administrative (e.g., disability or worker's compensation independent psychological examinations), or criminal proceedings.

Before closing this chapter, we should acknowledge an increasing number of anecdotal reports in some parts of the country that attorneys apparently have adopted a strategy in litigation and independent medical evaluation cases of attempting to remove certain experts from forensic practice in their locale by filing numerous, unsubstantiated ethical complaints against the experts. Such a strategy in itself appears to involve ethical violations (e.g., Standard 1.07, Improper Complaints) *if*, rather than attorneys, the complainants were psychologists. It is less clear that attorneys, who are governed by different principles, would be perceived as unethical in carrying out such obviously blameworthy acts.

The degree of concern regarding filing of disingenuous ethical complaints as a strategy to remove legitimate experts from appropriately influencing the outcomes of forensic cases has prompted the Board of Directors of the American Academy of Clinical Neuropsychology (AACN) to create a position paper on the subject (American Academy of Clinical Neuropsychology, 2003). Some highlights from this position paper are worth noting here. Ideally, an ethics committee or licensing board that receives an ethics complaint, the genesis of which is a forensic evaluation, would consider and be guided by the following points: (1) members of the investigating body should have no prior forensic experience either with the law firms or psychologists involved in the case identified by the complainant; (2) many ethical concerns originate within forensic proceedings because of the complexity of issues addressed and the all too human weakness of strong emotional responses that occur when professional opinions are challenged aggressively; most of these initial concerns disappear when the forensic proceeding is concluded, (3) investigations of ethical concerns should be set aside until the end of any adversarial forensic proceeding that could benefit the complainant; (4) members of an investigating body must consider possible self-interested motivations of complaining psychologists and/or attorneys who have vested interests in IME or other adversarial proceedings that are antagonistic to the complainee, (5) investigations of some complaints made to state ethics committees and licensing boards against neuropsychologists require expertise of specialists in clinical neuropsychology; forensic peer review experts should be selected from a different geographic region in order to minimize the possibility of any conflict of interest in local adversarial activities.

It is likely that the complex nature of forensic neuropsychology will continue to demand of practitioners a keen awareness of relevant ethical guidelines and their applicability to the case scenarios that commonly develop within adversarial proceedings. Fundamentally, ethical behavior in a forensic neuropsychologist is not simply an aspirational goal; ethical behavior is an essential component of an effective forensic expert, if he or she is to be relied upon to render an unfailingly objective opinion.

References

American Academy of Clinical Neuropsychology (2003). Official position of the American Academy of Clinical Neuropsychology on either complaints made against clinical neuropsychologists during adversarial proceedings. *The Clinical Neuropsychologist, 17*, 443-445.

American Psychological Association. (1992). Ethical principles of psychologists and code of conduct. *American Psychologist, 47*, 1597-1611.

American Psychological Association. (2002). Ethical principles of psychologists and code of conduct. *American Psychologist, 57*, 1060-1073.

Binder, L., & Thompson, L.L. (1995). The ethics code and neuropsychological assessment practices. *Archives of Clinical Neuropsychology, 10*, 27-46.

Committee on Ethical Guidelines for Forensic Psychologists (1991). Specialty guidelines for forensic psychologists. *Law and Human Behavior, 15*, 655-665.

Garner, B. (Ed. in Chief) (1999). *Black's law dictionary. Seventh edition*. St. Paul, MN: West Group.

Grote, C., Lewin, J., Sweet, J., & van Gorp, W. (2000). Responses to perceived unethical practices in clinical neuropsychology: Ethical and legal considerations. *The Clinical Neuropsychologist, 14*, 119-134.

Guilmette, T., & Hagan, L. (1997). Ethical considerations in forensic neuropsychological consultation. *The Clinical Neuropsychologist, 11*, 287-290.

Hansen, M. (2000). Expertise to go. *American Bar Association Journal, 86*, 44-52.

Lees-Haley, P., & Cohen, L.J. (1999). The neuropsychologist as expert witness: Toward credible science in the courtroom. In J. Sweet (Ed.) *Forensic neuropsychology: Fundamentals and practice* (pp. 443-468). Lisse, Netherlands: Swets & Zeitlinger.

Merriam-Webster (2002). *Webster's universal encyclopedic dictionary*. New York: Barnes & Noble Publishers.

Nagy, T. (2000). *Ethics in plain English: An illustrative casebook for psychologists*. Washington, DC: American Psychological Association.

Sweet, J., Grote, C., & Van Gorp, W. (2002). Ethical issues in forensic neuropsychology. In S. Bush, & M.L. Drexler (Eds.) *Ethical issues in clinical neuropsychology* (pp. 103-133). Lisse, Netherlands: Swets & Zeitlinger.

Sweet, J., King, J., Malina, A., Bergman, M., & Simmons, A. (2002). Documenting the prominence of forensic neuropsychology at national meetings and in relevant professional journals from 1990-2000. *The Clinical Neuropsychologist, 16*, 481-494.

Sweet, J., Peck, E., Abramowitz, C., & Etzweiler, S. (2003). National Academy of Neuropsychology/Division 40 (American Psychological Association) Practice Survey of Clinical Neuropsychology in the United States, Part II: Reimbursement experiences, practice economics, billing practices, and incomes. *Archives of Clinical Neuropsychology, 18*, 1-26.

Sweet, J., & Moulthrop, M. (1999). Self-examination questions as a means of identifying bias in adversarial assessments. *Journal of Forensic Neuropsychology, 1*, 73–88.

Weissman, H., & DeBow, D. (2003). Ethical principles and professional competencies. In A. Goldstein (Ed.) *Volume 11: Forensic Psychology, Handbook of Psychology, I.* Weiner (Ed. in Chief), (pp. 33-53). New York: Wiley.

Section 3

ETHICAL CHALLENGES IN NEUROPSYCHOLOGY IN MEDICAL SETTINGS

Introduction

Neuropsychologists provide a diverse range of services in acute medical settings. Although such diversity may allow for stimulating professional experiences, it may also contribute to ethical challenges (Wilde, Bush, & Zeifert, 2002). Such challenges do not always arise from a lack of awareness of ethical issues, but may result from two or more ethical principles conflicting with each other. For example, while the neuropsychologist may be quite aware of the value that most patient's derive from making decisions for themselves (Respect for People's Rights and Dignity), he or she may be in a position to recommend a reduction of such autonomy due to cognitive impairment in order to maximize the patient's safety (Beneficence). Challenges such as these tend to be common in many medical settings, and the authors of this chapter guide the reader through an understanding of such issues and steps to resolve them in the best interests of the patient, neuropsychology, and the medical setting.

Reference

Wilde, E.A., Bush, S., & Zeifert, P. (2002). Ethical neuropsychological practice in medical settings. In S.S. Bush & M.L. Drexler (Eds.), *Ethical issues in clinical neuropsychology*, 195-221. Lisse, NL: Swets & Zeitlinger Publishers.

Chapter 6

ETHICAL CHALLENGES IN NEUROPSYCHOLOGY IN MEDICAL SETTINGS, PART I

James B. Pinkston

Scenario 1

A neuropsychologist employed at a busy medical center is asked to perform a pre-operative neuropsychological evaluation of a patient who is a candidate for anterior temporal lobectomy for the treatment of medically intractable epilepsy. The patient is being treated on an inpatient basis and is currently undergoing continuous video-electroencephalogram (EEG) monitoring within the hospital's epilepsy monitoring unit. The patient is connected to the monitoring equipment via a series of EEG leads adhered to her scalp, face, and torso. The presence of these EEG leads is an ongoing and salient irritant and distraction to the patient. These leads also limit her movement and essentially confine the patient to her bed. It is probable that she will remain reclined on her bed for the evaluation. The patient will likely also have an intravenous line placed in the forearm of one arm. Furthermore, she is typically undergoing constant video recording and may be distracted by observing her scrolling EEG results on a large monitor next to her bed.

As in many institutions, this patient is in a joint room in which only a thin cloth curtain divides her bed from that of her roommate. This arrangement, coupled with being in a strange environment and the necessary monitoring by nurses during the night, results in sleep deprivation and concomitant somnolence. Also, the family members of the adjoining patient are in the room and are a source distraction during a portion of the evaluation. The patient is a minor and is mentally incompetent. Furthermore, the patient's parents or legal guardian are not immediately available. Finally, routine hospital tasks take place during the evaluation. These interruptions are comprised of visits by hospital staff including rounding neurologists and other physicians, visits by nurses, the bringing and removal of meals, and the activities of cleaning personnel. Such interruptions were partially prevented by careful planning and the support of the nursing staff, but they occur nonetheless and manifest themselves during time-sensitive measures and the presentation of memory tasks.

Compounding the distracting and limiting effects of the physical arrangement of the patient's room are the physiological changes occurring within her system. As part of the epilepsy monitoring procedure, the patient is being aggressively titrated off of all of her anti-epileptic medications in the hopes of producing a series of seizures for lesion or seizure focus localization. The progressive removal of these chemicals from her system may be affecting her cognitive functioning as her body rebounds from its habituation to the neurocognitive side effects of such medications. Furthermore, the patient experienced more than one significant seizure just prior to her neuropsychological evaluation and experiences a seizure during the neuropsychological evaluation. These seizures negatively impact her performance during the evaluation. One seizure during the evaluation was sufficiently severe to require that the patient receive PRN anti-epileptic medication, such as Diazepam, to stop an ongoing episode of status.

Relevant Ethical Issues

Elements of the above situation are relatively common and encompass several ethical issues. The relevant ethical considerations, as described in the 2002 APA Ethics Code, include privacy and confidentiality, informed consent, evaluation and assessment, and interpretation of test results.

Privacy and Confidentiality

Inpatient evaluations place significant limitations on maintaining the privacy of the patient during evaluation when rooms are shared or family members or others are present. These limitations should be discussed with the patient at the outset of the evaluation and as needed if cognitive status changes, and steps should be taken to limit breaches in confidentiality (Standard 4.02a,b). If at all possible, the patient should be evaluated alone, and care should be taken not to enquire into or discuss sensitive and personal information with the patient when such information may be overheard by a family member, fellow patient, or member of the hospital staff.

Informed Consent

Patients evaluated on an inpatient unit may be experiencing altered states of consciousness or impaired cognition due to a variety of factors, including neuropathology, other medical conditions, and medications. Furthermore, the guardian of minors or legally incompetent individuals may not be as readily accessible as in an outpatient setting. Given these factors, obtaining informed consent for the evaluation may require more effort on the part of the neuropsychologist than is required in some other settings. The neuropsychological evaluation and its purpose should be carefully explained in language readily comprehendible by the patient (Standard 3.10a & 9.03a). In addition, the legal guardian must be sought out for formal informed consent in the case of minors or individuals with limited or questionable competence (Standard 3.10b). In such cases, efforts should also be made to obtain the patient's assent (Standard 3.10b & 9.03b).

Assessment

Finally, the demands and less controlled environment inherent in an inpatient setting create several challenges surrounding the administration and interpretation of neuropsychological measures. The validity of many neuropsychological measures rests upon the assumption of a standardized assessment procedure. The capacity of these neuropsychological measures to make comparisons between a patient's performance and that of a representative normative group depends largely upon adherence to standardized instructions and conditions. Neuropsychological evaluation within the inpatient setting, with its distractions and physical demands, can place limits on the neuropsychologist's ability to adhere strictly to the standardized procedures of such measures. These limitations need to be taken into account when the neuropsychologist attempts to draw inferences about the patient's cognitive abilities based on her performance on such measures (Standard 9.06).

Although few measures are expressly normed for an inpatient setting, most standardized neuropsychological measures will likely still produce reliable and valid results in so far as the neuropsychologist is careful to take steps to control those untoward elements in the inpatient environment. In those situations in which, even after the neuropsychologist's attempts to impose sufficient control and adherence to standardization procedures, the demands of the inpatient setting are felt to confound the results of neuropsychological assessment, the neuropsychologist must account for those confounding influences. Specifically, the limits of the assessment must be identified and characterized (Standard 9.02b).

Case Resolution

The neuropsychologist in the above scenario fortunately had the opportunity later that day to administer those portions of the evaluation that were unable to be completed due to patient and environmental variables. Prior to the second session, the neuropsychologist was careful to prepare staff and visitors that interruptions should only occur for urgent matters. The second session went relatively smoothly. Nevertheless, the neuropsychologist indicated in his report those aspects of test administration that he believed were adversely affected by the setting, and he was careful not to over-attribute pathology in his interpretation of the data.

Conclusions and Recommendations

The 2002 Ethics Code does not deviate significantly from the general direction taken by the 1992 Ethics Code in regard to ethical considerations of privacy and confidentiality, informed consent, evaluation and assessment, and interpretation. Several modifications are noteworthy, however. The neuropsychologist is obligated to help the patient understand the limits of confidentiality as they pertain to all of the neuropsychologist's activities that impact the patent, rather than just the services provided to the patient. In regards to informed consent, the 2002 Ethics Code now admonishes the neuropsychologist to consider the "rights and welfare" of the patient and contains

wording that has been strengthened from the obligation to simply consider the patient's "preferences and best interests" as stated in the 1992 Ethics Code. The documentation of consent, permission, and assent, be it written or oral, is also expressly required. Finally, the 2002 Ethics Code contains revised wording that is slightly less specific and broader in its scope regarding the interpretation of test results and substantiation for assessment findings. Although these changes do not significantly alter the overall import of the Ethics Code, they do tend to broaden its scope because of the decreased specificity.

Not all neuropsychological evaluations are conducted within the predictable and controlled environment of the outpatient office. Frequently, neuropsychologists are called upon to perform evaluations of individuals who are being evaluated and cared for on an inpatient basis within a hospital. These evaluations may consist of pre-operative neuropsychological evaluation for epilepsy surgery, post-operative evaluation following cerebral spinal fluid drainage for the treatment of hydrocephalus, evaluation in the acute stages of recovery from traumatic brain injury or cerebral vascular accident, or evaluation of various other neurologic conditions for which the patient is being treated on an inpatient basis and for which answers regarding neuropsychological functioning are required. The neuropsychologist plays a valid and integral role in acute care and inpatient settings to assure the best possible treatment planning and care for the patient. However, such settings are not without their own unique challenges.

Confidentiality, informed consent, evaluation and assessment, and interpretation naturally continue to be important ethical considerations and rightfully receive significant attention within the Ethics Code. A neuropsychologist working within a medical center will not find significant changes impacting his or her work with the 2002 revision of the Ethics Code in this regard. However, he or she should be aware of some of the subtle changes in the wording pertaining to professional activities, patient confidentiality, and informed consent.

Scenario 2

A neuropsychologist at a large medical center is asked to provide education on the use of various neuropsychological tests and screening instruments to other members of the hospital staff. The request has come from prominent individuals within the medical department that encompasses the neuropsychology section. These professionals function as direct or indirect consumers of the neuropsychologist's services. Over time, they have come to appreciate the usefulness of the information provided in neuropsychological reports. In the eyes of these professionals, several of the neuropsychological measures used and reported on by the neuropsychologist are particularly relevant to the care of many of their patients. The neuropsychologist, therefore, has been asked to educate them in the administration of these measures so that they can use them in their individual practices to augment patient care.

Although well qualified in their respective areas, none of these professionals has had more than a cursory exposure to neuropsychological theory or application. To accomplish this education, the neuropsychologist has been asked to bring the materials and conduct a one-hour training conference. The professionals are aware that the neuropsychologist utilizes trained, non-licensed technicians in the administration of these measures. They believe that the proposed one-hour training will be sufficient to prepare them, as licensed professionals in their various fields, to both administer and interpret these measures.

Relevant Ethical Issues

This neuropsychologist is in a relatively common situation that threatens potential intradepartmental conflicts, and more importantly, poses ethical dilemmas. The relevant ethical considerations, as described by the 2002 Ethics Code, include the use of psychological assessment techniques by unqualified persons and maintaining test security.

Assessment by Unqualified Persons

The Ethics Code mandates that, except for training purposes, neuropsychologists do not promote the use of assessment techniques by those not qualified to use them appropriately (Standard 9.07). There are obvious reasons for this position. Rather than interpreting Standard 9.07 as an attempt to protect the guild of neuropsychology by excluding others from the use of such assessment techniques, this section is necessary to maintain the highest standards of patient care. Neuropsychology, in both theory and applied form, may appear deceptively straightforward and simple to the new initiate. However, as one gains more understanding and experience, as is often the case in specialized fields, one begins to appreciate the subtle complexities that go into the interpretation of evaluation results and the process of differential diagnosis. Certainly, the assertions put forward in neuropsychological reports should be based on more than the results of standardized testing alone. An understanding of the statistical properties of a given measure, the presentation and performance of the patient during testing, the patient's individual personal variables and life history, and many other factors must come to bear when arriving at the sound interpretation of neuropsychological test results. Although the synthesis required is not unique to neuropsychology, the application of these skills within a neuropsychological framework is not something one can learn or even adequately appreciate without extensive training and experience.

Maintaining Test Security

The concept of maintaining test security is applicable in this situation as well. Neuropsychologists in medical settings make reasonable efforts to maintain the integrity and security of test materials and other assessment techniques (Standard 9.11). Without an academic background and supervised experience in the use of standardized assessment measures, individuals will likely not appreciate the importance of maintaining test security. Although not likely to breach test security out of malice, other professionals may neglect test security by overtly, or inadvertently, indicating the correctness of a patient's responses during testing. Also, less rigorously trained individuals may acquiesce to patients' repeated demands for the correct answers to test items.

Case Resolution

In this scenario, the neuropsychologist finds himself presented with both a challenge and an opportunity. Whereas the pressure to appease the interest of intradepartmental colleagues is palpable, complying with their request potentially jeopardizes the test security of those instruments, risks lowering the standard of care, and therefore, is in opposition to the Ethics Code. However, the request for education was utilized as opportunity for increased understanding. The neuropsychologist used the forum to present rational arguments for why the sound use and interpretation of neuropsychological assessment techniques requires substantial training and supervision. Furthermore, the neuropsychologist presented information about the variety of referral questions that can be answered through neuropsychological evaluation and the important information, recommendations, and answers such evaluations can provide the referring physician.

Conclusions and Recommendations

Neuropsychologists are typically broadly trained within psychology and related fields and are accustomed to being flexible in their approach to solving problems. In medical settings the recognition of these traits may be the impetus behind the fact that neuropsychologists are frequently called upon to perform a variety of tasks. These duties may include educating the public, patients, other health care professionals, and physicians regarding issues pertaining to neuropsychological assessment. Such education can serve to improve patient satisfaction and overall quality of care. It can also function as a means of increasing interdepartmental understanding and recognition for the usefulness of neuropsychological evaluations, thereby increasing the flow of appropriate referrals. However, neuropsychologists are sometimes asked to provide education that, ultimately, may not be in the best interest of the profession or patient care.

Neuropsychological evaluation and the techniques utilized therein are appealing to many disciplines. However, the use of neuropsychological instruments and techniques requires substantial training and supervision to be performed competently. The APA Ethics Code affirms the importance of ensuring that individuals have sufficient background and experience before utilizing such techniques. In addition, the neuropsychologist is obligated to take reasonable steps to protect the integrity and security of such measures and techniques.

In this process of maintaining test security and ensuring appropriate use of measures, difficulty may arise in determining which measures are solely within the purview of neuropsychology. Rehabilitation therapists, neurologists, and others in medical settings frequently use standardized measures of cognitive and linguistic abilities to assess patients. Such measures may range from screening instruments such as the Mini-Mental State Exam to more sensitive measures of higher level functions. Some neuropsychologists may believe that certain measures do and should fall solely within the purview of psychology or neuropsychology, whereas many nonpsychology colleagues may disagree. The ability to negotiate this challenge becomes still more complicated when such measures have been used by other disciplines for years prior to the neuropsychologist's arrival at an institution.

To clarify this issue, test publishers have established requirements for various levels of education in order to purchase the tests that they sell (although the degree to which these requirements are enforced may vary). This information can be shared with those who are using tests without possessing the requisite credentials. In addition, some nonpsychology professionals may use tests that are in the public domain. Tactfully inquiring into their educational and training background in the appropriate use of such measures may reveal avenues through which the neuropsychologist can encourage the correct use, or nonuse, of the measures. Within a medical center, aspirations to ensure correct test use can often be met through the careful education of other interested professionals. Although this can be a particularly challenging and difficult issue to negotiate, neuropsychologists have an ethical obligation to try (General Principles: A, Nonmaleficence and Beneficence; and B, Fidelity and Responsibility; Standards: 1.03, Conflicts Between Ethics and Organizational Demands; 3.09, Cooperation with Other Professionals; 9.07, Assessment by Unqualified Persons; 9.11, Maintaining Test Security).

References

American Psychological Association. (1992). Ethical principles of psychologists and code of conduct. *American Psychologist, 47*, 1597-1611.

American Psychological Association. (2002). Ethical principles of psychologists and code of conduct. *American Psychologist, 57*, 1060-1073.

Chapter 7

ETHICAL ISSUES IN NEUROPSYCHOLOGY IN MEDICAL SETTINGS, PART II

Elisabeth A. Wilde

Scenario 1

A neuropsychologist has a faculty position at a university medical center. His time is split between clinical responsibilities on the rehabilitation floor and his own research in traumatic brain injury (TBI). He has years of experience with TBI patients and has worked hard to provide assistance to his patients and their families in obtaining medical, rehabilitation, educational, psychological, social, and financial resources that are available in the community. He learns of a small but enthusiastic non-profit organization whose mission is to provide education about head injury to a wide array of audiences (health care professionals, patients, caregivers and family members of patients, and large community groups) and to sponsor social events and support services for head injury survivors. In addition to his desire to help patients, he is interested in networking with other professionals who work with this population. He joins the organization and attends several events sponsored by this group. The neuropsychologist's interest and expertise are quickly recognized, and the board (comprised of physicians and rehabilitation professionals from different institutions in the community) proposes to make him a board member.

Not long after his election onto the board, the board is approached by an attorney specializing in personal injury litigation. This attorney reports that she has been very successful at helping injured individuals gain financial compensation for their suffering and has developed both an understanding of and sympathy for these individuals. She reports that she would like to donate a substantial sum of money to the organization since she believes in their objectives. She points out that this small organization has some good goals, but that its activities are constrained by its very limited financial resources. Furthermore, she points out that board members, who are all professionals volunteering their time and effort, are spending a great deal of their time doing things that could be handled by well-trained support staff. This would enable the board to better utilize their time and professional skills to benefit the organization and the public. She suggests that she help fund some additional activities as well as bankroll some full-time support personnel and perhaps provide the board members with "just a little compensation" for their time and devoted effort.

Relevant Ethical Issues

The Ethics Code provides basic guidelines that may be of some benefit in further considering the above situation.

Beneficence and Nonmaleficence (Principle A)

One of the primary motivations of the neuropsychologist for joining the head injury organization and serving on its board is his interest in further assisting those who have sustained head injuries and their families. Consistent with the principle of beneficence, he is volunteering his time to bring his experience and the perspective of neuropsychology to this group. His additional motivation to further his own professional development and contacts is not inconsistent with this principle; in fact, by doing so, he may be better able to serve his patients.

The neuropsychologist's actions are also consistent with the principle of nonmaleficence. That is, he is attempting to anticipate potential ethical conflicts that may arise through the attorney's proposed, and likely well-intentioned, actions. He is attempting to foresee potential harm to those with head injuries, their loved ones, and the organization and to bring potentially harmful actions to the attention of the other board members so that a course of action that is in the best interest of all parties can be pursued.

Multiple Relationships (Standard 3.05)

Admittedly, numerous scenarios involving multiple relationships arise where there is little foreseeable risk of harm to either party. In the above scenario, it may be that the neuropsychologist's position on the community board (despite his additional role as a treatment provider) is defensible if he is vigilant in his role as a board member to have limited and very well-circumscribed contact with any patients that he has previously treated. He may also need to carefully consider how to handle multiple relationships with

individuals who are or may become subjects in his research. Finally, the neuropsychologist may also need to consider his pre-existing obligation to the institution that employs him to ensure that his position as a board member for this organization would not lead to any foreseeable risk of exploitation or harm to the hospital. The ethics code acknowledges that not all dual relationships are to be avoided. What a loss it might be to his community if the neuropsychologist and other psychologists did not contribute a portion of their time and expertise to serve their community for little or no financial compensation. However, because of the enormous potential harm that can result from certain kinds of multiple relationships, this continues to represent an important ethical standard and deserves constant and careful consideration.

Conflict of Interest (Standard 5.06)

The introduction of the attorney's offer to the board may give rise to any number of possible "conflict of interest" complications down the road. For example, what if the attorney attends a social event her donation funds and socializes with several head injury survivors? Even without directly soliciting business at all, she mentions in the course of casual conversation that she is an attorney, and a patient-member of the organization later contacts her for legal advice and wishes to become her client. What happens if the neuropsychologist assumes a role as an expert witness (for either side) on a future case that the attorney is involved in? What happens if, in the future, the attorney needed (because of her own ethical obligation to "zealously" represent her client) to use information now available to her and/or the employees she is paying about the hospital, the board members, or the TBI survivors and their families to the detriment of any of these parties? Future events could result in possible conflict of interest complications even where the initial motives of both the benefactor and the board seem neutral and harmless. However, one can also easily imagine a host of future difficulties if the attorney's or any of the board members' motives for involvement with the organization were less honorable.

Case Resolution

The neuropsychologist discussed the situation with other appropriate faculty (particularly those with more forensic experience) and sought advice on how to best handle the situation; this enabled him to better anticipate future difficulties and possible conflict of interest complications. The neuropsychologist also immediately reviewed the hospital's Conflict of Interest policy, which required him to disclose his affiliation with the volunteer organization. He completed a statement that would be reviewed both by other senior faculty and the chair of his department to ensure that his activities would not compromise his obligations to the institution that employed him.

The neuropsychologist then consulted legal counsel for the hospital, explained the situation, and stated his concerns about protecting the institution from possible future harm. The attorney also outlined some preliminary concerns from the point of the view of the hospital's potential liability in light of the fact that many of the board members were affiliated with the hospital and many of the survivor-members had been treated there. He asked that the neuropsychologist provide him with a specific written proposal that could be reviewed in depth by hospital counsel before proceeding further with any agreement. He also recommended that the neuropsychologist have the proposal reviewed by an outside attorney or attorneys who could objectively discuss other concerns that the board may wish to consider regarding conflict of interest, liability for the community organization, and the financial and tax consequences of accepting the donation.

As the neuropsychologist was not familiar with the potential board member's/attorney's reputation, he decided to contact the State Bar Association regarding the individual's disciplinary history to ascertain if there were any notable past instances of breach of professional ethics or questionable past behavior. He realized that the absence of a disciplinary history certainly did not mean that there were no foreseeable risks in entering into a relationship with this individual, but rather regarded it as one small step in a long process of risk analysis. The neuropsychologist was also relatively unfamiliar with the professional and ethical obligations of attorneys, so he located and reviewed these guidelines in order to better understand and anticipate significant differences in professional and ethical obligations that may arise between professionals.

Finally, the neuropsychologist took an active role in informing the board about issues that required careful consideration to protect the TBI survivors and their family members involved in the organization, the board members, the institutions that the board members worked for, the organization itself, the individual board members, and the attorney as benefactor. He voiced his opinion that certain aspects of the proposal were probably inappropriate (e.g., financial compensation of the board members) and suggested aspects of the proposal which would have to be altered in order to be more acceptable. He also emphasized the need for ongoing dialogue, expert advice, and thoughtful consideration as the decision-making process commenced.

Conclusions and Recommendations

Situations in which there is an obvious line between right and wrong and/or a fairly predictable outcome are typically not the ones with which most neuropsychologists will ever struggle. Rather the more difficult decisions often occur in the midst of conflict between two competing values that are, at their core, essentially "good" things or scenarios where the outcome is particularly difficult to anticipate. The above scenario illustrates several such conflicts (e.g., between being actively engaged in acts of beneficence and avoiding conflict of interest) as well as underscores difficulties that may result from competing allegiances.

In the above situation, it is possible that the motive underlying both the benefactor's offer and the board acceptance of the offer is, at least on some level, quite philanthropic: perhaps everybody involved sees a need in this particular community of patients and professionals and just wants to help others. However, human interactions are rarely motivated by single forces, and several important future variables could easily create complications. In addition to legal and financial consequences for the organization and the individual board members, the neuropsychologist must also carefully anticipate the likelihood of ethical difficulties.

1. Familiarize yourself with institutional policy in each organization where you act in a professional capacity. Faculty or employees of a medical center or university may need to be particularly careful to make certain that they understand institutional policies regarding outside employment or consultation or any regulations that the university or hospital might have regarding service on community boards.

2. Where appropriate, establish a relationship with and seek the advice of legal counsel at the institution by which you are employed. Keep in mind that the hospital attorneys have a primary obligation to promote the best interests of the institution, but they may be able to offer helpful information regarding potential legal difficulties.

3. Recognize differences between ethical codes of different professions. While the ethics codes of many professions address "conflict of interest" in an attempt to protect clients/patients, institutions, or other parties from harm or exploitation, there may be subtle differences in emphasis across professional

codes that can create difficulties. In working in a multidisciplinary setting, work to educate non-neuropsychologist colleagues about potential differences that may impact perspective and decision-making.

4. Consult with other experienced neuropsychologists who can help you anticipate potential risks and benefits of involvement in various organizations. There may not necessarily be a single solution to a particular scenario, especially in situations such as the one illustrated above where the neuropsychologist may initially be operating with little specific information. Using caution and foresight in ambiguous situations may allow a neuropsychologist to avoid obvious major pitfalls. This may be particularly important in areas with increased risk for forensic involvement.

5. Consider the advantages of very specific and detailed written proposals and agreements. Again, particularly in situations that could conceivably involve forensic proceedings, this may facilitate more thorough consideration of difficult issues, which may help psychologists "strive to keep their promises and to avoid unwise and unclear commitments" (Principle C: Integrity). In addition, this documentation may serve as evidence of attempts to avert foreseeable harm.

Scenario 2

A neuropsychologist in a large hospital is called to perform a consult on one of the medical units to determine a patient's competence to make decisions regarding medical treatment and disposition planning. The patient is an 18-year-old woman with a complex medical history. The referring physician notes that this young woman has been hospitalized many times throughout her life for issues related to her condition and complications of treatment, yet recently hospitalizations have become even more frequent as a result of bacteremia and infections of the patient's permanent lines. The staff report that they have provided the patient and her mother with instructions regarding the care of her line ports and have stressed the importance of these procedures; they are concerned that the patient may have "learning problems" either as a direct result of her medical condition or as a result of her very limited and disrupted formal education.

As a result of her recent complications, the patient is now also faced with a transplant decision, and the staff note that she has been rather unwilling to discuss the potential benefits of this procedure. Each time they begin to explain the potential benefits of the transplant, which is currently available, she interrupts them, stating "You'll have to talk to my mom about this, but I doubt she'll go for it." As the patient is an adult with adequate cognitive capacity to make medical decisions for herself, the staff expresses frustration and concern about her deferring to her mother as well as the plan to discharge her back to her previous living situation at home. They report that the patient's mother did not come to visit for three days after the patient's admission. When she did arrive earlier that morning, she was obviously intoxicated, very unkempt, and notably hostile toward both her daughter and the hospital staff. In addition, it is clear that she has not quit smoking despite the continued danger that this presents to her daughter's health.

The neuropsychologist introduces herself and explains her role on the treatment team as an expert in cognitive functioning. She briefly explains to the patient that she would like to conduct some cognitive testing and ask her some questions regarding her preferences for disposition. The patient is initially cooperative through screening tests of general intelligence and academic achievement, but quickly evidences notable distractibility and decreased motivation as testing proceeds. Later in the session, she angrily refuses to continue the evaluation, stating that she cannot understand how this could possibly be relevant to her medical condition.

The neuropsychologist again explains that the treatment team is concerned about her well-being and how to help her seek appropriate assistance in managing her self-care. When the neuropsychologist asks the patient to describe proper hygiene procedures, the patient begins to cry and states "of course I know what I am supposed to do. I'm not stupid."

As the neuropsychologist talks further to the patient, it is clear that the patient seems indifferent to the severe consequences of failing to adequately follow recommendations regarding hygiene and the care of her lines. In discussing her recent string of infections, she states that she does not "see the point" in performing basic hygiene since she is "not going to be around people anyway." She also discloses that she has been intentionally placing large quantities of over-the-counter hypnotics and prescription pain medications in her line when she becomes bored or feels "hopeless" about her medical condition. She then demands that the neuropsychologist not disclose any of this information to her mother or her physicians.

Relevant Ethical Issues

Boundaries of Competence (Standard 2.01)

Neuropsychologists who perform capacity evaluations should have appropriate training and should have attained competence in determining which areas of cognition may be impaired, how impairment may impact the patient's functioning in different areas, whether impairment is likely to be transient or lasting, and the likely cause of the impairment. Second, neuropsychologists should have a solid and evolving understanding of specialized assessment tools utilized in the measurement of capacity and rely upon an evidence-based knowledge regarding the use of any other general neuropsychological assessment tools for this particular purpose. Third, they should work to develop an understanding of the particular form of capacity at issue, acknowledging that "competence" is not a unitary phenomenon nor is it static and permanent. In addition, the neuropsychologist should work to develop an understanding of forces and beliefs underlying the particular patient's (or family member's) values, concerns or behavior, especially those which are at odds with the recommendations of the medical staff. Finally, although most instances of capacity to live independently and capacity to make medical decisions are not formally contested in a legal arena, psychologists who participate in such evaluations should have an adequate understanding of state and federal legal requirements involved in determining competency and should "be or become reasonably familiar" with their role should a patient's situation result in or necessitate a formal legal proceeding.

Informed Consent (Standard 3.10 and 9.03)

In addition to information about informed consent that generally applies to all professional activities, Standard 9.03 further outlines specific elements that are to be considered in obtaining informed consent in assessment situations. These include "an explanation of the nature and purpose of the assessment, fees, involvement of third parties, and limits of confidentiality and sufficient opportunity for the client/patient to ask questions and receive answers." In routine assessments, covering these elements may be fairly straightforward; however, in situations such as the one above, providing even basic information about the nature and the purpose of the assessment may prove a more difficult task and may alter the patient's willingness to participate or provide some kinds of information about current level of functioning. The current Ethics Code provides a few exceptions to obtaining formal informed consent: assessment of decision-making capacity is one of these special situations (see Standard 9.03). However, valid assessment almost always requires some degree

of assent and willing participation, and, in some situations, providing some initial explanation as to the use and importance of the assessment results may, in fact, be helpful in encouraging the patient's best effort on formal testing.

Use of Assessments (Standard 9.02)

Neuropsychologists who become involved in evaluating a patient's medical decision-making capacity should have a solid understanding of current research regarding the use of standard neuropsychological instruments for this particular type of assessment. In addition to measures specifically aimed at determining the form of capacity at issue, cognitive and personality testing can be quite useful in determining patterns that may be reflective of certain cognitive or psychological disorders or in identifying areas of functioning which are likely to be problematic. However, using results of these more general tests for predictive purposes (i.e., determining future behavior) should be done with appropriate caveats and in context of other evidence that directly relates to the individual's capacity.

Interpreting Assessment Results (Standard 9.06)

Obviously the first major concern in interpreting the data gathered in the above scenario involves the patient's motivation and effort. Because this patient's effort was inconsistent, findings based upon formal cognitive functioning are quite limited. Furthermore, the patient's educational history may be a potential limiting factor in interpreting results of some cognitive tests. Finally, the neuropsychologist should also note situational factors that may be influencing a patient's performance. In this patient's case, the neuropsychologist may have scrutinized the possible effects of pain, medication, transient and long-term metabolic dysfunction, a suboptimal testing environment, and the inevitable interruptions that occur on an inpatient hospital unit to determine if any of these factors impacted the patient's performance. More importantly, however, the neuropsychologist in this case should consider the impact of the patient's current mood, the acute stress of the hospital stay, and her difficult family dynamics on her behavior.

Confidentiality, Minimizing Intrusions on Privacy, and Disclosures (Standard 4.01, 4.02, 4.04, and 4.05)

These standards emphasize the need to protect a patient's privacy and to limit disclosure of unnecessary sensitive information. In their attempt to be thorough in considering potential causes for cognitive or psychological disturbance, neuropsychologists may frequently uncover "sensitive information" even though they are not intending to be intrusive. Medical history and treatment, substance use history, educational history, and social history all provide important factors for the neuropsychologist to consider as part of many evaluations where there is not a detailed or specific referral question; however, these are also areas where sensitive information is likely to surface. In addition, most examiners must exclude the possibility of significant psychiatric issues and depression as contributing factors in cognitive disturbance, as well as gather information about "psychiatric" manifestations of certain physical disorders and medications. Furthermore, gathering information regarding the individuals' general ability to function in his or her job and home responsibilities is often essential in forming a context for the patient and as evidence regarding the manner and extent to which cognitive deficits are impacting day to day functioning. In addition, discussing the limits of confidentiality may seem straightforward in principle, but executing this may be more difficult in practice since introducing an assessment by cataloging an exhaustive list of people who may have access to the record may discourage patients from disclosing certain kinds of important information. Finally, in reporting results to the referral source, the neuropsychologist must use careful deliberation in walking what may be a fine line between disclosing "unnecessary" details and substantiating his or her conclusions and recommendations and illustrating the urgent need for further services.

Explaining Assessment Results (Standard 9.10)

Providing feedback to inpatients in medical settings may be particularly challenging for several reasons including the fact that the patient may be discharged from the unit or hospital shortly after the evaluation is completed. In addition, neuropsychologists in medical settings often assume a consultant role where the neuropsychological examination may only be a part of the diagnostic process; therefore, the neuropsychologist is in an awkward position to answer questions regarding diagnosis and prognosis, particularly if other parts of the evaluation are still pending. Furthermore, providing feedback can be time-consuming and difficult to coordinate if the patient is frequently in other parts of the hospital for procedures or treatment or family members are difficult to locate. Finally, providing adequate explanations to patients with more severe cognitive disturbance or explanations to ill-prepared family members can be challenging. Nevertheless, Standard 9.10 emphasizes that the neuropsychologist is ultimately responsible for providing information regarding the results of neuropsychological assessment.

Case Resolution

The neuropsychologist explained the limits of confidentiality in this situation, stating that if the patient disclosed information that led the neuropsychologist to believe that she was at significant risk for further self-harm, the neuropsychologist was legally obligated to take additional action and inform other appropriate persons, including her physicians and her mother. In addition, the neuropsychologist informed the patient that although she would limit some of the details of the patient's disclosure in her written report since her record would be potentially accessible to all treatment providers within the institution, her report would include a recommendation for further psychiatric evaluation and the general basis for that recommendation. The neuropsychologist explained to the patient that she was concerned about the significant risks that the patient was taking each time that she misused medications or failed to follow important hygiene precautions. The neuropsychologist attempted to gather more information about the patient's neuropsychological functioning to assess her risk for further self harm. She ascertained from the patient's responses that her behaviors had indeed led to acute life-threatening complications on several occasions despite the absence of a clear-cut intent to harm herself. The neuropsychologist explained the benefits of meeting together with the patient's mother present to further discuss the transplant decision and more long-term disposition plans. The patient was initially very reluctant, but ultimately agreed to this. The neuropsychologist also obtained the patient's permission to speak with her mother as part of the assessment process.

The neuropsychologist then met with the patient's mother in an attempt to gain a better understanding of the mother's behavior, the relationship between the patient and her mother, and the safety of the patient in her home environment. It quickly became clear that although the patient's mother was concerned about her daughter's well-being, her own coping difficulties rendered her unable to provide the level of support and supervision that her daughter currently required. At first, the patient's mother was defensive and insisted that her daughter return home. Gradually, however, the neuropsychologist was able to diffuse the mother's hostility somewhat, and the mother voiced her concerns about the family's limited financial resources and the cost of the transplant and subsequent treatment. She acknowledged some resentment

and concern regarding her daughter's dependent and seemingly attention-seeking behavior and explained that her absence was an attempt to force the patient to assume some responsibility. The neuropsychologist explained the benefits of individual and family therapy and explored the patient's mother's feelings about this recommendation.

The neuropsychologist created an evaluation summary that briefly restated basic demographic information and some limited information regarding the patient's decision-making ability based upon her interaction with the patient. She noted that although she had attempted formal testing to address the referral question regarding basic intelligence and the presence of a learning disorder, limiting factors including the patient's motivation precluded further meaningful interpretation of formal testing results. She suggested that the patient's mood, situational factors, and family relationship difficulties may represent significant barriers to effective and deliberate decision-making at this time, but that these factors should be explored in greater detail within the next few days. She recommended further consults by psychiatry and social work. In her oral reports to the primary service, the neuropsychologist used care in providing essential information to appropriate members of the treatment team, but emphasized to them the need to continue to treat the patient and her mother with respect and to use care in how they documented sensitive information.

With the patient's permission, the neuropsychologist scheduled a meeting where the patient, her mother, the attending physician, the social worker, and she met together to discuss the risks and benefits of the transplant as well as some solutions to her mother's financial concerns. In this setting, the patient was better able to display an ability to adequately comprehend the information provided to her, appreciate the consequences of having the transplant or not, and communicate a rational decision in regards to the transplant procedure. In addition, the group discussed a disposition plan that carefully balanced the need to foster autonomy with the need to ensure the patient's safety.

Conclusions and Recommendations

While psychiatrists are often utilized in determining issues of "capacity" to make medical decisions or to live independently, neuropsychologists are also frequently recruited when a patient's cognitive abilities are in question, since abilities such as understanding alternatives, manipulating information, and communicating preferences are requisite to decision-making. In addition to the need for expertise related to cognitive functioning alone, neuropsychologists may also offer additional forms of expertise. Because of the unique training related to understanding human behavior that many clinical neuropsychologists receive, they can often play an invaluable role in helping other medical professionals uncover more subtle psychiatric issues or better understand the contribution of a patient's psychological state to his or her medical condition or cognitive state. This may be particularly useful in making determinations about suspected conversion disorders or in helping to determine the contribution of situational or mood factors to a medical disorder. Some neuropsychologists may also receive significant training in therapeutic interventions used with individuals or family systems where there are dysfunctional forces or significant coping deficits. Finally, the neuropsychologist may be able to become uniquely attuned to important differences in perspective between the medical professionals and the patient or between the patient's family members. Neuropsychologists clearly provide an array of skills that may be very helpful in complicated situations such as the one described above.

1. Perform evaluations regarding decision-making capacity only with sufficient training and expertise to do so. Competence in this area of practice may require a thorough understanding of general issues related to cognitive disturbance and the use of neuropsychological assessment tools as well as some specific evidenced-based knowledge of the validity of using these techniques for this particular purpose. There are also instruments that have been specifically developed to address "capacity" in different areas of functioning, and the examiner should have at least some familiarity with the strengths and limitations of these instruments.

2. Discuss the limits of confidentiality with the patient as part of the introduction to the assessment or provide them with written information and an opportunity to ensure that they understand these limits. Optimally, this should include identification of the members of the primary service as well as other medical professionals in the future who may have access to the written report and insurance providers who may have access to the report and/or diagnostic codes and findings. The neuropsychologist may also wish to discuss with the patient what information the neuropsychologist has permission to share with family members and how this information will be communicated. Finally, the patient should be informed of other foreseeable limits to confidentiality including the use of records in a forensic proceeding or the need to execute appropriate intervention in situations of harm to self or others. It may be helpful to reassure the patient that care will be used in the written documentation of sensitive information. In addition to professional ethics, relevant state and federal laws must be considered.

3. Limit information in written and oral reports to that which is germane to the referral question and/or to that which is necessary to obtain further treatment. Keep in mind that a written report may be viewed by a diverse audience; document findings accordingly, carefully balancing both privacy and accuracy.

4. Understand and document any limitations of the assessment tools, the assessment process, the accuracy of the testing data, and the ability to interpret the data.
5. In capacity evaluations, strive to attain an appropriate balance between encouraging the patient's autonomy and self-determination and concerns for the patient's safety and well-being.
6. Foster a growing familiarity with resources in the hospital and community and, within reason, educate patients or help them gain access to the necessary services and expertise of other appropriate professionals. In addition to understanding services that a patient could take advantage of in an ideal situation, consider the practical barriers to obtaining services so that specific recommendations and referrals are helpful.

Section 4

ETHICAL ISSUES IN NEUROPSYCHOLOGY IN PSYCHIATRIC SETTINGS

Introduction

A primary difference between the neuropsychological assessment and treatment of individuals with psychiatric disorders and individuals with other neurological disorders is the *perception* of their competence (Gur, Moberg, & Wolpe, 2002). For example, the patient with neoplastic disease is considered to have the cognitive capacity to make medical decisions independently, whereas patients with psychiatric disorders tend to be considered unable to make similar decisions. Such stigma continues to underlie the way in which the public and some clinicians view those with psychiatric disorders. As a result, such preconceptions may interfere with appropriate neuropsychological assessment of decision-making capacity, with implications for the patient's ability to provide informed consent. The authors of this chapter take the reader into the world of psychiatric neuropsychology to examine the ethical challenges that are commonly encountered in such settings. The issues presented will likely be of value not only to those working in such settings but also to all neuropsychologists struggling to integrate similar ethical principles with challenging professional responsibilities.

Reference

Gur, R.C., Moberg, P.J., & Wolpe, P.R. (2002). Ethical issues in neuropsychology in psychiatric settings. In S.S. Bush & M.L. Drexler (Eds.), *Ethical issues in clinical neuropsychology*, 165–193. Lisse, NL: Swets & Zeitlinger Publishers.

Chapter 8

ETHICAL CHALLENGES IN NEUROPSYCHOLOGY IN PSYCHIATRIC SETTINGS, PART I

Paul J. Moberg

Scenario 1

A middle-aged Asian-American female was referred to a neuropsychologist by the court to conduct a competency evaluation due to her refusal of treatment for a life-threatening illness. The patient was undergoing treatment for a recent bout of serious depression and in the course of standard laboratory testing was diagnosed with lymphatic cancer. Despite the seriousness of her illness, her oncologist and the treatment team agreed that this cancer would be readily treated with surgical intervention and brief chemotherapy. With treatment, her odds of survival were felt to be approximately 99%; without treatment, she would not live for more than 9-10 months. The oncologist and surgeon spent 2-3 hours with this patient and her spouse describing the nature, course and outcome of her cancer. Treatment options were outlined, as were potential risks, etc. Following these sessions, the patient, despite demonstrating a very detailed knowledge and understanding of her condition and the positive and negative outcomes of her choice to pursue treatment, refused to undergo any type of medical intervention. Her husband was quite distraught by her choice and sought the assistance of

his family to alter her decision. After his failure to convince his wife to undergo treatment, he retained a lawyer who then petitioned the court to compel his wife to undergo treatment for her cancer. As a result of this petition, a neuropsychological evaluation was requested by the court to evaluate her competency.

At the time of the neuropsychological exam, the patient expressed concern that results of this examination would be used to challenge her wishes. Despite having raised this concern, the consulting neuropsychologist told the patient that this exam was "like any other clinical case" she saw and proceeded to evaluate the patient. Results of intellectual assessment revealed overall abilities in the High Average range, with evenly developed verbal and nonverbal skills. Academic abilities were generally commensurate with obtained IQ. Against this background, neuropsychological testing revealed only mild reductions in attentional skills and mild bilateral motor slowing on tests of fine motor speed and coordination. The remainder of her neuropsychological exam was intact, showing strong problem-solving, memory, visuoperceptual, and language skills. No tests or measures of emotional functioning or personality were obtained, nor were specific measures of decisional capacity administered. The neuropsychologist concluded that there was no data from her exam to indicate any neuropsychological deficit which was impacting the patient's judgment, reasoning or comprehension skills and that the patient was competent to make the decision not to seek treatment. No additional treatment was recommended. Notably, when asked in the interview why she was refusing treatment, the patient stated that she knew that she would certainly die without medical intervention, but related that she "did not care" whether she lived or died. She stated that she felt that death would be a better outcome than her current state (depression) and that she should have the right to make decisions about her own body. In addition, she related that she was a devout Buddhist, that she did not fear death, and that she would leave her fate "in the hands of Buddha".

Relevant Ethical Issues

There are a number of ethical issues that arise from this vignette. First, this evaluation was initiated by the court and, as such, fully explaining the purpose and scope of the neuropsychological examination and limits to confidentiality are even more important than they are in a regular clinical evaluation (see 2002 Standard 9.03, Informed Consent in Assessments; Standard 3.10, Informed Consent; and Standard 4.02, Discussing the Limits of Confidentiality). It is not, as the consulting neuropsychologist stated, "like any other clinical exam", as these results could indeed be used against the patient's wishes and would be made available to the court and anyone else involved in the proceedings.

Second, despite a precipitating episode of depression, no formal assessment of emotional state was given. Such affective disruption can clearly impact decisional capacity, just as neurocognitive dysfunction can. Given this fact, testing of this domain should have been included in the assessment, or limitations on the battery given

should have been outlined in the neuropsychologist's report (see 2002 Standard 9.06, Interpreting Assessment Results). Third, there is a small but emerging body of research specifically examining decisional capacity or competence (Carpenter et al., 2000; Charland, 1999; Marson, et al., 1995; Roberts & Roberts, 1999). Given this literature and the questions posed to the examining neuropsychologist, addition of tasks designed to specifically test capacity would be important to understand the patient's comprehension, judgment and reasoning behind the choices she had made (see 2002 Standard 9.02, Use of Assessments, subsections b and c below).

Lastly, her religious and cultural beliefs did not necessarily support the view that death was to be avoided, and when combined with her feelings of hopelessness and marked depression, made the choice of death seem reasonable to her. Inclusion of her belief system and cultural background into the assessment process would be important to ensure the examiner is not imposing a different (or their own) cultural or religious standard upon the case (see 2002 Principle E, Respect for People's Rights and Dignity; and Standard 2.01, Boundaries of Competence, subsection b).

Case Resolution

Despite there not being strong support for neuropsychological deficit that would render this patient incompetent, there was no direct assessment of her emotional state in the initial evaluation. The issue of very significant depression was quite clear, however, and upon reevaluation by another neuropsychologist, the impact of her psychiatric state on her reasoning was more fully elucidated. After this second evaluation, which included measures specifically aimed at her emotional state (MMPI-2, BDI-II, etc.), as well as targeting her ability to consent to treatment (i.e., MacCAT-CR), the second neuropsychologist concurred with the first evaluator's conclusion that there was not any significant neuropsychological deficit which was impacting her judgment and reasoning. He did argue, however, that despite her intact cognitive state, her depression and hopelessness were indeed impacting her decisional capacity. Specifically, it was argued that the decision to let her self die despite reasonably clear expectation of a cure and no significant residual deficits was not a decision that the "average" person would make. That is, despite intact *neurocognitive* functions, her *affective* state was coloring her decisional capacity and rendered her subsequent decisions questionable. Regardless, there was not significant evidence from the second neuropsychological evaluation to force the patient to undergo treatment against her will. In addition, the second neuropsychologist consulted with an Asian psychologist familiar with the Buddhist faith to address possible cultural and religious issues in her decision not to pursue treatment.

In the end, the second neuropsychologist recommended evaluation for pharmacologic treatment for her depression, as well recommending that she work with the Asian psychologist he consulted with concerning cultural and religious issues. He deemed that while her affective state was coloring her decisions, there was no clear suicidal ideation or other factors which would lead the court to compel her to undergo medical treatment. After a number of weeks working with her therapist, the patient eventually agreed to pharmacologic treatment for her depression (which up to that time she had refused). After a month of pharmacologic treatment in combination with ongoing psychotherapy, the patient's depression resolved and she decided to undergo treatment for her cancer.

Conclusions and Recommendations

As with most issues dealing with such complex ethical dilemmas, a purely neuropsychological focus does not always address other issues known to impact consent to treatment and other decision-making capacity in patients suffering from neuropsychiatric or neurologic disorder. Such "nonrational" factors include: (1) trust in the clinician, (2) experience of suffering, (3) coercion, (4) desperation, (5) altruism of the ill person or, (6) hope (Charland, 1999; Roberts & Roberts, 1999). A number of studies have shown that these factors also weigh heavily on the decision making processes of psychiatric patients, and need to be given as much attention as is given to neuropsychological and other clinical matters. Competence is a legal determination that implies an "all or none" capability; however, in clinical settings, a person may have the capability to make certain decisions (i.e., taking PRN medication) while not being able to make others (i.e., undergoing surgery and chemotherapy). It is, therefore, more appropriate to speak of "capacity" as opposed to competence. In addition to standard neuropsychological techniques, the neuropsychologist must be prepared to include measures that are designed to directly assess the question at hand. In this case, the inclusion of a measure or measures probing decisional capacity can be very helpful, and certainly assessment of the impact of her emotions on her decisions also warranted examination. Lastly, the inclusion of cultural and religious factors is also important to put the evaluation in the context of the individual's personal beliefs and traditions.

Scenario 2

A counseling psychologist was approached by a close friend whose adult son was experiencing significant psychiatric problems. The father, who was a psychiatrist, stated that his son had suffered from longstanding Bipolar disorder with primarily manic features, and that his son had recently decompensated. The father stated that his son was not thinking clearly and that he was concerned for his safety. He asked the psychologist to see his son in therapy to ascertain his condition. After 2-3 weeks of bi-weekly therapy, the therapist felt that the patient had not responded well to therapy and did not seem "to be following him" in their sessions. He then referred the patient for a neuropsychological evaluation.

After discussing the case with the psychologist, the neuropsychologist raised concerns that the therapist was conducting therapy with the son of his close friend, stating that he felt that this constituted a conflict of interest and that it would be most appropriate to transfer the patient's care to a more objective third-party. The psychologist agreed that his treatment of the patient was inappropriate, but that he cared for this young man and that he was "trying to help him out". Regardless, the psychologist agreed to discontinue treatment, and he transferred the patient to the care of a clinical social worker who had worked with the patient previously, coordinating care for his HIV as well as providing therapeutic services. The neuropsychologist agreed to see the patient for an assessment but informed the referring psychologist that all communication concerning the outcome and recommendations of the assessment would go to the case worker and/or the father of the patient. The patient's medical history was unremarkable with the exception of the fact that two and a half years prior to the assessment the patient had been diagnosed as HIV-positive. He had been undergoing medical treatment as well as practicing safe sex and making sure his potential sexual partners were informed of his condition. The patient reported to the neuropsychologist that he stopped taking his medication about two months prior and recently began "to see the light of his being". The patient presented with pressured speech, flight of ideas, tangential thinking, auditory hallucinations, delusions and thought-blocking. Specifically, he related hearing the voice of an "entity" which had instructed the patient that he was "the chosen one" and that he had special powers to heal others as well as "infinite wisdom". While acknowledging his HIV-positive status, the patient stated that he had been "blessed" by this entity which had "cured him" of his HIV. Given this belief, he

reported that he no longer took medication for this disease nor did he take any precautions to practice safe sex with his partners or inform them of his HIV-positive status. Indeed, the patient stated that he saw his "divine mission" to impregnate as many women as possible so that his "special abilities can be spread about the world".

After fully explaining the assessment process to the patient and obtaining consent, the neuropsychologist proceeded with his examination. Results of intellectual assessment revealed a Full-Scale IQ in the Average range, with verbal and nonverbal abilities in the same range with no marked scatter evident. Neuropsychological testing revealed significant impairment in attentional skills as well as deficits in higher level problem-solving and reasoning. Disinhibition and poor planning were also evident. Memory skills showed some encoding problems, but good retention of information that was already encoded. Results of the MMPI-2 revealed a single elevation on Scale 9 consistent with a manic presentation. The neuropsychologist felt that the patient would benefit from an inpatient admission to treat his current mania and to stabilize the patient both pharmacologically and therapeutically. The neuropsychologist also felt that there was not only imminent threat to the patient due to his untreated HIV$^+$ status, but also to other potential sexual partners of the patient who were at risk of contracting the virus from him. After receiving feedback and recommendations from the neuropsychologist, the patient stated that he saw nothing wrong with his functioning at this point and stated that he did not wish any treatment nor did he want any information about his assessment to be shared with his caseworker, father or anyone else.

Relevant Ethical Issues

Like case 1, there are a number of relevant ethical challenges posed in this vignette. First, the original referring psychologist treated the son of a close friend. This would constitute a conflict on interest (Standard 3.06, Conflict of Interest) and a multiple relationship (Standard 3.05, Multiple Relationships). A more appropriate response to the father's request would be to provide the contact information for qualified psychologists who could conduct such an assessment and treatment. The neuropsychologist correctly addressed this issue with the psychologist, relaying his concerns as well as the appropriate resolution to the matter (Standard 1.04, Informal Resolution of Ethical Violations). The second issue is that of confidentiality of the results from neuropsychological testing. While the patient refused to allow feedback to the referral source and significant others, he exhibited a number of behaviors and made statements that could be judged to pose a risk for harm to himself (i.e., untreated HIV and psychosis) and others (i.e., spread of HIV to others) (Standard 4.02, Discussing the Limits of Confidentiality, and Standard 4.05, Disclosures). Given this potential harm, a breach of confidentiality might be necessary to protect the patient as well as other potential sexual partners who might be unknowingly infected (Principles A, B, C, E).

Case Resolution

The neuropsychologist in this case felt that the patient posed a significant risk both to himself and others with regard to his psychosis and untreated HIV (harm to self) as well as possibly spreading the virus to others (harm to others). The neuropsychologist reviewed the consent information he obtained at the time of the assessment, and felt confident he had explained the procedures sufficiently as to when confidentiality could be breached. He subsequently contacted the patient's caseworker, informing her about his concerns and that he felt that the patient needed to be admitted to an inpatient neuropsychiatry unit for treatment of his acute symptoms. The caseworker brought the patient

into the local emergency room where he was committed to inpatient treatment, albeit against his wishes. During his initial stay on the unit, the patient was very angry with the neuropsychologist for breaking the confidentiality of the assessment and requested to see the hospital attorneys to lodge a complaint. The neuropsychologist went to court for the commitment hearing where the patient's complaint was heard and the consenting information was reviewed. The judge upheld the commitment and found that the neuropsychologist had acted within the bounds of his professional responsibility. With treatment on the inpatient unit, the patient's psychosis resolved, and his psychiatric status was stabilized. He began taking medication for his HIV once again and dropped any further complaints against the neuropsychologist.

Conclusions and Recommendations

This vignette supports the importance of recognizing professional boundaries, both in personal relationships and in dealing with other professionals. It also highlights that in addition to being a good *neuro*psychologist, each clinician should also utilize the basic *clinical* skills that are part of most neuropsychologists' training. Three national surveys of clinical neuropsychologists spanning the last ten years (Sweet & Moberg, 1990; Sweet et al., 1996; Sweet et al., 2000) have demonstrated that a majority of practicing neuropsychologists feel that a clinical psychology degree is the preferred training background for clinical neuropsychologists. This belief emphasizes the importance of being aware of as well as examining/interpreting, both neurological and "non-neurological" factors when assessing patients. The importance of integrating these ethical principles into neuropsychological practice has gained more attention recently (Bush & Drexler, 2002), and, as these vignettes indicate, a thorough knowledge of the new ethics code can help guide the practitioner to a course of action that is not only beneficial to the patient but also consistent with good ethical practices.

References

Appelbaum, P.S., & Grisso, T. (1996). *The MacArthur Competence Assessment Tool–Clinical Research.* Sarasota, FL: Professional Resource Press.

Bush, S., & Drexler, M.L. (Eds.) (2002). *Ethical issues in clinical neuropsychology.* Lisse, NL: Swets & Zeitlinger.

Carpenter, W.T., Gold, J.M., Lahti, A.C., Queern, C.A., Conley, R.R., Bartko, J.J., Kovnick, J., & Appelbaum, P.S. (2000). Decisional capacity for informed consent in schizophrenia. *Archives of General Psychiatry, 57*, 533-538.

Charland, L.C. (1999). Appreciation and emotion: Theoretical reflections on the MacArthur Treatment Competence Study. *Kennedy Institute for Ethics Journal, 8*, 359-376.

Marson, D.C., Cody, H.A., Ingram, K.K., & Harrell, L.E. (1995). Neuropsychologic predictors of competency in Alzheimer's disease using a rational reasons legal standard. *Archives of Neurology, 52*, 955-959.

Roberts, L.W., & Roberts, B.R. (1999). Psychiatric research ethics: An overview of evolving guidelines and current ethical dilemmas in the study of mental illness. *Biological Psychiatry, 46*, 1025-1038.

Sweet, J.J., & Moberg, P.J. (1990). A survey of practices and beliefs among ABPP and non-ABPP clinical neuropsychologists. *The Clinical Neuropsychologist, 4(2)*, 101-120.

Sweet, J.J., Moberg, P.J., & Westergaard, C.K. (1996). Five year follow-up survey of practices and beliefs of clinical neuropsychologists. *The Clinical Neuropsychologist, 10(2)*, 202-221.

Sweet, J., Moberg, P.J., & Suchy, Y. (2000). Ten-year follow-up survey of clinical neuropsychologists: Part I. Practices and beliefs. *The Clinical Neuropsychologist, 14(1)*, 18-37.

Chapter 9

ETHICAL CHALLENGES FOR NEUROPSYCHOLOGISTS IN PSYCHIATRIC SETTINGS, PART II

Allan Yozawitz

Scenario 1

The patient, a 14-year-old male psychiatric inpatient, was referred for a neuropsychological evaluation of what appeared to be a chronic learning disability and behavior problem. The patient had exhibited inadequate academic performance and disruptive behavior at school since first grade. Several special academic programs and school placements had been employed without apparent success. In the seven months prior to assessment, the patient was suspended from his seventh grade classes for belligerent behavior and a general attitude of insubordination. He subsequently received homebound instruction from a private tutor, and he reportedly was progressing better academically in response to that individualized training.

At the time of referral, the patient was in the process of a family court proceeding in response to an ungovernable petition filed by his guidance counselor. His prior legal history included a criminal trespass charge one year ago, a criminal possession of stolen property charge five months ago, and a burglary charge pending in family court. The patient's mother reported that her son was not a behavior problem at home, although she was aware of his fighting at school. She

acknowledged that the patient was not learning at school, but expressed confidence that he can learn when motivated. She noted nothing unusual about his developmental history or intellectual functioning that appeared different in comparison to her other children. However, school reports indicated that the quality of parental-child interaction was poor and that there was instability within the home environment.

Neuropsychological evaluation revealed a pattern of dysfunction in spatial synthesis, conceptual ability and abstract reasoning processes, visual memory, phonemic hearing, and right-sided tactile acuity. The manifestation of the patient's impaired spatial abilities included deficient visual-spatial and tactile-spatial integration as well as disturbed understanding of logical-grammatical constructions. The latter deficit appeared to be associated with the patient's poor social adjustment and delinquent behavior. Namely, individuals who manifest disturbances in understanding logical-grammatical constructions have difficulty comprehending sentences in which an action is transacted from one subject to another (e.g., the difference between "to take to someone" and "to take from someone") and in which there is an inverted position of the elements with respect to the action they describe (e.g., John was struck by Paul. Who was the bully?). Such neuropsycho-logically mediated semantic impairment, during critical periods of moral and social development, conceivably could alter its ultimate evolution within the individual.

This neuropsychological perspective needed to be communicated to family court not only to provide an understanding of why the patient may have repeatedly transgressed and failed to appre-ciate the nature of his wrongful acts, but also to initiate appropriate treatment interventions.

Relevant Ethical Issues

The ethical responsibility of the clinical neuro-psychologist was to advocate for treatment that would serve the patient's best interest and that of society more effectively than the punishment that already proved unsuccessful (Ethics Code's General Principles: A, particularly Beneficence; B, particularly Responsibility; & D, Justice). Were the clinical neuropsychologist to leave interpreta-tion of the neuropsychological report to the courts, it is conceivable that the saliency of the findings would either not be adequately understood or not acted upon. It is as much the responsibility of the clinical neuropsychologist to interpret findings to allied professionals, untrained in brain-behavior relationships, as it is for the clinical neuropsycho-logist to communicate findings to the patient (Standards 1.01, Misuse of Psychologists' Work; 3.09, Cooperation with Other Professionals; and 9.10, Explaining Assessment Results).

In addition, the importance of advocacy and treatment follow-up, illustrated by this case, warrants rereading Standards 10.09 (Interruption of Therapy) and 3.12 (Interruption of Psycho-logical Services). In so doing, these standards arguably could be perceived as acquiring new meaning with regard to their application to neu-ropsychological assessment in many contexts (particularly within psychiatric settings). Standard 10.09 states, "when entering into employment or contractual relationships, psychologists make

reasonable efforts to provide for orderly and appropriate resolution of responsibility for client/patient care in the event that the employ-ment or contractual relationship ends, with para-mount consideration given to the welfare of the client/patient." Standard 3.12 states, "Unless otherwise covered by contract, psychologists make reasonable efforts to plan for facilitating services in the event that psychological services are interrupted by factors such as the psycholo-gist's illness, death, unavailability, relocation, or retirement, or by the client's/patient's relocation or financial reasons." These Standards (10.09 and 3.12) may be supplemented with specific reference to the termination of assessment serv-ices. Support for this position can be found within General Principle B, Fidelity and Respon-sibility (viz., "Psychologists consult with, refer to, or cooperate with other professionals and institutions to the extent needed to serve the best interests of those with whom they work.").

Case Resolution

The clinical neuropsychologist's testimony in this case complemented the testimony of two psy-chiatrists, each of whom agreed that the patient's unpredictable behavior was related to brain dys-function combined with emotional disturbance. The testimony further indicated that the patient required a treatment program to develop improved self-worth and to heighten his motivation to achieve. As was explained to the court, such a program would focus on areas where the patient does well and avoid those in which he functions poorly. Because of the patient's aversion to structured settings and his difficulty establishing relationships with peers, it was recommended these interventions be provided in an individual-ized (1:1) format. Consequently, instead of con-tinuing to institutionalize this youth, the judge and the attorneys responsible for disposition recom-mended outpatient treatment that incorporated: (1) individualized educational programming within a stable environment, and (2) training to help the patient understand his problems and learn to control his reactions.

The neuropsychological testimony provided in family court on the patient's behalf generated a newspaper article that posed the question, "what can the family court do when no facility in the state is prepared to offer the care and treatment needed by a young teenager who, without appropriate treatment, seems likely to become a danger to the community?" In answer to that question, the judge in this case was able to tailor a unique program in accordance with recommendations advanced by the clinical neuropsychologist's testimony (even though no template for such a program existed within any of the state agencies potentially responsible for this individual's treatment). The patient was provided a secure supervised community residence with six other youths, psychotherapy twice per week on an outpatient basis, family counseling (for the patient's mother), and individualized (1:1) instruction in academics by the local school district at the residence. This disposition had the further advantage of keeping the patient in touch with his mother who was a relatively positive and supportive presence in the patient's life. Indeed, the patient never performed any violent acts at home.

At the conclusion of the previously mentioned newspaper article, the reporter noted that this case illustrated a different procedure in handling a family court proceeding in that both sides were pulling together as a team, rather than acting in an adversarial fashion, in order to find the best solution to the patient's behavioral problems. Additionally, had the clinical neuropsychologist not testified in this case, the judge would not have been empowered to persevere with agency administrators to extract the services from their institutions that were necessary to address the patient's needs. The family court judge exerted all the leverage of his office because of his conviction, developed after digesting expert testimony, that this was the only way to resolve the patient's problematic behaviors.

Conclusions and Recommendations

Consistent with the Ethics Code's General Principles and the highest ideals of ethical practice, clinical neuropsychologists should function as advocates for their patients in psychiatric settings, particularly when patients demonstrate limited ability to advocate for themselves or when their needs may have gone unnoticed or unappreciated by other health care professionals. For didactic purposes, one can conceptualize three forms of advocacy and treatment followup for clinical neuropsychologists in psychiatric settings.

The first form of advocacy involves medical follow-up. For example, for a patient with evidence suggestive of transient ischemic attacks, endocrine dysfunction (e.g., thyroid disorder), neoplasm, or seizure phenomenology, it is imperative that advocacy be directed at insuring the individual is referred to an appropriate medical specialist to further define the nature of these conditions and to implement treatment.

The second form of advocacy involves rehabilitative follow-up. It is incumbent upon clinical neuropsychologists to endeavor toward insuring that the deficits uncovered during evaluations are translated into active treatment utilizing the individual's strengths to circumvent and to develop deficient areas of functioning. This may take the form of providing specific guidelines for occupational, physical, or speech-language therapeutic intervention. It also may involve specific guidelines for academic and scholastic programming. The latter might include detailed recommendations regarding the nature of academic task instruction, type of class placement (e.g., self-contained vs. mainstreamed), and extent of instruction (e.g., 10 vs. 12 month programs).

The third form of advocacy involves judicial follow-up. It is often necessary for clinical neuropsychologists to stand behind their findings and recommendations in judicial proceedings involving their patients. This may involve hearings regarding medication over objection, discharge, cognitive capacity to stand trial for wrongful acts, and culpability for a wide range of crimes. The above case illustrated rehabilitative and judicial follow-up.

Advocacy and treatment follow-up typically are not recognized as applicable to clinical neuropsychological assessment regardless of setting. They are intrinsically codified, however, under General Principles A (Beneficence and Nonmaleficence), B (Fidelity and Responsibility), and D (Justice) and under Ethical Standards 1.01 Misuse of Psychologists' Work, 3.09 (Cooperation with other Professionals), 3.12 (Interruption of Psychological Services), 9.10 (Explaining Assessment Results), and 10.09 (Interruption of Therapy). The customary applicability of these Standards has been for the practice of psychotherapy, to insure that appropriate services are provided or maintained so that patients are not abandoned by their therapists or discharged prematurely without appropriate follow-up treatment (such as may occur in the context of the psychologist's unavailability or end of employment). The neuropsychological assessment of psychiatric inpatients, however, incorporates the same inherent need for continuity of treatment. There is no less clinical accountability for the practitioner performing neuropsychological assessment, exploring the roots of their patient's cognitive and emotional maladjustment to improve current functioning, than for the psychotherapist attempting to achieve the same clinical objective with a different method.

An essential ethical challenge for the clinical neuropsychologist in a psychiatric setting is to maintain advocacy and follow-through after the assessment to implement treatment recommendations. After all, the sine qua non of a clinical neuropsychological evaluation is its value in forming the diagnostic blueprint of an individual that ultimately will forge an improved outcome. Without appropriate advocacy and follow-through, clinical neuropsychological evaluations in psychiatric settings likely would be reduced to meaningless exercises.

Scenario 2

The patient, a 57-year-old female, was referred for neuropsychological assessment during her acute inpatient hospitalization. The evaluation was requested to explore the nature of her directional disorientation, which appeared to be of recent onset. The patient presented with a history of multiple and brief psychiatric hospitalizations, since she was 23 years of age, for treatment of recurrent affective episodes. A review of clinical records revealed that her symptomatology included situational and social anxiety, psychomotor agitation and restlessness, manic excitement, irritability, depressed mood, heightened religiosity, clinging dependency, muddled thinking, and elation. During one hospitalization, she received a series of ECT treatments. The patient never had been employed, and she always had resided with her mother. She was placed in a proprietary home following her mother's death seven months prior. Difficulty finding her way between that home and her outpatient treatment provider posed an immediate management problem that led to the current assessment. Medical history had been negative with the exception of a possible goiter during adolescence.

Neuropsychological evaluation revealed evidence of mild visual-spatial dysfunction, of nondevelopmental origin, that appeared to be secondary to her psychiatric dysfunction. A comprehensive psychodiagnostic assessment, employing a semistructured interview schedule, revealed a spectrum of behavior pathology that was suggestive of Bipolar I Disorder, Most Recent Episode Mixed, superimposed upon a Dependant Personality Disorder. Although the neuropsychological evaluation was helpful in indicating that the patient was not evidencing early signs of dementia as the cause of her directional disorientation, its greatest value was in redefining the nature of her psychiatric presentation.

A review of the patient's protracted history of psychiatric hospitalizations revealed that, despite ECT treatments, she never had been diagnosed with an affective disorder. The pre-dominant diagnosis across the years was paranoid schizophrenia. Consequently, she had never been treated with a mood stabilizer. It was incumbent upon the clinical neuropsychologist to diagnose bipolar disorder and to recommend adjustments of her medication regimen, in addition to further assessment of her thyroid functioning with a complete blood chemistry analysis. The clinical neuropsychologist, who was current with the neurology and the psychiatry literature, felt com-fortable specifically recommending treatment with a mood stabilizer.

Relevant Ethical Issues

The ethical challenges in this case, frequently confronting clinical neuropsychologists in psy-chiatric inpatient settings, pertain to (a) the moti-vation and ability to address clinical concerns beyond the cognition-focused referral question, and (b) the issue of whether or not to offer rec-ommendations for psychopharmacological treat-ment. The tenets underlying all ethical codes and practice standards in clinical settings are to avoid harm and to provide better care for patients. With that in mind, it is requisite for clinical neu-ropsychologists to do everything in their power to insure that every consideration for improving their patients' clinical care and management is made available to individuals who provide treat-ment (General Principles A, Beneficence and Non-maleficence; and B, Fidelity and Responsibility).

Clinical neuropsychologists with limited expe-rience in psychiatric settings cannot assume com-petence in such settings solely based on their training in the assessment of brain-behavior relationships in other contexts (Standard 2.01, Boundaries of Competence). Without a thor-ough understanding of psychiatric disorders and their cognitive manifestations, a clinical neuro-psychologist practicing or consulting in a psychi-atric setting would be violating the ethical standard of conduct pertaining to Boundaries of

Competence. In addition, a clinician who focuses solely on the referral question without consider-ing additional, often unexpected, findings would be violating the General Principle of Beneficence.

When aware of a treatment that may have potential benefit for their patient, it is impera-tive that clinical neuropsychologists make that information available in a professional manner. Several Ethical Standards are applicable for this purpose; note Standards 1.02 (Conflicts Between Ethics and Law, Regulations, or Other Governing Legal Authority), 2.01 (Boundaries of Compe-tence), 2.04 (Bases for Scientific and Profes-sional Judgments), and 3.09 (Cooperation With Other Professionals).

Standard 1.02 provides the ethical basis for clinical neuropsychologists making medication recommendations within their domain of com-petence (Standard 2.01) despite the fact that, in most states and situations, they are not licensed to prescribe medication. This position does not imply a lack of regard for the competence of our psychiatric colleagues; it simply reflects the operation of a team model for treatment that incorporates multidisciplinary perspectives into treatment planning in order to best serve each patient's treatment needs. Nevertheless, it is essential that these recommendations be tact-fully communicated, with adequate rationale, so that they are likely to be perceived by the pre-scribing psychiatrist as simply advice to either accept or reject. Indeed, Standards 2.01 and 2.04 require that recommendations be: (1) limited within the boundaries of an individual's educa-tion, training, and experience; (2) accompanied by appropriate literature citations; and (3) sup-ported by sustained competence through appro-priate continuing education. Moreover, Standard 3.09 requires that recommendations be provided to psychiatrists in a collegial manner to maximize the likelihood of their acceptance. After all, the patient ultimately suffers if potentially effective treatment recommendations are rejected because the clinical neuropsychologist does not adequately attend to the delicate nature of seemingly crossing traditional professional boundaries with novel suggestions.

Case Resolution

After 34 years of recurrent psychiatric decompensations, the patient was stabilized with the addition of lithium carbonate to her treatment. Were medication recommendations not rendered for fear of crossing professional boundaries, the patient likely would have endured additional episodic decompensations.

Conclusions and Recommendations

This clinical vignette illustrated the importance of affirmatively resolving the ethical challenge confronting clinical neuropsychologists about whether they should (a) address clinical concerns beyond the cognition-focused referral question, and (b) offer psychopharmacological recommendations, within their domain of competence, when aware that such treatment potentially may benefit their patient. It clearly was in this patient's best interest that the clinical neuropsychologist, after comprehensively assessing cognitive and emotional status and thoroughly considering diagnostic possibilities, conveyed the recommendation to her psychiatrist that she be treated with a mood stabilizer. It also was in her best interest that information about medications was conveyed in a nonthreatening and collegial manner that facilitated its acceptance. Of course, the latter approach did not guarantee acceptance. Notwithstanding, it was important for the clinical neuropsychologist to have brought all treatment knowledge to bear in this case by dispensing a complete range of recommendations as part of the evaluation.

Clinical neuropsychologists may, by virtue of their unique training in brain-behavior relationships and their familiarity with the neurological literature, have an additional perspective to offer psychiatrists when considering treatment options with psychotropic medication. For example, in the early 1980s, this clinical neuropsychologist's familiarity with the mood stabilizing benefit of temporal-limbic specific anticonvulsants led to an appreciation of its potential clinical applications beyond the treatment of complex partial seizures. In particular, treatment suggestions were offered at that time to consider these anticonvulsants for moderating affective instability in individuals manifesting temporal-limbic perturbations from postconcussion syndrome and from manic-depressive disorder. Some psychiatrist colleagues eschewed the advice to add these anticonvulsants to their patient's treatment; others solicited and applied that advice. As the literature would later reveal, that approach proved successful to the degree that temporal-limbic specific anticonvulsants (viz., carbamazepine and, subsequently, valproic acid/divalproex sodium) have come to be considered first line treatments for manic-depressive disorder.

Ethically conducted neuropsychological evaluations have their roots in competent training, appropriately supervised experience, and continuing education. Therefore, in following those parameters of ethical conduct, the practice of offering a complete range of neuropsychological recommendations for treatment that may include psychopharmacologic advice only can serve to benefit the public and the skill of allied professionals who utilize psychological knowledge in their work.

Performing neuropsychological evaluations in a psychiatric setting presents many ethical challenges. This section explored two of those ethical challenges which, when successfully addressed, are requisite practice standards for maximizing good clinical outcome.

Section 5

ETHICAL CHALLENGES IN NEUROPSYCHOLOGY IN REHABILITATION SETTINGS

Introduction

Brain injury rehabilitation can be as ethically challenging as it is professionally and personally rewarding. The interdisciplinary nature of most rehabilitation settings, the severity of many of the brain injuries sustained, the frequent existence of multiple co-morbidities, and degree of family involvement are just a few of the factors that contribute to professional and ethical challenges in neurorehabilitation. In additional, issues that may seem to be beyond the immediate influence of the clinician, such as legislation and institutional policy, affect the nature of neuropsychological services and must be considered in discussions of rehabilitation ethics.

Given the complexity of many of the ethical issues faced in neurorehabilitation, not all of the issues can be addressed in the four cases allotted for this chapter. Yet, the authors have done an excellent job presenting case illustrations that reflect some of the common and particularly challenging types of problems confronting clinicians. For additional reference, a brief list of suggested readings is provided.

References

Banja, J.D. (1999). Ethical dimensions of severe traumatic brain injury. In M. Rosenthal, E.R. Griffith, J.S. Kreutzer, & B. Pentland (Eds.), *Rehabilitation of the adult and child with traumatic brain injury, third edition*, 413-434. Philadelphia, PA: F.A. Davis Company.

Banja, J. (1999). Patient advocacy at risk: ethical, legal and political dimensions of adverse reimbursement practices in brain injury rehabilitation in the U.S. *Brain Injury, 13(10)*, 745-758.

Banja, J.D., Adler, R.K., & Stringer, A.Y. (1996). Ethical dimensions of caring for defiant patients: A case study. *Journal of Head Trauma Rehabilitation, 11 (6)*, 93-97.

Bush, S., Goldberg, A., & Johnson-Greene, D. (2003). Rehabilitation psychology ethics: Understanding and applying the 2002 APA Ethics Code. *Rehabilitation Psychology News, 30 (4)*, 13-15.

Hanson, S.L., Guenther, R., Kerkhoff, T., & Liss, M. (2000). Ethics: Historical foundations, basic principles, and contemporary issues. In R.G. Frank & T.R. Elliott (Eds.), *Handbook of rehabilitation psychology*. Washington, DC: American Psychological Association.

Malec, J.F. (1993). Ethics in brain injury rehabilitation: existential choices among western cultural beliefs. *Brain Injury, 7*, 383-400.

Malec, J.F. (1996). Ethical conflict resolution based on an ethics of relationships for brain injury rehabilitation. *Brain Injury, 10*, 781-795.

Rosenthal, M., & Lourie, I. (1996). Ethical issues in the evaluation of competence in persons with acquired brain injuries. *NeuroRehabilitation, 6*, 113-121.

Rosenthal, M. (1996). 1995 Sheldon Berrol, MD Senior Lectureship: The Ethics and Efficacy of Traumatic Brain Injury Rehabilitation – Myths, Measurements, and Meaning. *Head Trauma Rehabilitation, 11*, 88-95.

Swiercinsky, D.P. (2002). Ethical Issues in Neuropsychological Rehabilitation. In S. Bush & M.L. Drexler (Eds.), *Ethical issues in clinical neuropsychology*, 135-163. Lisse, NL: Swets & Zeitlinger.

Wong, T.M. (1998). Ethical issues in the evaluation and treatment of traumatic brain injury. In R.M. Anderson, T.L. Needles, and H.V. Hall (Eds.), *Avoiding Ethical Misconduct in Psychological Specialty Areas*, 187-200. Springfield, IL: Charles C. Thomas Publisher, Ltd.

Chapter 10

ETHICAL CHALLENGES IN NEURO-PSYCHOLOGY IN REHABILITATION SETTINGS, PART I

John DeLuca

Scenario 1

The patient, a doctor, is a 49-year-old white male who was referred for a neuropsychological evaluation by his neurologist to examine the extent of cognitive impairment and to outline intervention strategies as appropriate. About 4 months prior to his visit, the patient suffered a seizure following a fall in which he injured his head. He suffered bilateral frontal contusions and hemorrhage. He was unconscious for approximately four to five days, and lethargic and confused for a number of weeks afterward, with some degree of impaired insight regarding his condition. The patient has a long history of neurologic difficulties, including recurrent facial palsies and left-ear hearing loss since childhood. His condition resulted in total deafness while in medical school. He lost his sense of smell about 15-20 years ago, and subsequently began to demonstrate poor balance. Despite his physical limitations, he had become a successful endocrinologist with his own private practice. A few years ago he developed a frontal meningioma and meningiomatosis at the base of the skull, affecting the cranial nerves and spinal cord. The tumor

extended into the frontal lobes, resulting in two surgical attempts at removal. It was after his most recent surgery that the patient had a seizure, resulting in the above mentioned fall.

After the fall, the patient was unable to return to work due to significant cognitive impairment, and he was placed on disability. He demonstrated little to no insight into his condition, despite a large list of cognitive and behavioral problems outlined by his spouse, including: difficulties in sequencing or temporal processing of events, attention to detail, errors in making check deposits between family and business checking account), self-monitoring, significant personality changes (delusions, disinhibition, decreased initiation), and problem solving difficulties. There was no premorbid psychiatric history, or medical complications other than that mentioned above.

During the evaluation, the patient was alert and oriented ×3. He had a mild left facial weakness, and a marked ataxic gait. Language was coherent to casual conversation. His voice inflections and cadence were mildly exaggerated, likely due to years of being totally deaf. Although he did not use sign language, he was adept at lip reading. There was clear evidence of perseverative thinking and impaired judgment and self monitoring. Affect was appropriate, but appeared mildly depressed. Yet, he displayed a keen sense of humor. Functionally, he was independent with his ADL's, and spent most of his time watching TV and reading. Although he had recently begun driving again, his spouse reported several examples of dangerous driving incidences and impaired judgment.

The neuropsychological evaluation was performed on an outpatient basis in the neuropsychology office, four months after the patients' fall and injury. Test administration was modified in consideration of the patient's sensory deficits (see below), and such modification was noted in the ensuing report. The results of the evaluation revealed significant cognitive impairment, consistent with primarily frontal-executive system involvement. Several recommendations were made. Briefly, recommendations included: (1) A complete ophthalmologic evaluation because of his reading errors, and the prominence of the visual domain in interacting with the world; (2) A formal driving evaluation, with instruction to refrain from driving in the meantime; (3) Return to work was not recommended because of the severity of his deficits and the nature of his work (i.e., treating patients); (4) Supportive counseling, and (5) A neuropsychological re-evaluation in six months to one year.

Relevant Ethical Issues

Several ethical and practical issues are raised by this case. First is the issue of reasonable accommodations and consumer protection, both associated with the Americans with Disabilities Act (ADA). Students of psychology and neuropsychology are taught that strict adherence to standardized test administration is critical and that deviations could have detrimental consequences on the interpretation of the results obtained since the tests' psychometric properties were based on the strict administrative procedures. However,

there is also a literature in psychology on the need for departures from standard administration in order to obtain an accurate "evaluation" as opposed to accurate "testing" (see Caplan and Shecter, 1995 for a full review of these issues). A strict interpretation of the standardized administration of neuropsychological tests would have precluded an accurate assessment of the patient's true cognitive abilities. The modification of administrative procedures in order to obtain meaningful clinical information took precedence over the need to maintain standardization of administration.

Ethical principle 9.02a states that "Psychologists administer, *adapt* [emphasis added], score, interpret, or use assessment techniques, interviews tests, or instruments in a manner and for the purposes that are appropriate in light of the research on or evidence of the usefulness and proper application of the techniques". As such, psychologists are bound ethically to "adapt" the administration and testing scenario to the needs and abilities of the patient. However, it must be emphasized that this should be done cautiously and with full understanding of the implications (e.g., norms may not be valid) and impact that such adaptations may have on such special populations (Principle 9.02b).

A major clinical issue in the current case was the ability for the patient to return to work. The recommendation was that the patient should no longer work clinically in direct patient care, clearly an issue related to Consumer Protection issues. The neuropsychologist felt that the errors in judgment (in conjunction with actual examples of such errors already made) could potentially result in harm to a patient. Practically, this meant that the patient would have to sell his practice, an issue which the family and patient were debating for some time and looking to the neuropsychologist for practical answers. Indeed the patient did not agree with my assessment and resisted. However, the family was in full agreement. It was pointed out that this did not mean that the patient could not continue to function as a physician! The neuropsychologist indicated that Dr M. could still function in several capacities as a physician (e.g., such as teaching residents, delivering lectures, writing, consulting with other physicians on endocrinology issues of a patient, but not be responsible for direct patient care).

The second, and perhaps larger ethical issue, involves making recommendations regarding the work-related competency for an occupation for which the neuropsychologist does not have the requisite skills or authority. The same could be said for the recommendation in this case for the patient to not drive until further evaluated. Such issues involve the neuropsychologist's professional competence in making these specific recommendations. Even for areas with which the psychologist is familiar, such as standardized test administration, and has the expertise and knowledge of brain–behavior relations, the ecological validity of neuropsychological test results has been questioned by some (e.g., Sbordone, 1996). Binder and Thompson (1995) recommend that neuropsychologists acknowledge the "limits of certainty with which diagnosis, judgments, predictions can be made about individuals". However, a recommendation is not a mandate. The recommendation is made to the referring agent, who then chooses to use it as appropriate. The neuropsychologist should feel comfortable in making recommendations based on his/her area of expertise (e.g., understanding impaired cognition and its impact), in order to address the referral questions. In doing so, the neuropsychologist must continue to recognize the limits of one's education, training and experience, but does not have to hinder the ability to make specific and meaningful recommendations.

Case Resolution

Because the patient was totally deaf, many of the tests could not be administered using standardized procedures, thus requiring alterations. These included writing the directions down verbatim with slight alterations (e.g., "you will see" vs "I will read") or the patient read the directions aloud from the test manual (e.g., during the Category Test). For the California Verbal Learning Test and Paired Associate Learning Test, the words were presented visually on index cards for silent reading. Paragraph recall (i.e., Logical Memory) was evaluated by having the patient read each paragraph aloud. Interpretation and scoring otherwise remained in accordance with standardized procedures. The need to modify the procedures was documented in the report.

Regarding the recommendation of not returning to clinical practice, working with the referring physician and family, a plan was devised to have the patient return to work on a part-time basis under supervision by his peers. He was to provide lectures to residents and consult with practicing physicians. The patient reluctantly agreed. He was assigned to providing lectures to medical residents. He prepared long and hard for his first lecture which was a success. However, according to his spouse, it soon became apparent that he had great difficulty preparing for the lectures. He could not organize his lectures, and lacked initiative to prepare at all. After several "disasters", he was asked to stop his lecture activity. Regarding the medical practice, eventually, the family convinced him to put his practice up for sale. Unfortunately, his practice was sold for a fraction of what they thought it was worth.

Conclusions and Recommendations

1. *Obtain specific referral questions*. Make sure that referral questions are clear enough so that they can be addressed by your evaluation. Work with the referring agent and/or family to refine precisely what is needed from the evaluation.
2. *Develop and maintain competency*. Be familiar with the literature regarding general issues (e.g., assessment needs) relevant to patient populations that you work with.

3. *Practice only within your competencies.* Decline or refer out if you are not well trained with a certain population. Recognize limits to your competencies.
4. *Obtain supervision.* Where needed, do not hesitate in obtaining relevant supervision (e.g., working with the deaf) if this is in the best interest of the patient.
5. *State in your report any deviations from standardized procedures and give rationale for doing so.*
6. *Provide a statement regarding potential limits to the interpretation/conclusions/ recommendations.*
7. *Researchers should continue to develop neuropsychological instruments for use with specific populations or develop norms based on modified procedures.*

Scenario 2

The patient, a 79-year-old, right-handed male, was referred for neuropsychological evaluation by his neurosurgeon following discovery of an unruptured 8 mm anterior communicating artery (ACoA) aneurysm. Since there were no neuropsychologists on the neurology or neurosurgical services, the referral went to a neuropsychologist working in outpatient rehabilitation. The goal of the neuropsychological evaluation was to help determine the extent and source of the patient's apparent cognitive decline. The neurosurgeon was particularly interested in determining if the cognitive decline suspected was due to the effects of the ACoA or if there was a second source of cognitive decline in effect as well, namely Alzheimer's Disease. This determination was sought to aid in the decision of whether or not to pursue surgical intervention for treatment of the aneurysm (e.g., clipping of the aneurysm). Specifically, the neurosurgeon was trying to determine whether or not he should proceed with neurosurgery. At the time the patient presented to the hospital a few months prior to the current

evaluation, the patient's family reported their observations of a recent progressive decline in cognitive functioning (e.g., distractibility, difficulty doing two things at once, bookkeeping errors). They reported that he would get lost in familiar places, miss appointments, and erroneously recall time and date related information. Although the patient denied such difficulties (or any other cognitive problems), he acknowledged that his family was reporting these changes. The patient lived alone, spending most of his time at the family business (mostly "sitting around") and with his family, who lived nearby. However, the family reported increased apathy and general disinterest. He was independent in ADL's. Medical history was significant for Diabetes Mellitus Type II for 12 years, diet controlled; hypertension; peripheral vascular disease; and Benign Prostatic Hypertrophy. The patient reported that he completed five years of formal education, but received his GED while in the military, attaining a rank of First Sergeant.

The patient was alert, attentive and oriented ×3 throughout the interview and evaluation. Speech was fluent, with no overt word finding difficulties noted. Affect was appropriately variable to conversation content, but mildly euphoric. The patient easily engaged in conversation and appeared open and honest throughout the interview and testing. However, conversation was occasionally tangential, at times over-elaborative, with content that was mildly inappropriate at times.

The neuropsychological evaluation was conducted in an office in an outpatient rehabilitation clinic. Results of the evaluation revealed decline in specific areas of cognitive function from estimates of premorbid intellectual abilities. These deficits were consistent with frontal executive systems disturbance. Verbal intellectual capacities, language abilities, simple nonverbal visuoperceptual abilities, attention/concentration abilities, and measures of verbal and nonverbal new learning and memory were all consistent with estimated low average premorbid levels.

However, significant decline was observed in complex visuoperceptual tasks (likely due to a frontal/dysexecutive syndrome), organization abilities, abstract reasoning, mental flexibility, and complex problem-solving. In addition, the sensory perceptual examination was notable for multiple suppressions within the left visual field and left auditory field.

Following the examination, the neuropsychologist called a fellow neuropsychologist who had considerable experience working with a neurology and neurosurgery service. He then offered the following recommendations: (1) cognitive rehabilitation to help the patient compensate for his deficits; (2) given the nature and severity of executive dysfunction, driving should be curtailed if not discontinued; (3) the patient's family should closely monitor dangerous household activities, such as cooking, ironing, etc; (4) given the family's concerns about the patient's behavior and cognitive status, family education and therapy may be helpful, in dealing with the how to implement some of the above mentioned recommendations as well as provided needed support; (5) individual counseling for the patient if his emotional adjustment declines when he faced with limitations in his previous activities and with the increased supervision; (6) a neuropsychological re-evaluation in one year.

Relevant Ethical Issues

The primary ethical issue in this case example is that of practicing within the boundaries of one's education, training and expertise. In this case, the boundaries were both between and within disciplines. The 2002 Ethical standard 2.01 (Boundaries of Competence) states that "Psychologists provide services, teach, and conduct research with populations and in areas only within the boundaries of their competence, based on their education, training, supervised experience, consultation, study or professional experience." Standard 2.04 states that "Psychologists'

work is based upon established scientific and professional knowledge of the discipline". Although a major referral question for the neurosurgeon in this case was whether or not to treat the aneurysm via an invasive process (e.g., craniotomy to clip the aneurysm) this specific question was not one that the neuropsychologist could address specifically. That decision was not within the education, training or experience of a psychologist. However, an important referral question could be addressed. That is, based on the results of the neuropsychological evaluation, was the pattern of cognitive impairment consistent with the presence of the aneurysm (or related factors such as mass effect) or were the cognitive problems more likely associated with a totally different etiology such as dementia. This information was indeed provided and used by the neurosurgeon and family to come up with an ultimate decision regarding whether or not surgery was to be performed. The input provided by the neuropsychologist played an important role regarding this decision. However, the neuropsychologist made no explicit or implicit recommendations or suggestions about the surgical decision. During the evaluation, the patient and family both asked the neuropsychologist's opinion regarding surgery. However, the neuropsychologist made it clear that this question was not within their area of expertise, and directed them to the neurosurgeon.

The second but related aspect in this case is the boundaries of competence within the discipline of Neuropsychology. The neurosurgeon approached the neuropsychologist in this case because he knew that the neuropsychologist had specific experience (research and clinical) with persons with cerebral aneurysms (particularly of the ACoA). However, working primarily in rehabilitation with individuals who have documented brain injuries, the neuropsychologist had little experience with differential diagnosis involving dementia. If a neuropsychologist is asked to address a referral question for which they have little or no education, training or experience (e.g., working up the present ACoA evaluation having only worked with schizophrenia in the past), the neuropsychologist should then either refer the case to a neuropsychologist who has such experience, or seek supervision to ensure an appropriate and meaningful evaluation. Standard 2.01(c) states that "Psychologists planning to provide services … involving population … new to them undertake relevant education, training, supervised experience, consultation, or study".

Case Resolution

As indicated above, the pattern of relative strengths and difficulties for the patient was consistent with the presence of a dysexecutive syndrome marked by mental inflexibility, poor problem-solving, limited abstract reasoning, subtly impaired self-regulatory mechanisms, and poor organization and planning abilities. Such a circumscribed pattern of cognitive deficits is consistent with dysfunction of brain systems subserved by the frontal lobes or the frontal executive system.

Importantly, the observed pattern of test performance was *not* consistent with diffuse or generalized cognitive dysfunction typically associated with a dementia syndrome, such as one of the Alzheimer's Type. This was a specific rule out from the Neurosurgeon's referral question. While the possibility of an early dementia of the frontal lobe type (e.g., Pick's Disease) cannot be ruled out based on the pattern of test results, the observed pattern of results was not consistent with an advanced dementing syndrome of any etiology, once again addressing a key referral question. Alternatively, the observed deficits may have represented the effects of the aneurysm of the ACoA, with possible resultant frontal vascular ischemic compromise and/or mass effect. Still another diagnostic possibility, which cannot be entirely ruled-out, is that the pattern of results actually represented the long-term functioning of the patient, with perhaps undocumented or undiagnosed executive deficits. One possibility may

be an undiagnosed ADHD, a possibility that should be considered given a family history of ADHD. However, the overall pattern of performance, the family's observation of recent cognitive decline, and the presence of left unilateral visual and auditory suppressions would argue against a long-standing condition such as ADHD.

Given that the neuropsychological evaluation demonstrated fairly specific deficits, likely due to the effects of the ACoA and related mass effect, rather than an advanced dementing syndrome, surgical intervention remained a viable option for the patient and his family. After receiving the results of the evaluation, the neurosurgeon scheduled an appointment with the patient and his family, where he, along with the patient and family, decided not to pursue surgery to repair the aneurysm. Given the relatively minimal disruption of the patient's behavioral and cognitive symptoms in everyday life, his advanced age, as well as the relatively small probability that the aneurysm would actually rupture during the patient's lifetime, surgical intervention was not pursued.

Conclusions and Recommendations

1. *Obtain specific referral questions*. As with case one above, ensure that the referral questions are clear enough so that they can be addressed by your evaluation.
2. *Boundaries of competency*. Ensure that one has the education, training and skills needed to address the referral questions being asked. If not, either refer elsewhere or seek the appropriate supervision needed to ensure a competent and useful evaluation.
3. *Making recommendations*. Make recommendations that are within the boundaries of one's competency and expertise. Address questions with patients, family, friends and other professionals that are within one's area of professional training and experience.

References

Binder, L.M., & Thompson, L.L. (1995). The ethics code and neuropsychological assessment practices. *Archives of Clinical Neuropsychology, 10 (1)*, 27-46.

Caplan, B., & Schecter, J. (1995). The role of nonstandard neuropsychological assessment in rehabilitation: History, rationale, and examples. In L.A. Cushman & M.J. Scherer (Eds.), *Psychological Assessment in Medical Practice*. Washington, D.C.: American Psychological Association.

Sbordone, R.J. (1996). Ecological validity: Some critical issues for the neuropsychologist. In R.J. Sbordone & C.J. Long (Eds.), *Ecological validity of neuropsychological testing*, (pp. 15-42). Boca Raton, FL: St. Lucie Press.

Acknowledgement

The author expresses his thanks to Nancy Chiaravolloti, Ph.D. for her consultation on case 2 in this chapter, and for her overall comments on this chapter.

Chapter 11

ETHICAL CHALLENGES IN NEURO-PSYCHOLOGY IN REHABILITATION SETTINGS, PART II

Doug Johnson-Greene

Scenario 1

The patient is a 58-year-old gentleman with 12 years of formal education who was admitted for comprehensive inpatient rehabilitation following a right hemisphere middle cerebral artery stroke that occurred approximately two weeks earlier. Rehabilitation neuropsychology consultation was requested in order to provide recommendations relating to functional limitations and supervision needs following discharge from the hospital. The patient was employed full-time, lived alone, and had no significant psychiatric or substance abuse history. His medical conditions included diabetes and hypertension, which had remained untreated because of the patient's limited contact with health professionals. The patient was anxious to return home but otherwise expressed no specific concerns about other life domains. Prior to initiating a neuropsychological evaluation, the patient was given basic information about the nature of the tests he would be taking and an overview of the limits of confidentiality. In addition, on admission to the hospital he signed a treatment consent form that mentioned issues of confidentiality, but primarily provided details concerning the patient's financial obligations for his treatment.

Initial neuropsychological evaluation included basic measures of mood and the Cognistat (Neurobehavioral Cognitive Status Examination [NCSE]), which showed mild depression, mildly impaired calculations, moderately impaired delayed verbal memory, and severely impaired visuospatial skill. A more comprehensive 4-hour neuropsychological examination revealed mildly impaired auditory attention, learning, and delayed verbal memory, and severely impaired visuospatial skills (Rey Complex Figure Test). Based on these results, the patient was told to cease driving until further notice, which was also reported to the state Department of Motor Vehicles as mandated by law in the state where the patient resides. Upon learning the outcome of the evaluation the patient became angry and complained that he did not know that driving recommendations were going to be part of the evaluation. He subsequently stated that he would make a formal complaint to the state licensing board that he had not received adequate information about the purpose of the evaluation he had undergone.

Relevant Ethical Issues

There are several relevant ethical issues in the aforementioned case. First and foremost, the patient's informed consent for this evaluation was probably inadequate. The goals of the assessment were never fully explained at the outset of the evaluation, which was one of his complaints after the evaluation had been completed. Basic information was provided concerning the activities the patient would be asked to complete, confidentiality, and fees, but there was no discussion of the purpose(s) of the evaluation. In this case, the referral questions were to determine functional limitations and supervision needs, suggesting that these issues would be a primary focus of the evaluation and that recommendations concerning driving ability should have been anticipated. Operation of a motor vehicle is a basic activity of daily living for most persons and is one of the most common areas of concern among persons with neurological impairments because of the obvious safety considerations. Autonomy and self-determination can only be promoted if patients have a full understanding of the anticipated goals of an evaluation (Johnson-Greene, Hardy-Morais, Adams, Hardy, Bergloff, 1997). Ironically, some patients may refuse to be evaluated who could otherwise benefit from neuropsychological consultation, though obviously it is the patient's right to exercise this prerogative, assuming that they have decisional capacity. The 2002 Ethics Code specifically addresses informed consent in assessments in section 9.03(a) where it states that consent should include an explanation of the nature and purpose of the assessment. It should be noted that informed consent is not required where the purpose of the evaluation is to evaluate decisional capacity, but psychologists must still inform patients with questionable capacity about the nature and purpose of the assessment.

To summarize, there is an explicit requirement that neuropsychologists inform their patients about the nature and purpose of an evaluation (Johnson-Greene et al., 2003). Generic statements about the need to assess cognitive ability would probably be inadequate in most evaluative cases depending on the situation and the patient's capacity to understand and comprehend this information. As a final comment, the Ethics Code recommends discussion of the limits of confidentiality at the "outset of the relationship" (Standard 4.02b), but a timeline is only implied for informed consent at the outset of the relationship (Standard 3.10). It has been argued that respect for autonomy may need to be delayed while the patient is being educated about the nature of their disability and the need for services (Caplan, 1988).

A second issue in this case is confidentiality. Informed consent must include the limits of confidentiality and involvement of third parties under Standard 9.03(a) and in Standard 4.02. Where mandatory reporting requirements exist (Standard 4.05), such as those associated with the motor vehicle administration in some states, the limits of confidentiality and involvement of these agencies should be anticipated in neurological populations and discussed with patients as a possible limitation of confidentiality at the outset of an evaluation. As outlined in Standard 4.05(a), the disclosure is limited to the minimum necessary to achieve the purpose. Disclosing the patient's evaluative report in its entirety without their permission would not be ethical or appropriate, though one may be legally obligated to report that the patient has cognitive impairments associated with a stroke that may effect his safe operation of a motor vehicle.

A third and final ethical issue in this case pertains to the recommendation of driving cessation itself. According to Standard 9.02(a), psychologists use assessment techniques in a manner and for purposes that are appropriate in light of the research on or evidence of the usefulness and proper application of the techniques. Further, in Standard 9.02(b), when the validity and reliability has not been established, psychologists describe the strengths and limitations of test results and interpretation. The ecological validity of neuropsychological tests has yet to be established in many domains. At the present time the literature pertaining to prediction of driving safety as a function of the type and severity of neuropsychological impairments lacks strong support (Bieliauskas, Roper, Trobe, Green, & Lacy, 1998). This limitation would need to be reflected in the recommendation offered to this patient if by no other means than by coupling it with the need to procure in-vivo assessment of driving safety.

Case Resolution

The patient complained to the hospital's patient services representative and threatened, but did not follow through, with a complaint to the state licensing board. Hospital administrators reviewing the case gave the neuropsychologist a warning to more fully address issues relevant to informed consent, particularly potential implications of neuropsychological evaluation results. The patient reported that he would resume driving following discharge, whereupon the treatment team held a family meeting to emphasize the importance of its recommendation. After two additional weeks of acute rehabilitation, the patient returned home. The treatment team later found out that the patient had returned to driving without undergoing evaluation by the state department of motor vehicles, as was required by law.

Conclusions and Recommendations

1. This patient should have been given more complete information about the purpose of the evaluation, which in turn would have facilitated an informed decision about whether or not he wished to proceed. The fear of some neuropsychologists seems to be that patients will refuse evaluations if full and complete disclosure is made, though most patients appear to consent to evaluations despite receiving a comprehensive informed consent. The need to provide full and informed consent has direct implications for two important foundations of psychology (autonomy and self-determination).

2. Informed consent should have included a full disclosure of the limits of confidentiality, both those that are known and those that could be reasonably anticipated. Where there are mandatory reporting requirements to state agencies there should be disclosure of this possibility prior to commencement of a neuropsychological evaluation.

3. The recommendation to cease driving should have been associated with an opportunity to obtain an in-vivo test of driving safety since neuropsychological tests alone are relatively poor predictors of driving safety.

Scenario 2

The patient was a 67-year-old gentleman who was admitted to an acute rehabilitation center due to debility within the context of multiple medical problems. Medical conditions included hypertension, diabetes mellitus, end-stage renal disease, unexplained weight loss of sixty pounds in the past year, history of optic neuritis, and pneumocystis pneumonia. A neuropsychological evaluation revealed low average finger tapping and fine motor ability (Grooved Pegboard) and moderately impaired complex attention and processing speed (Connors CPT and Stroop). During the course of the clinical interview, the patient acknowledged that he had had inconsistent compliance with his anti-hypertensive medication and diabetes management. In consideration of the patient's medical problems and neuropsychological impairments, the patient was asked about HIV risk behaviors. He acknowledged occasional HIV risk behavior (unprotected sex) and fear that he may be HIV-positive, though he had apparently never been tested for HIV. He was concerned that this information be kept confidential, particularly the possibility that he was HIV-positive.

The next day, a rehabilitation team meeting was held in which multiple patients were discussed. This patient's care providers reported the findings from their initial evaluations. The rehabilitation neuropsychologist reported on the cognitive findings and opined that the findings were most consistent with the patient's suspected HIV-positive status. A report stipulating this information had already been written and placed in the patient's medical records. In attendance at the team meeting were quality assurance personnel for the hospital, professionals awaiting discussions of other patients, and a case manager for the patient's insurance company. At the request of his physician, nursing staff asked the patient later the same day to consent to an HIV blood test. The patient became irate that health care workers other than the psychologist were aware of the possibility that he was HIV-positive and refused to consent to the test. The following day, the patient's family members asked for an update and were told by the patient's resident physician, who had been absent the previous day at an educational seminar, that he had refused to consent to HIV testing. This was a significant surprise to the family, since they were not aware that the patient had a need for HIV testing. Finally, the patient was told that his insurance company was not approving additional days for acute rehabilitation. Team members speculated that since the case manager for the insurance company was at the team meeting, they may have recommended denial of additional rehabilitation days because of lingering questions about the patient's HIV status.

Relevant Ethical Issues

Confidentiality is one of the most problematic areas for psychologists in general (Pope & Vetter, 1992), and is particularly problematic in rehabilitation settings. The team-oriented approach that is common in rehabilitation settings is not usually conducive to maintaining confidentiality, though team members would undoubtedly underscore its importance. In rehabilitation settings professionals may feel compelled to offer information of a sensitive nature even when the patient articulates expectations of privacy. Compounding the problem is the fact that there are more professionals involved in patient care than just the core team, resulting in poorer communication between team members as illustrated by the above scenario. Lastly, there can be a lack of knowledge regarding appropriate ethical behavior across disciplines and how to achieve acceptable confidentiality. While some may not question the appropriateness of information or the role of those in attendance at team meetings, these issues are of primary importance in maintaining inappropriate disclosure of information.

Considerable vigilance is required to strive for acceptable standards of confidentiality, including awareness among team members of the pragmatics for achieving this goal. What information can you place in the medical record? What information can be shared at a team meeting? Who can ethically attend a rehabilitation team conference? These are all questions that must be answered before a professional standard of confidentiality can be ensured. Standard 4 of the 2002 Ethics Code outlines issues regarding privacy and confidentiality. In this case, the psychologist failed to discuss the limits of confidentiality as required in Standard 4.02. The psychologist may also have been remiss in including information that was not germane to the rehabilitation team and to persons not concerned with such matters (insurance case manager) as outlined in Standard 4.04.

Case Resolution

The insurance company denied authorization for further inpatient rehabilitation despite requests for additional time; however, outpatient rehabilitation services at another facility were approved (the patient refused to return to the same facility for outpatient services). The patient was discharged home and began outpatient rehabilitation, which included individual psychotherapy to address family concerns about his HIV status and the "betrayal" he experienced on the inpatient unit. The patient continued to deny requests for HIV testing, though he continued to experience ongoing AIDS-related health problems.

Conclusions and Recommendations

1. The psychologist should have discussed the limitations of confidentiality at the outset of the evaluation (Standard 4.02), particularly those that are inherent in the rehabilitation setting, such as limited discussion with other members of the patient's rehabilitation team.
2. When information was given about the HIV risk behaviors, the psychologist should have determined if this information was germane to the treatment team as a whole or should have been discussed only with the patient's attending physician for their consideration (Standard 4.04). More limited disclosure would have allowed the psychologist to have greater control over this sensitive information and would have potentially avoided inadvertent disclosures to the patient's family and insurance case manager.
3. Similar to item 2 above, the information may not have been germane in written reports placed in the medical record (Standard 4.04).
4. Lastly, it is inappropriate for an insurance case manager to have access to rehabilitation team conferences since their primary concern should be with financial matters and not clinical information per se. While the 2002 Ethics Code does provide for disclosure of information to obtain payment, it should be "limited to the minimum that is necessary to achieve the purpose" as defined in Standard 4.05, which would preclude an in-depth discussion of the patient at a team conference.
5. The number of persons with disabilities associated with severe chronic medical and neurological conditions has burgeoned, in part because the elderly constitute a progressively greater percentage of the population and advances in the medical field have increased survival rates following trauma. The goal of rehabilitation neuropsychology is to minimize the impact of neurological impairments through provision of cognitive assessment and treatment services, typically offered within the context of a multidisciplinary team. Neuropsychology and rehabilitation psychology are complimentary yet distinct disciplines, both of which share a common code of ethics designed to maximize patient welfare and to achieve resolution of unique and complex ethical dilemmas endemic to health care settings.
6. Ethical challenges have emerged from many sources, some of which are extrinsic to the patient–practitioner relationship and provide limited opportunities for proactive problem solving such as (a) scientific and theoretical advances in rehabilitation, (b) emerging legal mandates and precedents; and (c) financial pressures associated with managed care. Nonetheless, most common ethical dilemmas can be averted, or at least minimized, through emphasizing autonomy, nonmaleficence, and beneficence within the context of the provider-patient relationship, including frank discussion about the services the rehabilitation neuropsychologist intends to provide and their potential for untoward effects. Two common ethical issues in rehabilitation settings that have a direct bearing on patient-practitioner interactions are informed consent in persons with neuropsychological impairment and protection of confidentiality in a multidisciplinary environment. The previous two scenarios provided examples of the aforementioned areas of ethical conflict, as well as ways to avoid or negotiate such conflicts.

References

Bieliauskas, L., Roper, R., Trobe, J., Green, P., & Lacy, M. (1998). Cognitive measures, driving safety, and Alzheimer's disease. *The Clinical Neuropsychologist, 12*, 206-212.

Bush, S. Naugle, R., & Johnson-Greene, D. (2002). Interface of information technology and neuropsychology: Ethical issues and recommendations. *The Clinical Neuropsychologist, 16*, 536-547.

Caplan, A. (1988). Informed consent and patient–provider relationships in rehabilitation medicine. *Archives of Physical Medicine and Rehabilitation, 69*, 2-7.

Johnson-Green, D., Barth, J.T., Pliskin, N.H., Arffa, S., Axelrod, B.N., Blackburn, L.A., Faust, D., Fisher, J.M., Harley, J.P., Heilbronner, R.L., Larrabee, G.J., Ricker, J.H., & Silver, C.H. (2003). Informed consent in clinical neuropsychology practice: Official statement of the National Academy of Neuropsychology. Retrieved from http://www.nanonline.org/paio/IME.shtm 1/16/04.

Johnson-Greene, D., Hardy-Morais, C., Adams, K., Hardy, C., & Bergloff, P. (1997). Informed consent and neuropsychological assessment: Ethical considerations and proposed guidelines. *The Clinical Neuropsychologist, 11*, 454-460.

Pope, K., & Vetter, V. (1992). Ethical dilemmas encountered by members of the American Psychological Association: A national survey. *American Psychologist, 47*, 397-411.

Section 6

ETHICAL CHALLENGES IN THE NEUROPSYCHOLOGY OF PAIN

Introduction

Many of the individuals who present for neuropsychological evaluation following acquired brain injury are experiencing considerable pain, and many are being treated with analgesic medication or are self-medicating with alcohol or illicit substances. As the authors of this chapter describe, pain, its treatment, and associated factors may have an effect on cognitive functioning and neuropsychological test results. However, determining the exact nature and extent of that effect for any given examinee can be extremely challenging for those experienced in working with this population,

and may be impossible for those lacking such experience. As a result, professional competence in the ability to appropriately evaluate individuals experiencing acute or chronic pain is a primary ethical concern. In addition, since such evaluations are often performed in the context of personal injury litigation, the ability to maintain appropriate role boundaries and avoid engaging in multiple, conflicting relationships must be an area of focus for the examining or treating neuropsychologist. The authors examine these challenging ethical issues through the complexity of pain-related cases.

Chapter 12

ETHICAL CHALLENGES IN THE NEUROPSYCHOLOGY OF PAIN, PART I

Michael F. Martelli

Scenario 1

A neuropsychologist performed an independent examination, the examinee's third, upon referral from a worker's compensation insurance company. The examinee was three years status post an unwitnessed injury in which a 175-pound steel beam fell ten feet, striking the worker's head, breaking his hard hat and causing him to fall to the ground and experience an uncertain loss of consciousness and an uncertain period of altered consciousness. Notably, he had been working while diagnosed with "walking pneumonia". After his accident, he was taken to a company nurse but refused medical treatment and went home for the rest of the day and the weekend. He reportedly slept most of the weekend, and apparently assumed that his symptoms of dizziness, nausea, confusion and several blackouts were results of his pneumonia. After the weekend, he attempted to return to work for several days but continued to have intermittent symptoms and was sent home each day. During the first week, his symptoms failed to improve, and he developed intense headaches. After a "blacking out" episode, his wife took him to the emergency room.

The examinee's headaches, dizziness, nausea and variable and intermittent confusion continued, but while his symptoms abated somewhat, his headache severity persisted. He subsequently received continuing assessment and treatment that over the next two years included multiple physicians with multiple specialties, without significant benefit in terms of primary persistent chronic head pain symptoms, as well as family complaints of problems with information processing, memory and irritability and anger. He did not return to work and was placed on short-term and then long-term disability.

On two occasions, the examinee received inpatient psychiatric hospitalization after bouts of severe depression with homicidal and suicidal thoughts and "personality deterioration". These were associated with reports of difficulty coping with pain, aggressive outbursts and fear of hurting family members. Diagnostic assessments continued and a tentative diagnosis of posttraumatic epilepsy was made based on variable EEG assessments, while CT and MRI findings revealed acute right frontal lesion that resolved on CT but not MRI, along with some evidence of an additional older (pre-injury) lesion also in the right frontal lobe. Sleep studies corroborated patient and family report of significant sleep disturbance. Primary treatments, however, were focused on chronic pain management and adjustment related problems, with perhaps overly aggressive medication management. At the time of this examinee's most recent independent examination, he had been enrolled in a residential, dual focused chronic pain and brain injury rehabilitation program. He had made measurable overall progress, albeit against a backdrop of a sawtooth pattern of functioning, and was being transitioned to a modified intensive outpatient treatment program.

This third independent examination was scheduled by the worker's compensation insurance case manager after discharge from residential treatment. The insurance company refused authorization for outpatient treatment and made a settlement offer that was rejected by the patient, who refused to negotiate and insisted on continued treatment. The case manager selected and scheduled an independent examiner with no training, knowledge, experience or recognition in chronic pain disorders, despite recommendations from the treating physician and neuropsychologist for an examiner experienced with chronic pain disorders. Based on his record review and examination, this examiner diagnosed malingering and concluded that the examinee's behavior was best explained by sociopathy, opining that continued medical treatment was unnecessary and would not be beneficial.

Upon receipt of this independent examiner's report by the worker's compensation case manager, all workers compensation medical and wage benefits were immediately discontinued. The previously supportive employer terminated the patient upon recommendation of their attorney. The worker's compensation case manager informed the treating practitioners of the results of the independent examination and instructed them to discontinue all treatment and medications. Without medical benefits or compensation payments, the patient paid out of pocket for a reduced medication regimen and limited outpatient treatment. He appealed the case. Although he was granted social security disability benefits, he accrued increasing debt and interest charges from borrowing to pay bills. He also experienced drastically increased personal and family stresses, a significant interruption in his treatment, and complication of his symptoms and course. He deteriorated in physical, neuropsychological, and interpersonal status. After one year of enduring numerous insurance company attorney delays for an appeal hearing, he won the appeal and all benefits were restored.

The unqualified diagnosis of malingering and the conclusions and recommendations listed in the report were offered based on seemingly supportive evidence from interview, neuropsychological examination, and medical record review. Despite the appearance of providing sufficient support, a critical review of the examination and report revealed both a selective review that excluded more prominent disconfirmatory evidence, and several critical conceptual and methodologic errors.

With regard to this evaluation, the diagnosis of malingering, which had significant consequences for harming this patient, is considered problematic for several reasons. The examination was conducted by a professional in a subject area outside his expertise. The examiner conducted a very brief interview with selective medical record review. The examiner performed an incomplete review or consideration of historical information, including critical disconfirmatory information. The examiner failed to adequately consider differential diagnostic factors. The examiner did not include any of the many appropriate pain complaint response bias measures. And, the examiner offered a strong and unqualified opinion without appropriate recognition of the numerous important conceptual and methodological limitations.

Relevant Ethical Issues

Competence

Performance of an examination, especially a more demanding medicolegal examination for which chronic pain is the primary complaint, despite lacking specific training, experience and competence in this area violates General Principles A, B and D. These relate to efforts regarding promoting benefit and avoiding harm (A), managing conflicts of interest to avoid harm (B), and protecting fairness and justice through precautions against insufficient competence and experience (D). It also fails the specific obligations prescribed in at least standards 2.01 (services only within boundaries of competence, education, experience), 2.04 (basing judgments on knowledge of the discipline) and 3.04 (avoiding potential harm).

Assessment

In this case, the examiner conducted a brief and insufficient interview based on report content, listing of one hour by the examiner, and wife report of it actually lasting thirty minutes or less. The examiner also failed to obtain and/or adequately review sufficient premorbid medical, work, military records, the records of the most recent treating rehabilitation neuropsychologist, or family records. Notably, evidence from pre-injury military, employment records and family report indicate an adaptive history that is inconsistent with sociopathy and malingering. He played on an army baseball team even with a fractured fibula, had very good work performance reviews, an average of fifteen hours overtime per week for the six months prior to his injury, and was working with pneumonia at the time of his injury; positive family functioning reported by family and coworkers is notable for absence of behavioral or emotional problems or conflicts. Therefore, in addition to violating Principles A, B, C (Integrity: ensuring accuracy), and D, the examiner also violated Standard 3.04 (avoiding potential harm), in addition to obligations relating to assessment.

Standard 9.01 (Bases for Assessments) requires that opinions be based on sufficient information and techniques to substantiate findings. Further, the failure to include appropriate, direct measures of pain response bias that could support a diagnosis of malingering additionally deviates from obligations in Standard 9.02 (Use of Assessments) relating to use of appropriate techniques with demonstrated utility (9.02a) and

established reliability and validity (9.02b). For example, Martelli, Zasler, Nicholson, Pickett, & May (2001) list numerous indicators of response bias in pain symptom report. This examiner did not use any, and instead, made leaping generalizations about malingering of pain on the basis of measures of cognitive response bias. Further, the failure to acknowledge and report any of the multiple limitations in procedures and methodology transgresses Standard 9.06 (Interpreting Assessment Results), which prescribes the taking into account limitations of interpretations.

Even greater concern must be raised in light of the additional observation of apparent confirmatory bias and selective medical record review. Notably, all evidence potentially consistent with malingering was considered much more strongly than the preponderant contradictory opinions and evidence. The examiner was notably vigilant to secondary gain while completely ignoring (assessment of) secondary losses (e.g., life disruption of strong premorbid coping style for deriving reinforcement, self esteem and identity, and coping with stress through traditional male role activities at work and home). The examiner also failed to mention or consider important reactive contextual factors (e.g., credible perception of insurance company "games"). This, again, transgresses Standard 9.06, which requires taking into account the situational and personal factors that might affect or reduce the accuracy of interpretations.

The examiner demonstrated conspicuous predilection for dichotomous sociopathic explanations for behavior, at virtually every point in inferential reasoning. Posttraumatic organic and reactive explanations for behavior were summarily discounted. For example, irritability and anger outbursts were attributed to sociopathy. However, the combination of negative premorbid history and neuroimaging evidence of a right frontal insult, especially when combined with evidence of a high association between chronic pain disorders, anger, and violence (e.g., Bruns, Disorbio, & Hanks, 2003), were not considered through differential diagnostic review, apparently due to a combination of bias and lack of competence in chronic pain. Further, no apparent consideration was made that true organic impairment can co-occur with exaggeration or malingering. Finally, the examiner engaged in unethical behavior by offering strong and unqualified opinions despite lack of expertise in the subject area (Standards 2.02 and 2.04); by performing an inadequate assessment (Standards 9.01 and 9.02); and through his failure to express resulting limitations of the assessment procedures (Standard 9.06), interpretations, and the resultant potentially harmful consequences of the conclusions. These behaviors also clearly infringed on General Principles A (avoidance of harm) and D (Justice), which prescribes taking "precautions to ensure that their potential biases, the boundaries of their competence, and the limitations of their expertise do not lead to or condone unjust practices."

Conflict of Interest

Finally, conducting this evaluation seems to breach Principle A (managing conflicts of interest to avoid harm) and Standard 3.06 (Conflict of Interest). The latter proscribes taking on professional roles when objectivity, competence or effectiveness might be impaired, or where it might risk harm. Because this examiner accepted an evaluation outside of his areas of competence and the area where he conducts clinical assessments, motivation and desire for more lucrative medicolegal work presumably influenced his judgment and decision, resulting in compromised competency of procedures, non-objectivity, and harm. The enticing financial incentives in medicolegal work are being increasingly recognized as underappreciated threats to objectivity (e.g., Martelli, Bush, & Zasler, 2003; Martelli, Zasler, Nicholson, Hart, & Heilbronner, 2001, 2002; Martelli, Zasler, & Grayson, 1999). In summary, the neuropsychologist's behavior violated, on multiple counts, the spirit and the letter of the Ethics Code.

Case Resolution

After the examinee's worker's compensation benefits were discontinued, his attorney procured a copy of the "independent examination" report. His treating physician and his neuropsychologist prepared a lengthy letter addressing justification for continuing treatment and concern for potential harm that could result from treatment termination. As part of this justification, the numerous methodological problems with the report on which the insurance company based its decision were outlined in detail. Recommendations were made for continued treatment at least until an independent examination was performed by a qualified expert. The letter, which included references to all of the concerns delineated in this scenario, was copied to the independent examiner, along with an note expressing concern that the issues raised in the letter addressed several apparent ethical breaches and that discussion seemed necessary.

When the insurance company refused to reconsider their decision, the patient's wife, after collaboration with the patient, family, attorney and state board of disability rights, appealed the decision and began completing a formal complaint against the examiner with the state licensing board. Because of the family decision to file formal complaint, no further contact or action was taken by the treating doctors, and the examiner also made no attempt at contact.

Conclusions and Recommendations

In this scenario, a neuropsychologist performed an independent examination and diagnosed malingering in an individual who was experiencing chronic pain and persistent cognitive sequelae following a blow to his head. This diagnosis produced significant negative consequence for the subject in terms of health care access, finances, relationships within the family, and general functioning. However, the assessment methodology, interpretations, conclusions and recommendations offered in the independent examination report clearly failed to satisfy several aspirational guidelines and several specific Ethical Standards outlined in the 2002 APA Ethics Code. An inadequate evaluation that transgressed numerous ethical standards served as the basis for a diagnosis that produced significant life consequences and the penultimate ethical breach – the careless and unjustified infliction of harm.

Martelli and Zasler (2001), in one of the major volumes on pain management, addressed ethical issues relating to competency and offered a checklist summary of guidelines for evaluating professional expert qualifications in chronic pain. This checklist was employed to rate the neuropsychologist in this scenario. The neuropsychologist's score of 0 of 48 was included in the letter written to the insurance company, and copied to the neuropsychologist, to argue against the acceptance of the malingering diagnosis and termination of benefits. A successful appeal took one year to reverse the insurance decisions that were based on the deficient examination of the neuropsychologist, at a considerable psychological cost to the individual and his family.

The positive changes in the 2002 Ethics Code more specifically define competence and emphasize disclosing limitations and promoting more just, equitable and transparent practice. The qualifications summaries offered by Martelli and Zasler (2001) in the areas of both chronic pain and brain injury (available at http://villamartelli.com) can assist in specifically assessing extent of competency and in prescribing activities to increase or maintain professional competency in the neuropsychology of pain.

Scenario 2

An experienced, well-known and respected neuropsychologist who specializes in forensic neuropsychological assessment agrees to perform an injury related clinical evaluation on a local chiropractor. The neuropsychologist had received treatment at the chiropractor's office over at a five-year period and had even been treated directly by him on at least couple of occasions. The chiropractor was seen for a neuropsychological evaluation one week after being hurt accidentally while shopping at an industrial construction store. He was struck in the head by a malfunctioning metal spring-loaded security camera and was knocked to the floor. He sustained a loss of consciousness of approximately fifteen minutes, experienced a three-hour period of posttraumatic amnesia (PTA), and sustained a back injury, per emergency room records. He was released from the emergency room several hours after arrival. The neuropsychological report, which was copied to the client's attorney, indicated twenty-four hour period of PTA based on interview of the patient's wife, and reported significant cognitive deficits, significant emotional distress, and head and back pain. Despite a reasonable neuropsychological battery, only very weak checklist measures of pain and emotional status were administered, along with a single measure of response bias. A diagnosis of mild to moderately severe traumatic brain injury (TBI) was given. Emotional distress and pain were not considered as possible influences on neuropsychological test findings. However, pain and distress were offered as explanations for a borderline performance on the symptom validity measure. No recommendation or referral for psychotherapy, or any strategies for reducing emotional distress, were offered. The neuropsychologist followed the patient and reported in a note a couple of weeks later that he was limiting scope of treatment to assessment and individual and family consultation to avoid a "dual relationship" that would be incurred with psychotherapy provision.

Several months later, the neuropsychologist (NP1) made a referral to another neuropsychologist after the patient's insurance changed to a company for which he was not a provider. Up to that point, no recommendation was made for reducing emotional distress. The patient was seen by the second neuropsychologist (NP2), an experienced TBI specialist, and evaluated two more times over a two year period. He was also referred to a psychiatrist for pharmacologic treatment of depression and to a multidisciplinary chronic pain management clinic. He subsequently underwent corrective back surgery.

A third neuropsychologist (NP3) was retained by the defendant's attorney to do an independent exam (IE) as a personal injury trial date approached. He was retained with the understanding from an initial record review that NP1, who was a friend, had withdrawn from treatment. NP3, on record review of repeated previous testing found indices of reduced motivation, inconsistent and improbable performances, somatic hypervigilance, and even observations that pain interfered with attention during testing and interview. On independent examination, he found that the chiropractor demonstrated: (a) Failure on several less well known response bias indicators; (b) stark inconsistencies throughout the evaluation; (c) clearly disruptive pain behavior that interfered inconsistently with attention during simple interview and testing (e.g., scores up to twice as impaired on similar tasks when he appeared to be having exacerbation of pain); (d) significant emotional distress, including interview-elicited evidence of a fairly extreme persistent rumination about perceived mistreatment from his injury and need to seek justice for the wrong; and (e) generalized severe impairments worse than usually seen in severe TBI and without evidence of any improvement across time. A report was issued that reported persistent neuropsychological deficits being due primarily due to an interaction of emotional distress, chronic pain, and motivation to exaggerate impairment. Aggressive psychological intervention was recommended.

After completing the independent examination, and while reviewing additional records, NP3 learned that NP1 had recently been retained by the plaintiff's attorney and performed a complete forensic examination that included reviewing of all records. He testified in a deposition that the patient was permanently disabled with severe neuropsychological impairments due to the TBI. His test performance was deemed valid, despite some suspicious symptom validity test scores, because he consistently scored in the same poor range across all testings post injury. Moreover, NP1's deposition testimony asserted that he had known the patient pre-injury, understood his personality and cognitive functioning, had good comparative data, and therefore had special qualification for more validly assessing post injury changes. In response to questioning about why a recommendation for psychotherapy and/or pain management was not made, he asserted that it was because he knew the patient's personality was consistent with a need to appear normal and feared suggestion of psychotherapy might make him "worse".

Relevant Ethical Issues

Multiple Relationships

There are several important ethical problems in this complex scenario. The most salient problem is the engagement in a multiple relationship that initiated a host of subsequent breaches related to assessment and conclusions. NP1 chose to initiate a clinical relationship with a person with whom he had a pre-existing professional relationship. Standard 3.06 (Conflict of Interest) proscribes taking on a professional role when personal (or scientific, professional, legal, financial, or other) interests or relationships could be expected to impair objectivity or expose the client to risk of harm. Similarly, Standard 3.05 (Multiple Relationships) proscribes entering into a multiple relationship if the relationship might reasonably impair objectivity, competence, or effectiveness in performing psychological duties, or otherwise risk harm to the person. No reasonable exceptions to compliance with these standards existed in this case, and several other competent neuropsychologists were readily available, including some with much more pain experience. No indications were given that the multiple relationship was considered even potentially problematic, and the report did not indicate any potential limitations or dangers as a result of this preexisting relationship. Only in later notes was the issue of multiple relationship conflicts raised, but only regarding the provision of psychotherapy. A subsequent report indicates that NP1 reasoned that because neuropsychological assessment and consultation services were "objective", multiple roles presented no conflict.

NP1's reasoning and interpretation of ethical standards regarding multiple relationships is clearly problematic. Perhaps only in an ideal world, if one assumes that two neuropsychologists could produce exactly the same interview and test results, would we expect all neuropsychologists to reach identical conclusions. In the real world, there is frequently disagreement about even the same test results, situations are often complex, and lawsuits involving mild brain injury are frequently accompanied by widely discrepant findings and opinions. In this case, examination of the assessment findings and recommendations from NP1 strongly suggest that this experienced and competent neuropsychologist's objectivity was significantly compromised by the multiple relationships. This lack of objectivity was manifest in inadequate assessment procedures, an uncritical diagnostic approach, and uncritical judgment that compromised his findings and the welfare of the patient in several ways, especially in terms of delayed treatment and prolonged disability. Hence, in addition to Standard 3.06 (Conflict of Interest), Standard 3.04 (Avoiding Harm) seems to have been breached. The spirit of the Ethics Code was also violated in terms of Principles A (striving to promote benefit and avoid harm), B (managing conflicts of interest to avoid harm), C (promoting accuracy and truthfulness), and D (protecting justice and fairness and avoiding bias).

Further, suspicion must be raised that the failure to recommend treatment reflects not only nonobjectivity and poor judgment due to contradictory

relationship role influences, but also the conflicting interests of the examiner. Chart notes indicating examiner intention to avoid a "dual relationship" by not providing psychotherapy indicates an awareness of need for this treatment. A failure to make a referral to someone with whom there would not be a dual relationship suggests the possibility that such a referral was avoided for one of more of the following reasons: (a) overemphasis on brain injury interpretations of cognitive symptoms to justify report findings and/or reach findings favorable to the familiar client's preference for organic explanations of difficulty and/or his lawsuit; (b) avoidance of exposing NP1's questionable dual relationship and reasoning regarding it; and/or (c) avoiding the possibility of losing income (both existing clinical income and anticipated more lucrative future medicolegal income) by referring to someone not hampered by a dual relationship. These likelihoods are supported by the following events: (a) when the client's insurance was changed to a network to which NP1 did not belong, a referral to another provider was made, and that provider initiated both psychological treatment and specialty pain management referrals; (b) NP1 became re-involved when he could again be reimbursed, by providing even higher paid medicolegal assessment and testimony; and, (c) NP1 asserted, at both points of his service provision with this client, that his previous relationship was advantageous (i.e., providing more pre-injury baseline information for comparison), without consideration of disadvantages (e.g., nonobjectivity from a previous non-clinical relationship or nonobjectivity from a previous clinical relationship).

NP1 failed to prevent his own personal interests from competing with those of his client. By entering into risky multiple relationships with role conflicts (3.06), he clearly compromised his professional objectivity, competence, and effectiveness (3.05), and did not take reasonable steps to avoid harm (3.04). By accepting this client a second time for medicolegal evaluation, NP1 expanded the ethical conflict resulting from multiple roles and interests. The following potential sources of bias existed: (a) a preexisting personal relationship that included having received health care treatment services at this persons office, and even by him, which could reasonably be expected to affect objectivity in a clinical evaluation of that person; (b) the preexisting personal relationship that could reasonably be expected to affect objectivity in a medicolegal evaluation; (c) the preexisting clinical treatment relationship that could reasonably be expected to affect objectivity in a medicolegal evaluation; and (d) apparent financial interests which initially, as a clinical assessment provider, seemed to compromise patient need for treatment, and later, as a highly paid expert, ignored precautions against possibility of nonobjectivity from both previous personal and clinical relationships (the fact that the former most likely contributed to the latter is also consistent with financial interests that conflict with appropriate assessment and treatment). NP1 failed to adequately consider and safeguard against potential conflicts and negative consequences of his decisions, and hence failed to take any precautions to avoid the harm that seems to have resulted. This harm included compromised objectivity and ineffectiveness in assessment, diagnosis and treatment planning that complicated recovery and contributed to prolonged distress and disability.

Assessment

In terms of NP1's initial assessment, numerous problems are evident. Inadequate checklist versus objective measures of emotional status and pain were employed. No measures of emotional status or pain complaint veracity were administered, and on the one measure of cognitive symptom exaggeration employed, a borderline score was produced but minimized and attributed to pain and emotional distress. These problems breach requirements in Standard 9.02 (Use of Assessments) regarding both failure to use appropriate techniques with demonstrated utility,

reliability and validity, and failure to indicate resulting limitations.

In terms of diagnostic opinions, the requirement in Standard 9.01 that opinions be based on sufficient information and techniques to substantiate findings was not met. Not only were insufficient measures employed, but there was then no consideration that pain, emotional status or motivation may have influenced neuropsychological test performance (e.g., Hart, Martelli, & Zasler, 2000; Hart, Wade, & Martelli, 2003; Martelli, Zasler, Nicholson, & Hart, 2001; Nicholson, 2000). The inconsistency in interpreting pain and distress as causes of a suspicious score on a very easy symptom validity test, yet not considering that they could affect performance on much harder neuropsychological measures is glaring evidence of bias. Further, pain and distress were not even considered as possible barriers to adjustment that required prompt and aggressive treatment. The failure to recommend prompt treatment to someone presumed to be in acute emotional distress and pain violates the primary bioethical principle of beneficence and nonmaleficence (APA, 2002; Beauchamp & Childress, 2001; Martelli, Zasler, & Johnson-Greene, 2001).

Case Resolution

After learning that NP1 had become re-involved as an expert with his former health care provider and then clinical patient, NP3 called NP1 to express concerns about apparent conflicts of interest and multiple relationships. With regard to accepting the subject as a clinical patient, he minimized how well he knew the subject and explained his rationale. He noted that he had consulted a colleague (a clinical psychologist/ psychotherapist) who agreed that neuropsychology was objective, that having a pre-injury baseline of cognitive and personality functioning was a unique advantage, and that avoiding psychotherapy would avoid a conflict. Regarding re-involvement for medicolegal examination, NP1 explained that the subjects attorney requested a re-evaluation and that he was only performing clinical duties.

In a subsequently scheduled meeting, NP3 delineated the ethical concerns. NP1 did not express complete agreement, and even questioned whether NP3's opinions were conflicted by his involvement as an expert "from the other side" of an adversarial court proceeding. NP1 nevertheless noted the following: (a) He did not fully critically consider, explicitly indicate, or explicitly make efforts to safeguard against potential conflicts inherent in such an examination, invited questioning of his objectivity, and did not indicate the potential conflicts or limitations in his reports; he admitted that if another neuropsychologist had conducted an evaluation under similar circumstances, he probably would have been suspicious; (b) this was the first evaluation of someone with whom he had a pre-existing relationship, and he would not perform a similar evaluation in the future, and he would be on guard more generally to issues relating to conflicted interests; (c) neuropsychologists are not always objective, and certain situations require greater scrutiny – e.g., he periodically uses the Sweet and Moulthrop (1999) self-examination questions, and these could have been used in this situation and perhaps should be used more frequently; and, (d) he would request a withdrawal from testifying in the legal case.

NP1 subsequently reported that a discussion between his business attorney and the retaining plaintiff's attorney determined that he would risk legal action if he withdrew from expected involvement in the plaintiff's case. Problem-solving discussions between NP1 and NP3 were planned. Prior to further discussion, a settlement was reached, obviating the need for decisions about NP1's continued involvement in the plaintiff's legal case.

Overattribution of post-injury problems to brain injury despite weak evidence reduced the credibility of the patient's complaints and misdirected treatment. Further, not recommending psychotherapy or pain management early after injury diluted recognition of the importance of these problems, delayed treatment and almost certainly protracted distress, complicated recovery, and prolonged disability. The small settlement that was awarded hardly seemed desirable compensation for the apparently harmful initial assessment and treatment of this patient that likely would not have happened absent the multiple conflicting relationship influences.

Conclusions and Recommendations

In the present scenario, the neuropsychologist employed poor judgment by entering into multiple relationships with multiple contradictory professional, personal and financial influences. He did not make reasonable efforts to consider the potential negative effects on his objectivity and effectiveness or the potential harm to the patient. He performed an inadequate assessment that very poorly assessed and poorly addressed the role of pain and emotional distress factors, as well as motivation, and overattributed problems to brain injury. He failed to (a) indicate any of the many potential limitations or qualify any opinions, (b) protect against compromising objectivity, (c) employ more reliable and valid instruments for pain and emotional assessment status, (d) appropriately interpret instruments, and (e) protect against the harm that eventuated.

NP1's inadequate assessment and treatment recommendations delayed appropriate treatment of pain and emotional distress symptoms, complicated recovery, and almost certainly protracted distress and disability. Whether by coincidence or subtle reinforcement, his initial involvement increased the likelihood of his seeing this patient later for lucrative work in his preferred specialty of forensic neuropsychology.

It should be considered an extremely difficult and underappreciated challenge to resist the highly reinforcing incentives associated with lucrative medicolegal work in an otherwise increasingly restrictive reimbursement environment. Although these incentives often exert an overt influence, it may be the more subtle and less conspicuous reinforcement that is the more dangerous threat, and there is increasing evidence that bias is as prevalent in forensic examiners as is it is in personal injury claimants (e.g., Martelli, Zasler, Nicholson, Hart, & Heilbronner, 2001).

The changes to APA Ethics Code help address the problem of inappropriate examinations by tightening standards in the areas of competence, validity and objectivity, consideration and indication of limitations, attention to individual factors, protections against harm, promotion of more equitability and justice, and transparency (Adams, 2003). Clearly, more attention is needed in order to parallel the increasing prominence of forensic neuropsychology specialists and services, particularly given the high frequency of pain complaints by personal injury litigants and those seeking disability benefits. It may be incumbent upon neuropsychologists to seek out additional readings that provide strategies for protecting against these potent yet often subtle threats to objectivity (e.g., Martelli, Bush, & Zasler, 2003; Sweet & Moulthrop, 1999).

References

Adams, K.M. (2003). It's a whole new world; or is it? Reflections on the new APA Ethics Code. *Division 40 Newsletter, 21 (1)*, 5-18.

American Psychological Association (1992). Ethical principles of psychologists and code of conduct. *American Psychologist, 47*, 1597-1611.

American Psychological Association (2002). Ethical principles of psychologists and code of conduct. *American Psychologist, 57 (12)*, 1060–1073.

Beauchamp, T.L., & Childress, J.F. (2001). *Principles of biomedical ethics* (5th ed.). New York: Oxford University Press.

Bruns, D., Disorbio, J.M., & Hanks, R. (2003). Chronic nonmalignant pain and violent behavior. *Current Pain and Headache Reports, 7*, 127-132.

Hart, R.P, Martelli, M.F., & Zasler, N.D. (2000). Chronic pain and neuropsychological functioning. *Neuropsychology Review, 10 (3)*, 131-149.

Hart, R.P., Wade, J.B., & Martelli, M.F. (2003). Cognitive impairment in patients with chronic pain: The significance of stress. *Current Pain and Headache Reports, 7*, 116-126.

Martelli, M.F., Bush, S.S., & Zasler, N.D. (2003). Identifying and avoiding ethical misconduct in medicolegal contexts. *International Journal of Forensic Psychology, 1*, 1-17.

Martelli, M.F., & Zasler, N.D. (2001). Promoting ethics and objectivity in medicolegal contexts: Recommendations for experts. In R.B. Weiner (Ed.): *Pain management: a practical guide for clinicians* (6th ed.), (pp. 895-907). Boca Raton, FL: St. Lucie Press.

Martelli, M.F., Zasler, N.D., & Grayson, R. (1999). Ethical considerations in medicolegal evaluation of neurologic injury and impairment. *NeuroRehabilitation: An Interdisciplinary Journal, 13 (1)*, 45-66.

Martelli, M.F., Zasler, N.D., & Johnson-Greene, D. (2001). Promoting ethical and objective practice in the medicolegal arena of disability evaluation. In R.D. Rondinelli & R.T. Katz (Eds.), Disability Evaluation. *Physical Medicine and Rehabilitation Clinics of North America, 12 (3)*, (pp. 571-584). Philadelphia: W.B. Saunders.

Martelli, M.F., Zasler, N.D., Nicholson, K., & Hart, R.P. (2001). Masquerades of Brain Injury. Part I: Chronic pain and traumatic brain injury. *The Journal of Controversial Medical Claims, 8 (2)*, 1-8.

Martelli, M.F., Zasler, N.D., Nicholson, K., Hart, R.P., & Heilbronner, R.L. (2001). Masquerades of brain injury. Part II: Response bias in medicolegal examinees and Examiners. *The Journal of Controversial Medical Claims, 8 (3)*, 13-23.

Martelli, M.F., Zasler, N.D., Nicholson, K., Hart, R.P., & Heilbronner, R.L. (2002). Masquerades of brain injury. Part III: Limitations in response bias assessment. *The Journal of Controversial Medical Claims, 9 (2)*, 19-21.

Nicholson, K. (2000). Pain, cognition and traumatic brain injury, *NeuroRehabilitation, 14*, 95-104.

Martelli, M.F., Zasler, N.D., Nicholson, K., Pickett, T.C. & May, V.R. (2001). Assessing the veracity of pain complaints and associated disability. In R.B. Weiner (Ed.), *Pain Management:* *A Practical Guide for Clinicians* (6th ed.), (pp. 789-805). Boca Ratan, FL: St. Lucie Press.

Sweet, J.J., & Moulthrop, M.A. (1999). Self-examination questions as a means of identifying bias in adversarial assessments. *Journal of Forensic Neuropsychology, 1*, 73-88.

Chapter 13

ETHICAL CHALLENGES IN THE NEUROPSYCHOLOGY OF PAIN, PART II

Keith Nicholson

Scenario 1

The patient was involved in a motor vehicle accident some three years previously when his car was rear-ended by another vehicle. Whereas there was a brief lapse of awareness for events (perhaps only a matter of a few seconds) and he felt "stunned" immediately after, he was not sure if there was any direct head trauma, and there was no indication of bodily trauma other than some whiplash related soft tissue injuries. He was moderately distraught at the scene of the accident, but there was then little pain or other apparent problems and he declined an offer to be taken to hospital by ambulance. He slept poorly that evening and the next morning awoke with severe neck, back and especially headache pain. He attempted a return to work as an accountant but continued to suffer from severe pain problems, sleep disturbance and daytime fatigue, followed soon thereafter by onset of psychoemotional difficulties including depressive and anxiety related problems, as well as becoming irritable and withdrawn. He also soon noticed marked problems with aspects of cognition, especially concentration, memory and speed of processing, but also word finding, problem solving, visuospatial difficulties, etc. He stopped working completely within days of the accident. He underwent extensive medical assessment including neuropsychological evaluation

and several brain imaging techniques (CT, MRI, SPECT, qEEG).

The results of comprehensive medical evaluation revealed no structural but some apparent functional abnormalities. With regard to neuropsychological evaluation, very poor performance in multiple areas was noted, as compared to his assumed good premorbid ability level. The conclusion of several examiners retained by the plaintiff's attorney, including more than one neuropsychologist, was that there had been a traumatic brain injury (TBI) and that the patient was continuing to present with a post-concussive syndrome, such insult proffered as an explanation for his many problems. When seen by specialists retained by the defense attorney, including more than one neuropsychologist, it was variously concluded that there had been no physical injury, including no head or brain injury, and that difficulties were either functional (and therefore suggested to be spurious, temporary or not as serious as if there were an actual brain injury) or associated with poor effort and malingering. Description of functional factors in the neuropsychological (or other specialist) reports was typically vague and only sometimes detailing what specific functional factors were thought to be relevant. The patient became involved in a long medicolegal process, the outcome of which was not deemed satisfactory for any of the parties involved.

Relevant Ethical Issues

Several questions concerning ethical issues or standards of practice are raised by this scenario. Ethical standard 2.04 (Bases for Scientific and Professional Judgments) is considered to be of primary importance in this and many other cases in which ethical issues may be of concern. This principle states that "Psychologists' work is based upon established scientific and professional knowledge of the discipline". However, many (or most) areas of applied psychology with human subjects involve issues in which there is not a simple, clear-cut or unambiguous basis in scientific or professional knowledge. The core problem of this scenario is why the patient is having difficulty. Although he did very poorly on neuropsychological testing and was apparently having marked difficulty in his everyday life, there was conflicting opinion about why this may be.

There has been longstanding controversy about the etiology or nature of the post-concussive syndrome (e.g., Lishman, 1988) or the nature of neuropsychological deficits following even more significant TBI. It should be realized that headache is the primary problem in virtually all surveys of the post-concussive syndrome and that post-traumatic headache is extremely common following head injury with or without evidence of brain injury (Nicholson, 2000a; Martelli, Grayson & Zasler, 1999). There is now ample evidence that headache or other pain may markedly interfere with aspects of performance, especially those functions traditionally considered to be vulnerable to the effects of traumatic brain injury (Nicholson, 2000a). In addition, several problems are often associated with chronic pain including sleep disturbance and psychoemotional difficulties that can also markedly impair aspects of performance. In contrast, critical medical characteristics associated with TBI in this scenario would suggest that any such injury was very mild (if indeed there was any TBI whatsoever), or that the degree of difficulty encountered by the patient on formal assessment or in his everyday life would not likely be accounted for by such injury. Given the available scientific evidence, it may be considered unethical to diagnose as brain injury what is more likely an effect of pain or related problems. In this context, Ethical Standard 3.04 (Avoiding Harm) should be mentioned, given that inappropriate or erroneous diagnosis of TBI may have serious iatrogenic effects.

It should also be realized that pain (acute or chronic) may have an actual effect on brain function, potentially involving widespread cortical and subcortical areas, as demonstrated by various functional imaging techniques (Nicholson, 2000b). There may well, therefore, be a neuropsychological deficit associated with discernible impairment of brain function in cases of chronic pain. However, not all persons who suffer from chronic pain have cognitive problems. In addition, not all persons who sustain some head trauma or other bodily injury go on to develop chronic pain problems. It remains unclear what person or other factors may co-determine development of, or vulnerability for, development of cognitive dysfunction associated with chronic pain and related problems. It is also unclear what the pathophysiology of many (or most) chronic pain problems may be although psychosocial factors may be most important in the etiology, maintenance, severity or exacerbation of such problems. These and other issues would suggest that a better understanding of the neuropsychology of pain is required (Nicholson, 1998).

Several issues related to Ethical Standard 2.01 (Boundaries of Competence; a, b, and e) are raised by this scenario. Ethical standard 2.01 (a) admonishes psychologists to only provide services "within the boundaries of their competence, based on their education, training, supervised experience, consultation, study or professional experience". Given that pain is a primary problem not only in many cases involving head injury but also other presenting problems, neuropsychologists dealing with such populations should be well aware of relevant issues if not an expert in pain assessment and chronic pain problems. Similarly,

Ethical Standard 2.01 (b) directs psychologists to have or obtain the appropriate training to ensure competence if an understanding of other factors is essential for effective implementation of their services. In this regard, the identified factor of "disability" is especially relevant given that the psychology of chronic pain and related problems certainly involves an understanding of disability issues. Ethical Standard 2.01 (e) may be especially relevant to this scenario. This standard indicates that "in those areas in which generally recognized standards for preparatory training do not yet exist, psychologists nevertheless take reasonable steps to ensure the competence of their work and to protect clients/patients, students, supervisees, research participants, organizational clients and others from harm". It is suspected that most training programs in neuropsychology have provided little about the neuropsychology of pain, the psychology of chronic pain more generally, or even the possible effects of pain and related problems on neuropsychological test performance. Similarly, Ethical Standard 2.03 (Maintaining Competence) requires psychologists to undertake efforts to develop and maintain their competence. Again, given that pain and related problems may be central to a client's presentation, neuropsychologists need to be aware of such issues and the relevant literature.

Ethical Standard 3.06 (Conflict of Interest) is applicable to this scenario as it involves defense or plaintiff neuropsychologists conducting medicolegal assessments, and as the opinion of either may well have been influenced by issues of financial compensation. Whereas there has been considerable interest in the effect of compensation on client presentation, there has been little attention devoted to how this may affect professional opinion. Although there is little empirical research related to this problem (Martelli et al., 2002), many neuropsychologists may be aware of colleagues who appear to be influenced by who is paying the bill.

Several of the Ethical Standards pertaining to Assessments are raised by this scenario. In particular, Ethical Standard 9.01 (Bases for Assessments, a and b) indicates that psychological opinion is based on information and techniques sufficient to substantiate their findings and that psychologists provide opinions only after they have conducted examinations adequate to support their statements or conclusions. If pain and related problems may be a part of a client's presentation, this needs to be determined and appropriately assessed. Ethical Standard 9.02 (a and b) states that psychologists use appropriate assessment instruments whose validity and reliability have been established for use with members of the population tested. However, the validity of most neuropsychological tests has not been established with chronic pain patients. Again, it remains unclear what effect chronic pain may have with an individual client, many chronic pain patients not presenting with such problems. Finally, Ethical Standard 9.06 (Interpreting Assessment Results) applies given that psychologists need to take into account various test factors or characteristics of the person being assessed in their interpretation of results, and as pain may be such an important characteristic or factor.

Case Resolution

As this was a medicolegal case, the differing opinions were mediated in that context (i.e., neuropsychologists being asked to provide rebuttals to other opinions in their reports or testimony), and the outcome was unsatisfactory to both sides.

Conclusions and Recommendations

Neuropsychologists need to be aware of many possible issues in the provision of assessment, treatment, consultation or other services. Whereas this case scenario has stressed the possible confounding effects of chronic pain and related problems on presentation during neuropsychological assessment, it has also been stressed that many questions remain and that there are often not simple clear cut answers to many clinical questions/issues. Indeed, it is this author's understanding that scientific or professional knowledge is not any static set of rules or universal truisms but that science is really a matter of working toward a better approximation of the nature of reality. It is questionable whether there are any simple laws of psychological science that may dictate the behavior of a practitioner, providing any simple algorithm of what to do in what circumstances. In this context, it may often be questionable what constitutes acceptable professional judgment versus what constitutes professional dogma. There is certainly much of the latter in psychology and several other scientific endeavors.

Neuropsychologists are urged to give consideration to the possible effects of pain and related problems as a determinant of neuropsychological status. It is also noted that whereas pain is widely suggested to be a multidimensional experience and a biopsychosocial phenomena, it appears that very often practitioners (neuropsychologists or others) adopt an either-or view of things, i.e., either pain is a "real" physical and biomedical phenomena or it is a "psychological" phenomena and only in the patient's "head" or "mind". Neuropsychologists should be careful not to fall into the pitfalls of mind-body dualism. Finally, it is expected that as a better understanding of the neuropsychology of chronic pain becomes explicated, many potential associated ethical dilemmas will be resolved.

Scenario 2

The patient was at work when he fell from a scaffold, hitting the right side of his body, with traumatic injuries involving primarily the right side of his head, shoulder and upper extremity. He was unresponsive for approximately five minutes having a very brief period of retrograde and a somewhat longer period of anterograde amnesia. He was admitted to hospital where an undisplaced skull fracture with a small contusion of the left posterior parietal area was identified on initial imaging, the later having completely resolved on a subsequent study. He continued to have marked problems with post-traumatic headache and was also subsequently diagnosed with a complex regional pain syndrome (formerly RSD) of the right upper extremity. He developed a moderately severe right sided hemisensory loss. He was started on opioids but continued to complain of severe pain (e.g., 9-10/10 on the verbal analogue scale where "0" = "no pain" and "10" = "the worst that pain could ever be") and doses were quickly escalated to very high levels. Nonetheless, pain severity ratings remained high. He complained of debilitating cognitive problems and was seen for neuropsychological assessment on request from his family physician who observed that there had been marked deterioration from premorbid status.

Results of a clinical neuropsychological assessment confirmed that there were widespread problems. The very poor performance on right sided manual motor tasks was interpreted as indicative of left hemispheric involvement. As this case involved worker's compensation, the patient was seen by a neuropsychologist retained by the Worker's Compensation Board who attributed poor test performance to the interfering effects of pain, other psychoemotional problems, or poor effort. The right sided hemisensory deficit was considered to be a "non-organic" sign suggestive of abnormal illness behavior. When seen for repeat neuropsychological assessment (his third) by a neuropsychologist retained by the plaintiff's attorney, an effect of opioid medication on test performance was apparent. He initially performed reasonably well on several tasks, but as the day progressed and he continued to take medication, he became more stuporous with slurred speech. He was referred to a multidisciplinary pain management program for further assessment of pain, including administration of sodium amytal procedures (Mailis & Nicholson, 2002), which suggested operation of factors at a psychophysiological interface. When seen again following stabilization of medications and participation in the multidisciplinary pain management program, there was dramatic improvement in the patient's test performance, with scores generally within expectation.

Relevant Ethical Issues

Many of the issues raised by this scenario are similar to those of the previous scenario and, more generally, are similar to other cases of neuropsychological assessment of patients presenting with chronic pain. An understanding of such issues will help to prepare the neuropsychologist for successful negotiation of the most common ethical challenges encountered when working with this population. As with the previous case, Bases for Assessment (Standard 9.01) is considered. Prior to making a diagnosis, each of the neuropsychologists should have performed an adequate examination that included measures of pain and other possible problems. Where such data was unavailable, the neuropsychologists should have discussed the limitations with which confidence could be placed in their diagnoses (Standard 9.06, Interpreting Assessment Results; Standard 2.04, Bases for Scientific and Professional Judgments).

Neuropsychologists have a responsibility to "take reasonable steps to avoid harming" those that they evaluate and treat (Standard 3.04, Avoiding Harm). By inadequately assessing the potential impact of pain or incompletely considering limitations of the test data, the neuropsychologists could have made diagnostic errors that could result in inappropriate treatment or inappropriately discontinued treatment. The neuropsychologist working with patient populations that present with pain who does not adequately assess the potential interaction of pain-related issues and cognition may be practicing outside his/her boundaries of competence (Standard 2.01). For the competent neuropsychologist, the tendency to consistently offer strong opinions in the direction supporting the referral source may reflect a philosophical congruence between the neuropsychologist's belief in the nature of cognitive impairment with certain populations and the nature of the referrals received. However, if that tendency is due to an intentional failure to consider alternative explanations that may be inconsistent with the goals of the referral source, a lack of truthfulness must be considered (Standard 5.01a, Avoidance of False or Deceptive Statements). Neuropsychologists working with individuals who are experiencing pain, particularly in medicolegal contexts, must strive to maintain objectivity, considering each patient individually.

Case Resolution

Given that this was a medicolegal case involving Worker's Compensation, conflicts of opinion were addressed within that context. Whereas one or more of the neuropsychologists conducting assessments may have suspected that previous examiners were biased in their interpretations of the examination findings, such bias did not seem to warrant confrontation or formal complaint. Nevertheless, informal action to educate the previous examiners and assist them from making the same mistakes in the future would be consistent with ethical behavior (Ethical Standard 1.04). Such action, taken after resolution of the case, would likely be best received if offered in a spirit of collegiality rather than confrontation, and might consist of sending them relevant articles with a cover letter mentioning the concerns.

Conclusions and Recommendations

This case introduced the issue of opioid medication and the effect taking such medication may have on neuropsychological test performance. Whereas opioid medication may result in performance deficits, it should also be recognized that appropriate opioid medication may result in enhanced performance due to amelioration of pain-related deficits (Chapman, Byas-Smith, & Reed, 2002). Of course, various other medications commonly used for treatment of chronic pain (e.g., anti-convulsants) may also result in significant performance deficits, and neuropsychologists need to be aware of these possibilities. This scenario also made mention of hemisensory deficits, with one neuropsychologist suggesting that this was associated with a functional overlay. However, hemisensory deficits have been shown to be associated with particular cortical and subcortical abnormalities on fMRI (Mailis et al., 2003), indicating a neurobiological substrate possibly associated with psychological factors. As previously emphasized, the neuropsychology of chronic pain and associated deficits needs further explication. Neuropsychologists need to be aware of these and related issues for provision of the most ethical and responsible services.

References

American Psychological Association (1992). Ethical principles of psychologists and code of conduct. *American Psychologist, 47*, 1597-1611.

American Psychological Association (2002). Ethical principles of psychologists and code of conduct. *American Psychologist, 57*, 1060-1073.

Chapman, S.L., Byas-Smith, M.G., & Reed, B.A. (2002). Effects of intermediate and long-term use of opioids on cognition in patients with chronic pain. *The Clinical Journal of Pain, 18*, S83-S90.

Lishman, W.A. (1988). Physiogenesis and psychogenesis in the "post-concussional syndrome". *British Journal of Psychiatry, 153*, 460-469.

Mailis, A., Giannoylis, I., Downar, J., Kwan, C., Mikulis, D., Crawley, A., Nicholson, K., & Davis, K. (2003). Altered central somatosensory processing in chronic pain patients with "hysterical" anaesthesia. *Neurology, 60*, 1501-1507.

Mailis, A., & Nicholson, K. (2002). The use of sodium amytal in the assessment and treatment of functional or other disorders. *Physical Medicine and Rehabilitation: State of the Art Reviews, 16*, 131-146.

Martelli, M.F., Grayson, R., & Zasler, N.D. (1999). Post traumatic headache: Psychological and neuropsychological issues in assessment and treatment. *Journal of Head Trauma Rehabilitation, 1*, 49-69.

Martelli, M.F., Zasler, N.D., Nicholson, K., Pickett, T.C., & May, V.R. (2002). Assessing the veracity of pain complaints and associated disability. In R.B. Weiner (Ed.), *Pain Management: A Practical Guide for Clinicians*, 6th edition, (pp. 789-805). Boca Raton, FL: St. Lucie Press.

Nicholson, K. (1998). *The Neuropsychology of Pain*. Special Presentation. 1998 National Academy of Neuropsychology Annual Meeting. Washington, D.C.

Nicholson, K. (2000a). Pain, cognition and traumatic brain injury. *NeuroRehabilitation, 14*, 95-103.

Nicholson, K. (2000b). At the crossroads: Pain in the 21st Century. *NeuroRehabilitation, 14*, 57-67.

Section 7

ETHICAL CHALLENGES IN PEDIATRIC NEUROPSYCHOLOGY

Introduction

To what extent should pediatric patients be involved in the informed consent process? Are there differences in confidentiality requirements for children and adolescents compared to adults? Should recommendations against third party observers of neuropsychological evaluations be extended to the evaluation of children? How can neuropsychologists interpret test results in the face of limited age-based norms for many standardized tests and limited data on neuropsychological profiles for many pediatric disorders? What is considered sufficient education and training for the practice of pediatric neuropsychology? In one of the few writings on the ethics of pediatric neuropsychology, Fennell (2002) began to examine these issues, emphasizing that the answers to these questions may vary somewhat depending on the arena of practice (e.g., hospital, school, forensic). In the current chapter, the authors continue to explore the ethical issues that may be unique to, or uniquely understood and applied in, the context of pediatric evaluation and treatment. Understanding the systems within which the child lives and interacts, within which the neuropsychologist works, and from which legislative decisions emerge are important to meeting the needs of consumers of pediatric neuropsychology.

Reference

Fennell, E.B. (2002). Ethical issues in pediatric neuropsychology. In S.S. Bush & M.L. Drexler (Eds.), *Ethical issues in clinical neuropsychology,* 75-86. Lisse, NL: Swets & Zeitlinger Publishers.

Chapter 14

ETHICAL CHALLENGES IN PEDIATRIC NEUROPSYCHOLOGY, PART I

Eileen B. Fennell

Scenario 1

A sixteen-year-old female sustained a severe closed head injury in a motor vehicle accident three months before the request for a neuropsychological examination was made by her attending physician. The patient had sustained both chest and head injuries in the accident and had been in a coma for four weeks prior to a gradual return to full consciousness. Acute MRI scans revealed multifocal intraparenchymal hemorrhages of the frontal poles, both left and right temporal lobes, and scattered subcortical areas. The neuropsychological examination revealed intellectual functioning within the average range but evidence of problems in sustained attention, verbal and visual delayed memory, and verbal fluency to both phonemic and semantic criteria. Motor slowing was also present bilaterally. The patient's behavior was notable for an impulsive response style, some jocularity, and increasing problems with distractibility as she fatigued. Premorbid intellectual functioning was described as above average, with academic functioning above grade level. The patient was described as a socially outgoing young woman who had been dating since age fifteen. Several weeks after the initial assessment, the neuropsychologist was advised by the patient's mother that the patient had recently had a sexual contact with a former boyfriend. The parent was distressed, feeling that due to the patient's brain injury, the patient had been taken advantage of by the boyfriend. Nursing staff reported that the patient had talked to them about her sexual activity, and they raised concerns about whether a complaint should be lodged with either the State Child Protection Team or with the State Attorney's Office. It was at this point that the neuropsychologist was consulted.

Relevant Ethical Issues

The previous scenario raises several relevant ethical issues. First, who was the client? The neuropsychologist had been approached by medical personnel to whom the events had been disclosed by the patient. Second, the competency of the patient to consent to the relationship was raised by both medical personnel and the parent who had learned about it from the nursing staff. Third, what were the limits of confidentiality of the patient under the circumstances? Fourth, what was the appropriate role of the neuropsychologist in these circumstances? Finally, what resolution would be in the best interests of the patient?

Examining the 2002 Ethics Code, it seems that several sections were of relevance in this situation.

Issues of Third-Party Requests for Service (Standard 3.07), Use of Confidential Information (Standard 4.07), Use of Assessments (Standard 9.02), and Discussing the Limits of Confidentiality (Standard 4.02) all are pertinent. Further, the obligation of the neuropsychologist to follow state statutory requirements in reporting potential abuse and/or neglect of children was at issue (Principle A, Beneficence and Nonmaleficence). Finally, determining the appropriate role of the neuropsychologist in this case was also an issue (Principle B, Fidelity and Responsibility).

Because of the complex issues in this scenario, initial consultations with colleagues were sought to clarify how best to proceed in response to the request of the nursing services (Standard 4.06). In accordance with the 2002 Ethics Code, patient identification was protected, and the discussion centered around defining the role of the neuropsychologist as consultant to the staff and the need to obtain specific clarification on requirements for reporting the incident to the Child Protection Team, as this information had only been divulged to the nursing staff. Further, the need to obtain parental permission to, once again, be involved in the patient's care was discussed, as well as the rights of a sixteen-year-old to consent to such an assessment was discussed. Of particular concern was the issue of the limits of confidentiality given the content of the patient's disclosure and whether such limits were waived given potential statutory requirements to report, especially if the patient's competency might be challenged.

Case Resolution

Standard 3.07 (Third Party Requests for Services) of the Ethics Code suggests that defining the role of the neuropsychologist, identifying who was the client, and determining the probable use of the services, was needed. In this scenario, Cooperation with Other Professionals (Standard 3.09) to provide appropriate and effective care

to the patient was clearly an issue as well. An overriding concern was determining whether a report was needed to the Child Protection Team, and which parties should file the report (nursing staff, parent, neuropsychologist). Ultimately, a report was called in by the nursing staff to whom the patient had disclosed the event. In this instance, state regulations clearly limited the patient's confidentiality, and the nursing staff was advised to inform both the patient and her parent of the need to call in the report. The parent then requested a consultation with the neuropsychologist to discuss her concerns regarding the patient's behavior. The neuropsychologist suggested that the parent might want to directly discuss the event with the patient in order to better understand the history and the circumstances of what happened and to provide any needed guidance for the future. Ultimately, the case was cleared by the Child Protection Team, and counseling sessions were arranged for the patient and her family to include education on sexuality in teenagers and head-injured patients. At the parent's request, no criminal charges were filed.

Conclusions

Under the guiding principles related to benefiting those with whom neuropsychologists work and taking care to do no harm, a central concern in the above scenario was the impact of the disclosure of the patient's sexual activity on her own life, on her relationship with her parents, on the individual with whom she had been intimate, and on the potential for future harm due to possibly compromised judgment as a result of her brain trauma. At the same time, the need to follow statutory requirements on reporting possible abuse was present. Consultation with colleagues, with professionals on the Child Protection Team, and with the staff involved provided guidance to the professionals involved. As information developed, the need for more details about the event became evident, as well as the need to provide follow-up care to the patient and to her family. Resolution of the case allowed the family to move on to focusing on continued recovery for the patient and developing clearer understanding of both the impact of brain trauma on behavior and the developmental stresses of adolescents.

Scenario 2

A pediatric neuropsychologist agrees to assess a child who purportedly sustained a head injury at a recreational facility. After examining records relating to the injury, including a prior neuropsychological examination requested by the plaintiff's attorney, the neuropsychologist set a tentative date for the examination. Subsequently, the neuropsychologist was informed that, according to a prior state circuit court ruling, the examination would be required to be videotaped and a court reporter would be present to record the examination. The defense attorney was unsuccessful in persuading the judge at a hearing that the presence of a third-party observer and videotaping would negatively impact the neuropsychological assessment.

Relevant Ethical Issues

Pediatric neuropsychologists who engage in forensic work are increasingly confronted with this type of scenario in which the court requires the videotaping of an examination and/or the use of a court reporter to develop a transcript of the entire exam. Both the National Academy of Neuropsychology (NAN, 2000) and the American Academy of Clinical Neuropsychology (AACN, 2000) have published position papers regarding the potential negative impact this may have on the assessment process. The 2002 Ethics Code is relevant to this issue given Standards 9.04 (Releases of Test Data) and 9.11 (Maintaining Test Security). Another issue relates to the competence of the

neuropsychologist in appreciating both the impact of a visible observer on a child's behavior and how this might change with age and the potential impact of deviation from standardized test administration procedures (Standard 2.01, Boundaries of Competence).

Case Resolution

The neuropsychologist refused to conduct the examination under the conditions stipulated by the court. Discussions with other neuropsychologists led to information on how others had responded to these conditions, such as requesting that test data or the exam not be allowed to be part of the public record or the case. However, individuals whose practice was primarily in the pediatric age group indicated that they typically refused to conduct an assessment under these conditions. Most often cited was the potential impact of the extra person and recording equipment in the examination room, particularly with younger children.

Conclusions

A particular concern to neuropsychologists whose professional practice primarily involves children is the failure of the courts to recognize that children's behavior can be affected by being observed or being filmed. As a result, the typical circumstances of an assessment are changed when requirement of videotape and court reporting are added. Thus, the standard of care changes and may impact the results of the examination. From the perspective of equality of care and treatment to clients, suggested by Principle E (Respect for People's Rights and Dignity), it would appear that such legal standards may lead to different assessment circumstances in certain forensic situations. It may also lead to avoidance of forensic work by individuals who by specific training and expertise might best be qualified to examine individuals in civil and/or criminal proceedings.

The newly published Ethics Code, like the 1992 edition, is designed to provide a benchmark to the neuropsychologist for appropriate conduct. Neuropsychologists whose primary clientele are children and/or their families must decide how certain sections of the 2002 Code are to be interpreted in applying these standards to their practice. For example, it is not unusual for a parent to request an evaluation of their minor child (Standard 3.07, Third Party Requests for Services) for school placement in special services (Lorber & Yurk, 1999). In that instance, the parent, by law, is the individual who is requesting the service for their minor child and from whom consent for the assessment is obtained (Standard 9.03, Informed Consent in Assessments). However, in many settings consent or assent is also obtained from the child. Similarly, written release of information may be obtained from *both* the parent and a child over the age of eight years. This practice would also apply in instances of the initiation of therapy (Standard 10.01) with a family in which there are minor children (Fennell, 2002). Informed consent for minors to participate in research (Standard 9.03) is typically governed by the specific requirements of the Institutional Review Board governing the conduct of research but in that setting contains similar requirements of both consent for older minors and assent for younger children. For those whose practice occurs in a hospital setting, a consultation request for assessment of a minor may be initiated not by the parent but by an attending physician who is treating the minor child. Consent for this assessment must still be obtained from the affected parties (parent and child) but requires the neuropsychologist to fully explain their consultative role to the parent (Standard 3.07) as well as the limits of confidentiality (Standard 4.02) that may exist with regard to access to the report in medical records. This is particularly relevant to the new patient privacy protection required under HIPAA regulations.

References

American Academy of Clinical Neuropsychology (2000). Statement on the presence of third party observers in neuropsychological assessments. *The Clinical Neuropsychologist, 15*, 433-439.

American Psychological Association (2002). Ethical principles of psychologists and code of conduct, *American Psychologist, 57*, 1060-1073.

Fennell, E.B. (2002). Ethical issues in pediatric neuropsychology. In S.S. Bush & M.L. Dresler (Eds.), *Ethical Issues in Clinical Neuropsychology*, (pp. 75-86). Lisse, NL: Swets & Zeitlinger, Inc.

Lorber, R., & Yurk, H. (1999). Special pediatric issues: Neuropsychological applications and consultations in schools. In J. Sweet (Ed.), *Forensic Neuropsychology*, (pp. 369-418). Lisse, NL: Swets & Zeitlinger, Inc.

National Academy of Neuropsychology Policy and Planning Committee (2000). Presence of third party observers during neuropsychological testing: Official statement of the National Academy of Neuropsychology. *Archives of Clinical Neuropsychology, 15*, 379-380.

Chapter 15

ETHICAL CHALLENGES IN PEDIATRIC NEUROPSYCHOLOGY, PART II

Alan L. Goldberg

Scenario 1

A neuropsychologist's services were contracted by a school district to provide neuropsychological services involving one child after the child underwent resection of an intracerebral tumor. The neuropsychological evaluation was sought because the child's parents disagreed with the results and recommendations from the school district's evaluation, thereby triggering a request for an independent educational evaluation. The neuropsychologist was chosen by both the school district and the parents. While the district set parameters on the evaluation, the parents' health insurance agreed to pay for a more extended battery of tests. The parents signed a release so that all neuropsychological assessment results could be shared with the school district.

The neuropsychological services were to include an interview of a child and parents, record review, testing, and participation in an Individualized Education Program (IEP) meeting with the school district. While the neuropsychologist was also an attorney, the purpose of the neuropsychologist's involvement was to educate those involved with the child's education about the neuropsychological sequelae of the tumor resection and potential implications for learning.

Historical information was obtained during the initial interview, to which the parents brought copies of medical records. The parents provided rich information about their child's behavior and learning style subsequent to tumor excision.

A battery of tests was administered to the child over three testing sessions. The child exhibited a somewhat unusual pattern of deficits, resembling site-specific damage to the dorsolateral frontal-subcortical circuit. It became quite clear that there were discrepancies between the child's intellectual assessment scores, achievement test scores and actual performance when higher order demands were placed on her. These included learning and memory problems, as well as problems with executive functioning. Although many of her problems appeared to be related to frontal systems functioning, surgical records indicated that the tumor was well encapsulated and entirely within the cerebellar region. Leiner, Leiner, and Dow (1991) and Daum and Ackermann (1995) have begun to theorize on contributions of the cerebellum to higher cognitive functions. Use of sophisticated scanning techniques has revealed an interrelatedness of the cerebellum and anterior association cortex (Desmond et al., 1996). Chafetz et al. (1996) reported declines in attention, declines in rote verbal memory, and lateralized impairments consistent with the contralateral relationship of the cerebellum with the cerebral cortex in general, and with prefrontal cortex in particular. Deficits in planning were also reported by Grafman et al. (1992) in patients with cerebellar lesions. More recently, Greve et al. (1999)

reported language processing and verbal memory deficits in a client with cerebellar lesions.

A ten-page report was generated by the neuropsychologist, and included 4 pages of recommendations. This report formed the basis for fine-tuning of the child's educational programming through additional consultation between the school district and the neuropsychologist. As stated above, the neuropsychologist also agreed to participate in an IEP meeting at the school. The meeting involved regular educators, special educators, a speech-language pathologist, a school psychologist, an occupational therapist, the school principal, the school district's director of special education, and the school district's in-house legal counsel. The parents understood that they could invite anyone they desired to the IEP meeting (Individuals with Disabilities Education Act [IDEA], 20 U.S.C. §1414). The parents invited a civil rights attorney, an advocate from the state advocacy and protection agency, and an advocate from a parent support and advocacy group. Review of past IEPs revealed that many goals were not well operationalized and that progress on learning objectives was difficult to measure. This meeting resulted in a user friendly IEP with clearly stated objectives and measurable goals.

Relevant Ethical Issues

General Principles

Beneficence and Nonmaleficence (Principle A)
The neuropsychologist was clear to strive to benefit the child and school district with objectively collected data. The welfare and rights of the district and the child needed to be considered.

Fidelity and Responsibility (Principle B)
The neuropsychologist's professional role and obligation needed to be clarified, and management of conflict of interest was important.

Integrity (Principle C)
The neuropsychologist had to strive to fulfill obligations both to the district and to the family, while avoiding unwise or unclear commitments.

Justice (Principle D)
The principle states (in part) that "Psychologists recognize that fairness and justice entitle all persons to access to and benefit from the contributions of psychology and to equal quality in the processes, procedures, and services being conducted by psychologists." This principle may be particularly important in cases such as this in which clients may have limited ability to advocate for themselves, such as with children and those with brain injuries.

Respect for People's Rights and Dignity (Principle E)
This principle is particularly important as it acknowledges the special vulnerabilities that may impair autonomous decision making of clients. In working with individuals with acquired brain injuries, special safeguards may be necessary to protect the rights and welfare of the examinees and their families.

Ethical Standards
Of particularly relevance was the fact that part of the evaluation was being done at the behest of the child's school system, and paid for by the school system, while another part was done at the parents' request, and was paid for by private insurance. The neuropsychologist was careful to obtain full informed consent from the family and district and to discuss the fact that all information was being collected in order to plan the child's best educational program. The nature of the relationships was discussed with the family and the school district, and consent was received from both parties (see Standards 3.05, 3.10 and 3.11). Note that the 2002 Code clarifies when multiple relationships exist, and that they may be ethical.

Multiple relationships were also at issue concerning the neuropsychologist's professional degrees as both licensed psychologist and attorney. In order to avoid potential problems, the neuropsychologist clearly defined the role as that of a neuropsychologist. The child's family chose to hire a separate attorney to provide legal advice to them. While the potential multiple relationships (neuropsychologist and attorney, neuropsychologist for district's and for parents' interests) could have led to violations of the APA Ethics Code (see Standard 3.05), it was believed that while acting in the neuropsychologist role, the neuropsychologist was not entering into a relationship that could reasonably be expected to impair effectiveness, and the child was not believed to be in danger of exploitation or harm. The neuropsychologist did not act in legal capacity in this case. Law and psychology have separate rules of conduct and different rules concerning confidentiality and privilege. It was felt that the blurring of roles would provide insurmountable conflict for the neuropsychologist. Although most neuropsychologists will not face this exact conflict, the need to avoid potentially harmful multiple relationships and to clarify the professional expectations is relevant to all clinicians.

Case Resolution

It was only after conducting extensive testing and interviewing that data were assembled to help the neuropsychologist understand the child's problems and help educators understand the child's educational needs. A positive program was then established for this child. Her program, however, continued to need to be closely monitored and tailored over time. This plan was in keeping with Graham and Goldberg's (1995) final step in a 6-step process to guide and develop successful educational programs for students with acquired brain injuries. That final step involved regular follow-up and modification of programming as necessary.

Given the developmental level of this child, and the level of adjustment of the individuals in her family, some recommendations were made in the evaluation report which could best be carried out in the future. These include sex education, counseling for the child (and counseling was also recommended privately to the parents for themselves), referral to vocational rehabilitation specialists, and neuropsychological reevaluation.

Conclusions and Recommendations

A free and appropriate public education is guaranteed to children with disabilities by the Individuals with Disabilities Education Act (IDEA). Under the IDEA, standard procedures are in place to ensure that children with disabilities are able to receive appropriate services from public schools. The IDEA states, "The State must demonstrate that all children with disabilities residing in the State, including children with disabilities attending private schools, regardless of the severity of their disabilities, and who are in need of special education and related services, are identified, located, and evaluated and that a practical method is developed and implemented to determine which children with disabilities are receiving needed special education and related services" (20 U.S.C. §1412). There must be a referral for evaluation, assembly of an evaluation plan and evaluation team, and determination of eligibility before an Individual Education Program team is convened. The IEP team consists of the parents, at least one regular education teacher, at least one special education teacher, a representative of the local education agency (LEA) who is qualified to provide or supervise the provision of specially designed instruction to meet the unique needs of children with disabilities, is knowledgeable about the general curriculum, and is knowledgeable about the availability of resources of the LEA. At the discretion of the parents or the LEA, other individuals who have knowledge or special expertise regarding the child may be invited to attend. The contents of the IEP are clearly defined in the statute. Special education services cannot be provided until the entire aforementioned process has occurred, and an IEP is in place (IDEA, 20 U.S.C. §1400 *et seq.*).

School participation of students with acquired brain injuries (including tumors) who do not appear to fit into established special educational programs has created numerous questions related to educational needs, physical site adjustments, counseling, assessment, and placement (Graham & Goldberg, 1996). Given the time consuming processes required for entrance into special education programming, at times, schools may choose to start students back in school with modified programming authorized by the Rehabilitation Act of 1973 (Section 504). (As an aside, some authors believe that planning for reintegration into the school setting should begin as close to the time of hospital admission as feasible [Clark, 1997; Graham & Goldberg, 1996]) Section 504 provides that "No otherwise qualified individual with handicaps in the United States ... shall solely by reason of her or his handicap, be excluded from the participation in, be denied the benefits of, or be subjected to discrimination under any program or activity receiving Federal financial assistance" (29 U.S.C. §794). Section 504 defines a "handicapped individual" in very broad terms. Many more students can be afforded protections and modifications to programs under Section 504 than under the IDEA (Ekstrand & Brousaides, 1996). Procedural requirements under this act are also far less time consuming than those of the IDEA.

Unfortunately, there are times when students are placed back in school with 504 protections, and changes in their needs are not closely monitored. Such was the situation in this case. The 504 plan allowed her to return to school quickly, but the school district became complacent, and never followed through on a formal IEP, until challenged by the parents at the start of the following school year. School districts, many of which are working under tight budgetary constraints, need to be prodded at times in order to allow children to receive the needed services.

This child's first IEP was very loosely structured and did not adequately address the child's needs. Goals were written in a subjective manner, and compliance with the plan was difficult to monitor. For these reasons, the second IEP was requested. Authors have noted that children with acquired brain injuries have very special needs, and that outside consultants may be required (Cohen, 1996; Nordlund, 1996). While the current revision of the IDEA includes a category of Traumatic Brain Injury (TBI), the definition of TBI is narrow, and students with brain tumors are not included, making planning even more perplexing for educators (these students often qualify for services under the category of "Other health Impaired"). School staff may also need help in deciphering medical reports from well-meaning service providers (including neuropsychologists) who may be unfamiliar with how to translate evaluation results into functional educational goals (Cohen, 1996). It must also be remembered that childhood brain injury is different from neurological insult in adults. Developmental processes are interrupted by injury, and evaluations reflect both recovery processes and developmental progression (Lehr, 1990). Furthermore, many cognitive-intellectual problems "slip through the cracks" following injury to the brain. Children often recover basic skills of mobility, age-appropriate self-care, basic language, and display recovery of pre-injury learning even though new learning may be impaired (Farmer et al., 1997).

This child's program was developed through active collaboration between the neuropsychologist and family, advocates, attorneys, and educators. The psychologist's involvement led to cooperation between the various parties, and prevented significant expenditures of time and money on Due Process Hearings. Knowledge and understanding of law and psychology practice, knowledge of educational systems, and knowledge of community resources helped the neuropsychologist in advocating for the child's needs, while adhering to the APA Ethics Code.

Scenario 2

A neuropsychologist's services were contracted by a rehabilitation facility to provide evaluation and treatment services for a 16-year-old female, who was injured in a motor vehicle accident. The patient and her boyfriend were on their way to his junior prom when the car was hit broadside by another vehicle that ran a red light. The boyfriend was killed in the accident. The patient hit the windshield, and was ultimately ejected from the car. She had bilateral frontal subdural hematomas and multiple areas of brain contusion. She was comatose for seven days, and then began responding. She was in an agitated state (Rancho Level IV) when transferred to the rehabilitation facility ten days after injury. Previously a high school cheerleader, the patient had multiple facial scars and a tracheostomy in place at the time of transfer. She remained in the facility for three weeks, during which time she began to walk with the aid of a cane, and she regained the ability to talk, although her speech was dysarthric, breathy, and slow. Response latencies were long. She returned to her home community, with enrollment in a special education program. The neuropsychologist was again involved as an evaluator and consultant after discharge.

The patient was seen for re-evaluation fourteen months after her discharge from the hospital, in the private practice of the neuropsychologist. Her parents had divorced, allegedly due to the stresses from the daughter's behavior. Her father was transferred out of state to a new military duty location. She was living with her mother, who was having a very difficult time controlling the patient, who often was out all night partying. Although the patient remained in school, she had no formal plans for after her graduation. She had become quite sexually active, resulting

in two abortions and treatment for chlamydia and syphilis.

The neuropsychologist discussed informed consent issues with the patient and her mother and then began the evaluation with a clinical interview. During the interview, she indicated that she had a 23-year-old boyfriend, and that they were sexually active. She stated that they "sometimes" used condoms, but that they were often unavailable when they were ready to have "spontaneous" sex. Further interview suggested many other times when disinhibition, poor judgment, and poor planning led to adverse consequences in the community. Formal testing, unsurprisingly, indicated significant frontal lobe inefficiency, but average intellectual function. Findings were suggestive of an orbitofrontal syndrome, complete with disinhibited, impulsive behavior, poor judgment and insight, distractibility, inappropriate euphoria, and emotional lability (Cummings, 1985).

At the conclusion of the evaluation, during a feedback conference with the patient and her mother, the neuropsychologist suggested the possibility of a group home living environment for the patient. Such settings, it was explained, offer supervision, and structure, both of which the neuropsychologist believed necessary for the young woman's optimal safe functioning. The neuropsychologist also indicated the need to report the patient's boyfriend under child abuse reporting statutes.

Relevant Ethical Issues

The primary ethical, and legal, issue in this case centered around the sexual relationship between the patient and her boyfriend. Legal considerations are presented first.

Legal Issues
All fifty states have passed some form of a mandatory child abuse and neglect reporting law in order to qualify for funding under the

Child Abuse Prevention and Treatment Act (CAPTA) (Jan. 1996 version), 42 U.S.C. 5101, *et seq.* The Act was originally passed in 1974, has been amended several times and was most recently amended and reauthorized on October 3, 1996 by the Child Abuse Prevention and Treatment and Adoption Act Amendments of 1996 (P.L. 104-235). Discussion of mandatory reporting laws for each of the fifty states are available online at the following sites: http:// www.smith-lawfirm.com, http://caresnw.org/state.htm, and http://www.calib.com/nccanch/statutes/index.cfm. Legal information about this case is specific to Arizona law, but should be viewed as an example of how to problem solve in an ethically responsible manner.

The duty to report statute applicable when dealing with sexual contact with a minor in Arizona can be found under the Arizona Criminal Code. ARS 13-3620 is entitled "Duty and authorization to report nonaccidental injuries, physical neglect and denial or deprivation of necessary medical or surgical care or nourishment of minors" (quite a mouthful). How many of us would think to look for this statute? The statute says, in part:

> Any psychologist whose observation or examination of any minor discloses reasonable grounds to believe that a minor is or has been the victim of injury, sexual abuse pursuant to section 13-1405, sexual assault pursuant to section 13-1404, sexual conduct with a minor pursuant to section 13-1405, sexual assault pursuant to section 13-1406, molestation of a child pursuant to section 13-1410, commercial sexual exploitation of a minor pursuant to section 13-3552, sexual exploitation of a minor pursuant to 13-3553, incest pursuant to section 13-3608 or child prostitution pursuant to section 13-3212 ... shall immediately report or cause reports to be made of this information to a peace officer or to child protective

services in the department of economic security ... A report is not required under this section for conduct prescribed by sections 13-1404 and 13-1405 if the conduct involves only minors age 14, 15, 16, or 17 and there is nothing to indicate that the conduct is other than consensual. Reports shall be made forthwith by telephone or in person forthwith and shall be followed by a written report within 72 hours" (The statute goes on to specify content of a written report).

It is of interest to note that under 13-1405, sexual conduct with a minor (under 15) is a class 2 felony. Sexual conduct with a minor who is at least 15 is a class 6 felony (but class 2 if the person is the minor's parent, stepparent, adoptive parent, legal guardian, or foster parent). A defense to prosecution is if the victim is 15, 16, or 17 and the defendant is less than 19 or attending high school and is no more than 24 months older than the victim, and the conduct is consensual. However, there may still need to be a report. A defense is something that is used at trial, and the judge or jury may or may not decide to accept it. Note that in the case under discussion, the young woman was 16, and her boyfriend was 23 years of age. Under the aforementioned statutes, reporting was necessary.

Ethical Issues

Under the APA Ethical Principles and Code of Conduct, several principles are important to mention in deciding whether a report is necessary, given that in some situations outlined above, reporting is not mandatory. Principle A (Beneficence and Nonmaleficence) is one such principle. It states (in part), "Psychologists seek to safeguard the welfare and rights of those with whom they interact professionally." Principle E (Respect for People's Rights and Dignity) is another important principle in a case involving sexual conduct with a minor. In working with individuals with acquired brain injuries, special safeguards may be necessary to protect the rights and welfare of the examinees and their families.

Ethical Standards 1.02 (Conflicts between Ethics and Law, Regulations, or Other Governing Legal Authority), 1.03 (Conflicts Between Ethics and Organizational Demands), and 4 (Privacy and Confidentiality) were (or could have been) involved in the case. Issues of confidentiality, privacy, and disclosure were at odds with the laws mentioned above. Adherence to state law was necessary, and the situation required breaking confidentiality and disclosing information to state agencies. For many practitioners, issues of reporting need to be discussed with the facility in which they are employed. Since the young woman was seen for reevaluation in a private practice setting, Standard 1.03 did not apply. Having been informed of the possible exceptions to confidentiality during the informed consent process (Standard 3.10, Informed Consent; Standard 9.03, Informed Consent in Assessments), the patient and her mother should have been prepared for, or at least aware of, the need for the neuropsychologist to report the sexual relationship to the appropriate agency.

When ethical responsibilities conflict with law, neuropsychologists should make known their commitment to the APA Ethics Code, and take steps to resolve the conflict in a responsible manner. If the conflict is unresolvable via such means, neuropsychologists may adhere to the requirements of the law, in keeping with basic principles of human rights (Standard 1.02, Conflicts Between Ethics and Law, Regulations, or Other Governing Legal Authority).

Case Resolution

The patient's mother understood the seriousness of the legal issues discussed during the feedback session. She also agreed to contact the insurer

and state agencies for funding and programs to provide additional structure for her daughter, since she was unable to provide such structure herself. As is typical in individuals with frontal lobe disorders, the patient was able to understand and discuss the consequences of her actions, but was unable to inhibit her behavior on her own.

Conclusions and Recommendations

When neuropsychologists receive information concerning sexual conduct with a minor, it can be a daunting task for the neuropsychologist to decide whether or not to report. The neuropsychologist may weigh the benefits of reporting against the possibility of alienating the patient and turning her against psychological or neuropsychological services, from which she would likely benefit in the future. The professional may want to take into consideration the psychological maturity of the minor, issues of psychopathology, developmental disabilities, intellectual level of the minor, and also physical health. Issues related to physical health might include whether the minor has had a brain injury, or whether endocrine problems contribute to sexual acting out by the minor. Issues of sexually transmitted diseases may also need to be taken into account. With ambiguous cases, it may be beneficial to engage the patient and the family in making a determination of a responsible course of action to safeguard the patient. Social supports in the community (e.g., clergy) should also be considered and consulted as needed. Clearly, in the case at hand, the brain injury, frontal disinhibition, and STDs needed to be considered in the interests of the patient's safety and health.

The bottom line is to use common sense and sound clinical judgment. Consult with colleagues, ethics committees, and psychological associations for help. Know the law, or consult an attorney for help in understanding the law as it applies to clinical practice.

References

American Psychological Association (1992). Ethical principles of psychologists and code of conduct. *American Psychologist, 47*, 1597-1611.

American Psychological Association (2002). *Ethical principles of psychologists and code of conduct.* http://www.apa.org/ethics/code.html

Cares Northwest (2002). Directory of state reporting agencies. http://caresnw.org/state.htm *Child Abuse Prevention and Treatment Act (CAPTA)(Jan. 1996 version)*, 42 U.S.C. 5101, *et seq.*

Chafetz, M.D., Friedman, A.L., Kevorkian, C.G., & Levy, J.K. (1996). The cerebellum and cognitive function: Implications for rehabilitation. *Archives of Physical Medicine and Rehabilitation, 77*, 1303-1308.

Clark, E. (1997). Children and adolescents with traumatic brain injury: Reintegration challenges in educational settings. In E.D. Bigler, E. Clark, & J.E. Farmer (Eds.), *Childhood traumatic brain injury: Diagnosis, assessment, and intervention* (pp. 191-211). Austin: Pro-Ed.

Cohen, S. (1996). Practical guidelines for teachers. In A. Goldberg (Ed.), *Acquired brain injury in childhood and adolescence: A team and family guide to educational program development and implementation* (pp. 126-170). Springfield, IL: Charles C. Thomas Publisher.

Cummings, J. (1985). Behavioral disorders associated with frontal lobe injury. In J. Cummings (Ed.), *Clinical Neuropsychiatry* (pp. 57-67). Orlando, FL: Grune & Stratton.

Daum, I., & Ackermann, H. (1995). Cerebellar contributions to cognition. *Behavioural Brain Research, 67*, 201-210.

Desmond, J.E., Gabrieli, J.D.E., Sobel, N., Rabin, L.A., Wagner, A.D., Seger, C.A., & Glover, G.H. (1996). An MRI study of frontal cortex and cerebellum during semantic and working memory tasks. *Society for Neuroscience Abstracts, 22*, 111.

Ekstrand, R., & Brousaides, E. (1996). Special education law. In A. Goldberg (Ed.), *Acquired brain injury in childhood and adolescence: A team and family guide to educational program development and implementation* (pp. 55-89). Springfield, IL: Charles C. Thomas Publisher.

Farmer, J.E., Clippard, D.S., Luehr-Wiemann, Y., Wright, E., & Owings, S. (1997). Assessing children with traumatic brain injury during rehabilitation: Promoting school and community reentry. In E.D. Bigler, E. Clark, & J.E. Farmer (Eds.), *Childhood traumatic brain injury: Diagnosis, assessment, and intervention* (pp. 33-62). Austin: Pro-Ed.

Grafman, J., Litvan, I., Massaquoi, S., Stewart, M., Sirigu, A., & Hallett, M. (1992). Cognitive planning deficit in patients with cerebellar atrophy. *Neurology, 42*, 1493-1496.

Graham, L., & Goldberg, A. (1996). Organizing a consultation system for brain injured students. In A. Goldberg (Ed.), *Acquired brain injury in childhood and adolescence: A team and family guide to educational program development and implementation* (pp. 119-125). Springfield, IL: Charles C. Thomas Publisher.

Greve, K.W., & Stanford, M.S. (1999). Cognitive and emotional sequelae of cerebellar infarct: A case report. *Archives of Clinical Neuropsychology, 14*, 455-469.

Individuals with Disabilities Education Act. 20 U.S.C. §1400 *et seq.*

Lehr, E. (1990). *Psychologial management of traumatic brain injuries in children and adolescents.* Rockville: Aspen Publishers.

Leiner, H.C., Leiner, A.L., & Dow, R.S. (1991). The human cerebro-cerebellar system: Its computing, cognitive, and language skills. *Behavioural Brain Research, 44*, 113-128.

National Clearinghouse on Child Abuse and Neglect Information (2002). http://www.calib.com/nccanch/statutes/index.cfm

Nordlund, M. (1996). Consultation models. In A. Goldberg (Ed.), *Acquired brain injury in childhood and adolescence: A team and family guide to educational program development and implementation* (pp. 113-118). Springfield, IL: Charles C. Thomas Publisher.

Rehabilitation Act of 1973, 29 U.S.C. §§706, 791-795.

Smith, S. (2002). *Mandatory child abuse reporting.* http://www.smith-lawfirm.com.

Section 8

ETHICAL CHALLENGES IN GERIATRIC NEUROPSYCHOLOGY

Introduction

Researchers and practitioners in geriatric neuropsychology are faced with many challenges that neuropsychologists working with younger populations may not experience or may experience to lesser degrees. For example, the elderly as a group tend to have more medical problems than younger individuals, thus requiring more medications, both of which have the potential to impact cognition. In addition, decrements in cognition are associated with the "normal" aging process. Estimates indicate that prevalence rates for dementia for those over 85 years of age are between 25% and 50% (American Psychiatric Association, 1997). With base rates that high for dementia, and with others experiencing Mild Cognitive Impairment, patients, families, and other referral sources may not get the easy answer they are looking for to the question, "Is it Alzheimer's or just normal aging?"

The ability to integrate issues of age-related cognitive decline with the many other risk factors for cognitive impairment related to aging with known neurological injury requires a high degree of professional competence specific to geriatric neuropsychology. It also requires reliance on neuropsychological measures that may lack adequate representative normative data.

The elderly often face decreases, either sudden or incremental, in their autonomy. As a result, involvement in the informed consent process to the degree possible takes on added importance, and the need to balance their right to privacy with the need to ensure their safety becomes a necessary and challenging task. These issues and many others result in ethical challenges. In a previous chapter by Morgan (2002) and in the current text, the authors illustrate and examine many such ethical challenges facing neuropsychologists working with geriatric individuals and their social systems. Their insights offer neuropsychologists a blueprint for addressing ethical challenges when they arise with this population.

References

American Psychiatric Association (1997). Practice guideline for the treatment of patients with Alzheimer's disease and other dementias of late life. *American Journal of Psychiatry, 154* (Suppl.), 1-39.

Morgan, J.E. (2002). Ethical issues in the practice of geriatric neuropsychology. In S.S. Bush & M.L. Drexler (Eds.), *Ethical issues in clinical neuropsychology,* 87-101. Lisse, NL: Swets & Zeitlinger Publishers.

Chapter 16

ETHICAL CHALLENGES IN GERIATRIC NEUROPSYCHOLOGY, PART I

A. John McSweeny

Scenario 1

A 67-year-old Hispanic female who received an apparent head injury resulting from a fall is referred for a neuropsychological evaluation by her primary-care physician. Although the patient does not speak English well, she is accompanied to the first appointment with the neuropsychologist by her husband who does speak English. The husband serves as interpreter for his wife and also provides additional history. The patient and her husband are recent immigrants from a South American country. There are several bruises on the wife's face and arms, which the husband also states are the result of his wife's fall.

A somewhat abbreviated but otherwise standard neuropsychological evaluation is conducted with the husband again serving as interpreter. The results are below average for the patient's age and educational level (sixth grade), particularly with respect to language-based tasks. The neuropsychologist is aware of the language issues in the evaluation and so writes the report providing tentative conclusions. However, he does suggest that patient's cognitive functioning is abnormal and that the impairment may be secondary to early dementia, a head injury, or a combination of the two etiologies. He also notes the difference between the verbal and nonverbal performances and raises the issue of possible hemisphere-specific injuries.

The patient is referred back to her primary-care physician for follow-up with a recommendation for a re-evaluation in six months to determine her course of recovery or possible decline.

Relevant Ethical Issues

Beneficence

This case presents an ethical issue that is familiar to neuropsychologists who work with patients of all ages. The patient's history, which cannot be verified independently of the husband's report and translation of his wife's report, combined with the presence of visible bruises on the patient's arms and face, provides for suspicion of spousal abuse. A quick review of the 2002 APA Ethics code does not reveal a specific standard that applies to this situation. However, General Principle A (Beneficence and Nonmaleficence) may apply in a somewhat indirect fashion. It is clear that the neuropsychologist should recognize that the wife may be at risk for physical abuse. In addition, given her limited competence with English and the likelihood that she is unfamiliar with the legal and support systems in her adopted country, she probably has few options to seek help on her own. Accordingly, the neuropsychologist has an ethical obligation to further assess the situation and take appropriate action.

Competence

The second major ethical issue in this case involves the patient's linguistic and cultural background. There are several ethical standards from the 2002 Ethics Code that potentially apply. Standard 2.01 (Boundaries of Competence) would certainly apply. The neuropsychologist is required to provide services only in those areas in which appropriate education, training, and experience have been received. The neuropsychologist's unfamiliarity with Spanish is evident by his use of the husband as an interpreter. Artiola and Mullaney (1998) have taken the position that patients should always be tested in their own language by someone who understands the subtleties of the patient's culture. The circumstances of the present case make it clear that the neuropsychologist does not meet this standard.

Human Differences

General Principle E (Respect for People's Rights and Dignity) applies to the present case in a very direct fashion. Neuropsychologists must be aware of and respect differences in the cultures, roles, and individual aspects of those who they evaluate and treat and take such factors into account when working with members of different groups. Standard 2.01(b) (Boundaries of Competence) reinforces the points made by Principle E and specifies that where knowledge in the discipline has established that an understanding of such differences is essential for effective service implementation, neuropsychologists must possess or obtain the appropriate skills or make an appropriate referral. Of course, there are situations in which neuropsychologists may need to perform evaluations which lie at the edge, or perhaps even slightly over the edge, of their boundaries of competence. These would include situations such as emergencies and locations where there are no neuropsychologists competent to assess the patient in his or her own language. In these situations, adaptations such as the use of interpreters may be employed, but the limitations of the results should be discussed fully in any report (Standard 9.06, Interpreting Test Results).

Incidentally, it should be obvious that the use of family members as interpreters in neuropsychological evaluations is undesirable for several reasons. First, there may be information that the patient does not wish to share with other family members or in the presence of family members. This is certainly possible in cases of suspected abuse. Second, family members may add to, delete from, or otherwise edit their interpretations of what both the patient and the neuropsychologist are saying. Finally, family members may not be competent in the language of the examiner and thus may not transmit instructions to the patient accurately. If an interpreter is to be used it should be someone with native fluency in both the examiner's and the patient's language, preferably a certified medical interpreter.

Assessment

Standard 9.02 (Use of Assessments) also applies in a specific fashion to the present case. This standard requires neuropsychologists to base their choice of procedures and measures on evidence of the usefulness and proper application of the techniques for the examinee. Such evidence would include established reliability and validity with members of the population being evaluated, taking into account the examinee's language preference and competence. The neuropsychologist in this case apparently used standard test instruments that presumably were normed on North American English-speaking populations and are thus inappropriate for use with a Spanish-speaking person from another region of the world. Again, it is recognized that neuropsychological instruments in languages other than English may not be readily available. Fortunately, this situation appears to be changing with the publication of several neuropsychological tests in Spanish that have been normed with North American Hispanic populations, although ironically such tests may also have not been ideal in the current case given the patient was not a North American native.

A final issue in this case concerns whether the techniques used in the evaluation and the results they provided are sufficient to draw conclusions about brain function. This is the concern of Standard 9.01(a) (Bases for Assessments). Neuropsychologists are to base the opinions contained in their reports on appropriate and sufficient information and techniques. The neuropsychologist in this case did not draw firm conclusions about hemisphere-specific brain impairment, but it is questionable whether the techniques he utilized would justify even suggesting regional impairment. Similarly, suggesting early dementia also seems inappropriate given the limitations of conducting an evaluation of a non-English-speaking person using an interpreter with instruments normed with English-speaking North Americans.

Case Resolution

The neuropsychologist was informed that the patient's primary care physician received the report, but no other information was exchanged about the case. The patient did not return for the recommended 6-month follow-up. An attempt was made to contact her with one phone call and one letter, but there was no reply to either. The neuropsychologist considered the case closed and never heard anything else from, or about, the patient.

Conclusions and Recommendations

This case represents the ease with which inadequate work can be performed with unknown ramifications for the patient and no apparent consequences for the clinician. With regard to suspicions of spousal abuse, neuropsychologists should contact a person with some expertise in handling such matters. If the neuropsychologist is employed in a hospital or agency, there may be a designated individual, often a social worker, whom the neuropsychologist can consult with. If the neuropsychologist is in private practice, he/she may wish to discuss the situation with a trusted colleague who may know the resources and legal context associated with spousal abuse in the neuropsychologist's community, which can vary considerably. It may be legally required to report suspected spousal abuse to authorities in some states, whereas in others reporting suspected abuse without the patient's permission might constitute a violation of privacy.

Regarding concerns about language and culture, it tends to be best if the neuropsychologist can refer the patient to a competent neuropsychologist who has native fluency in the patient's preferred language and who has access to and experience with materials for assessing such individuals. If this is not possible for reasons of geography or resources, the neuropsychologist may need the weigh the costs and benefits of not conducting any assessment versus conducting an assessment that might provide inaccurate or misleading results. As an alternative, the neuropsychologist may wish to work closely with a member of related discipline, such as a clinical psychologist, neurologist, or psychiatrist, who is fluent in the patient's preferred language and who can conduct an extended mental status exam. Using an interpreter is also possible but has limitations given that instructions and answers may not be accurately transmitted and the test materials may not be appropriately normed.

The following recommendations are offered:

1. Determine, preferably in advance, the local legal requirements and strictures with respect to reporting suspected child and spousal abuse.
2. Identify and consult colleagues within psychology and other disciplines who have expertise in abuse issues.

3. Identify colleagues within neuropsychology and related disciplines who have native fluency in other languages and are able to perform assessments within those languages based on their training, experience and access to appropriate materials and techniques. Refer patients to these persons or collaborate with them in the assessment process as appropriate.

Scenario 2

A 79-year-old female was referred for a neuropsychological evaluation by her primary care physician in order to make a differential diagnosis between depression and dementia. She had generally been known as a social person who was active in the community. Recently she had become less socially active and more dependent on immediate family members, including her husband and son. To some extent, her decline in social activity could be attributed to multiple medical problems.

The evaluation revealed very mild cognitive impairment but not dementia. In addition, the results of the interview and a depression checklist were consistent with a clinically significant depression. Indeed, the patient complained in detail about being lonely. She felt abandoned due to no longer being able to participate with her family and friends as she had previously had the ability to do.

The neuropsychologist met with the patient for a feedback session following the evaluation and discussed the results and the patient's concerns at length. The primary recommendation was for the patient to accept a referral to a mental health professional for treatment of her depression and to consult her primary-care physician regarding appropriate strategies for the prevention of dementia. In addition, the neuropsychologist suggested that the patient join a "Senior Center" where she could participate in social activities. However, the patient refused this suggestion, noting that she had limited transportation

and that she didn't want to be around "those old people." During the feedback session the neuropsychologist and the patient discovered a common ethnic and linguistic heritage. The patient seemed quite pleased with this discovery and related that she had not had the opportunity to talk to someone in the language of her parents after they had died several years before. This led to a discussion of their common experiences as the descendants of immigrants from a small European country. For example, they noted the difficulties they had with living in a society that had customs and expectations that diverged so greatly from the customs and expectations of family members. The neuropsychologist shared that this was still a relevant issue for her as it affected her relationship with her own children. After this discussion, the neuropsychologist repeated her recommendations and closed the feedback session.

Sometime after the feedback session, the patient called the neuropsychologist and stated that she wished "just to talk". Although the neuropsychologist's practice did not include psychotherapeutic services, she agreed to see the patient once more. At the follow-up session the patient reported that she had seen a psychiatrist but was unhappy with her treatment because the psychiatrist "just wanted to give me medication." The psychiatrist had referred the patient to another mental-health professional who provides psychotherapy but the patient indicated her dissatisfaction with this practitioner as well because she wasn't a psychiatrist. The patient emphasized how unhappy she was in general but how pleased she was to have the opportunity to talk to someone with a common ethnic heritage, who reminded her of her nieces who now lived some distance from the patient's home. The patient offered to help the neuropsychologist improve her fluency in their ancestral language and then left a box of home-cooked cookies "to share with your staff."

Shortly after the feedback session, the patient contacted the neuropsychologist again and again complained of her unhappiness and her desire to come in "just to talk" once more. The neuropsychologist demurred but did encourage the patient to reconsider her decision to reject mental health treatment. A day later the patient left a phone message for the neuropsychologist stating that she had wanted to thank the neuropsychologist for her assistance and for being an upstanding example of their ethnic community. Several days later, a package arrived for which the neuropsychologist had to sign a receipt. When she opened it she found an antique cameo necklace, broach, and bracelet. In addition, there was a note thanking the neuropsychologist for her assistance and "being the daughter I never had".

Relevant Ethical Issues

The primary issue here is one of multiple relationships. The neuropsychologist, by attempting to be "friendly" in the context of recognizing a common ethnic and linguistic bond with an emotionally needy patient, has inadvertently entered a second, nonprofessional relationship with the patient. It is evident from the case that the neuropsychologist did not actively seek this relationship but did acquiesce, to some extent, to the patient's active attempts to establish a more personal relationship. In addition, the fact that the patient and the neuropsychologist had faced common problems related to their ethnic heritage in their personal lives helped form the secondary, non-professional relationship, at least in the mind of the patient.

The primary standard from the 2002 Ethics Code that applies is 3.05 (Multiple Relationships). This standard requires psychologists to avoid entering into two or more roles with the same person, or someone close to the person with whom the psychologist has a relationship, if the potential for exploitation or harm exists. Sources of harm may include decreased objectivity, competence, or effectiveness in performing professional functions. It might be argued that Standard 2.06 (Personal Problems and Conflicts) could

also potentially apply, given that the neuropsychologist shared how her ethnic background had caused her problems, which extended into the present. According to Standard 2.06, psychologists are required to avoid initiating an activity if there is a substantial likelihood that their personal problems will interfere with their professional responsibilities. The neuropsychologist no doubt thought she was simply "being human" in sharing her experiences with the patient, but it appears that the patient, motivated by her own emotional needs, interpreted the sharing as an overture to developing a nonprofessional relationship.

Finally, Standard 6.05 (Barter with Clients/Patients) could apply if the neuropsychologist decided to accept the gift of the jewelry as a "thank you" for her services. However, the neuropsychologist had not initiated the gift receipt, so unless she failed to return the gift, this standard would not be relevant.

Case Resolution

After the neuropsychologist received the gift of jewelry and the note from the patient, she decided to consult with her colleagues in the clinic geriatrics and dementia program where she worked. As a result of her consultations, the neuropsychologist decided to return the gift via registered mail with a note indicating that she appreciated the patient's intentions but that accepting the gift would violate her ethical standards. In addition, the neuropsychologist emphasized that her relationship with the patient was a professional one and that her services had, for the present time, been completed. The neuropsychologist again encouraged the patient to follow through on her recommendations for mental health treatment and suggested that she contact her geriatrician or the social worker at the clinic for a referral to another psychotherapist, given that she was unhappy with the first practitioner that she consulted. The patient later contacted the neuropsychologist to apologize for "getting you in trouble." The neuro-psychologist assured the patient that she was not "in trouble" but she stated that she wished to keep her relationship with patient at a professional level despite their common ethnic/linguistic heritage.

Conclusions and Recommendations

In the evaluation of the patients' emotional func-tioning, neuropsychologists may find it beneficial to assess the potential for transference issues to emerge that may affect their expectations about the nature of the relationship and the services provided. Neuropsychologists should make clear that their relationships with patients should remain at a professional level and that such boundaries are in the best interest of the patients. In situations where the boundaries between "being human" and multiple relationships may be unclear,

neuropsychologists should discuss the issue with colleagues who can look at the situation objectively and provide advice.

Acknowledgment

The author would like to express his appreciation to Lisa Keaton, M.S.W., Geriatric Social Worker at the Medical College of Ohio Center for Successful Aging, for her assistance with the second case.

Reference

Artiola i Fortuny, L., & Mullaney, H.A. (1998). Assessing patients whose language you do not know: Can the absurd be ethical? *The Clinical Neuropsychologist, 12 (1)*, 113-126.

Chapter 17

ETHICAL CHALLENGES IN GERIATRIC NEUROPSYCHOLOGY, PART II

Joel E. Morgan

Scenario 1

It seems that you are contacted by an attorney; he got your name from a lawyer for whom you worked before who recommended you highly. He asks how much you know about, "memory problems in the elderly". You explain that you have had considerable experience in geriatric assessment, and he explains the case to you. The attorney is a Federal Public Defender. He tells you about the defendant (your examinee). Seems he was indicted for having stolen hundreds of thousands of dollars from the union of which he was in charge. But this allegedly happened 25 years ago and now he claims he doesn't remember. You are asked to determine his competence to stand trial and you accept the case, after all the appropriate arrangements have been made.

The examinee is a 78-year-old widower in poor health. He comes to the appointment accompanied by his "kid brother", a youngster of 74! They are nervous, and the younger brother does a lot of the talking. He tells you that the examinee is in poor health; he is diabetic, overweight, has hypertension, and a history of one mild MI. He is on many medications. He has no psychiatric or frank neurologic history. You review the medical record provided by the attorney as part of the discovery package, which corroborates what you have been told. There is a report of a recent MRI which indicates, "... multiple minute areas of white matter disease throughout frontal subcortical regions ... likely consistent with cerebrovascular disease ..." It is signed by a neuroradiologist that you know and respect.

The examinee's brother then proceeds to explain that the examinee has no idea what this whole thing is about, that when the examinee was the union boss, he took care of the union members – whatever they needed – an operation for this one's wife; braces for that one's kid; help with college expenses for X and Y's mom in the nursing home. Whatever the members needed, he was there. No one asked any questions; he helped them all. You are informed that the union members loved the examinee, "... he took good care of them ... he never took a penny for himself – he lives like a pauper – always has." He is quick to point out that none of it – "... not one cent, doc, was for himself – you should see how he lives – he has nothing – never has. He is not interested in himself; only wanted to help the guys." He is a H.S. graduate who worked his way up the union ladder, having been a police officer for many years, then eventually union rep, and finally union boss. The examinee nods his head. Soon you ask the examinee's brother to leave and proceed with the examination and testing.

Test Results

Neuropsychological examination soon indicates that the examinee is not the most cooperative of subjects. He performed in the questionable range on symptom validity tests, scoring above chance but below the "cutoff" on the TOMM (32 Trial 1; 40 Trial 2) and the Victoria Symptom Validity Test (20/24 "easy"; 14/24 "hard"). You give him the VIP. "Hey doc, this is hard. I never seen ones like this before ..." He ultimately has a "Careless Response Set", but not intentional failure.

You observe that he is rather unwell. He is obese with labored breathing, lethargic, and has slow processing. He nearly dozed off in the middle of testing! You check his medications for poly-pharmacy but see nothing there. You think to yourself, "... this sure is consistent with vascular dementias ..."

You are finally able to complete the battery. He scored between the borderline range and average range on all tests. "Hmmm ...," you think, "that doesn't look like a 'dementia' – exactly." His scores on anterograde memory tests are universally borderline. But he seems to remember what he learns and rapid forgetting is not observed. Effort was variable; he seemed to put in less effort on more difficult tasks.

In between appointments with him, you have a chance to fully review the enormous discovery file provided to you by his counsel. Seems he is accused of embezzling over $300,000 of union funds! The FBI had been gathering information, including banking records, on him for years. But it was true that he had no significant assets of his own; no offshore bank accounts; no other residences; no lavish lifestyle; he drove a 1993 Buick with 120,000 miles on it; his clothes were circa 1990 – J.C. Penny-style; nothing! In fact the FBI stated no motive for his alleged embezzlement. But FBI accountants' reports indicated that he kept very bad records; deposits and withdrawals were not properly annotated. The books *did* look bad, real bad!

Now that you have completed your formal neuropsychological assessment, you decided to interview him in depth; you ask him detailed questions about what he did or did not remember vis-à-vis his handling of union funds. You think this was a crucial step in your assessment of his competency. But you wonder to yourself, "Well, if there is a dementia on board, it seems relatively mild, especially considering his probable premorbid abilities. ... He is exhibiting only borderline anterograde memory loss and holds on to what he learned ... but is it really possible that he could have such limited recollection of what happened and his handling of union funds? That would suggest a more severe retrograde memory loss ... hmmmm ..."

The examinee and his brother come for the interview. The brother wants to be in the room to help the examinee. You say "no" of course. "But he's old, Doc. He doesn't remember." You explain to the brother that you need to see that for yourself. You'll speak to the brother alone later.

You have prepared many questions to ask the examinee. It doesn't seem to matter what you ask about those years as union boss, he seems to remember very little – and – he is very vague. But you get the sense that he really isn't exaggerating – he genuinely seems not to remember. As a well-trained neuropsychologist, you also prepared a number of questions about current events of that era (Jimmy Carter's presidency, assassination attempt on Reagan, etc). He has only vague recollection of this stuff, as well. You're really trying to figure this out ... you've determined that he has mild cognitive impairment – maybe barely meeting criteria for dementia, mild at that ... but his retrograde/long-term memory is disproportionately poor. He has limited reasoning ability as well – and has a hard time with novel problem solving. Executive functions such as set shifting, switching, planning and initiation are all borderline/mildly impaired. He does exhibit cognitive slowing rather consistently. But does this actually meet the criteria for "INCOMPETENCY TO STAND

TRIAL" in the legal sense? Are you *really sure* he isn't exaggerating?

Your Conclusions/Opinion

Not that you don't do this with every case, but you really think this one through carefully. After careful data analysis and bringing everything in, you diagnose the examinee with a mild dementia syndrome, consistent with a vascular etiology. But even more importantly in terms of the referral – you determine that he is competent to stand trial, *and can assist his attorney to a reasonable extent*. Although it is true that he claims not to remember important historical details of bank transactions and other information, in the eyes of the law he is competent *enough* to stand trial.[1] Surely you have concerns that the material evidence gathered by prosecution might overwhelm the examinee's reasoning and memory abilities, but in the eyes of the law you feel he has sufficient mental capacity. Besides, to be perfectly honest with yourself, you aren't 100% sure he isn't exaggerating, are you?

Relevant Ethical Issues

This is a somewhat more complex case than one might suspect on the surface. From the forensic perspective, the ethical neuropsychologist must be certain to operate from a perspective of "clinical-scientific" neutrality, despite which side has retained you. What that boils down to is taking the attitude that you will do your best, not to *help* retaining counsel, but to make sure that you, "Tell it like it is and let the chips fall where they may" (Standards 3.06, Conflict of Interest, & 3.07, Third Party Requests for Services). In essence, while you are hired by counsel, and technically

counsel is your client, it would be unethical to color your opinion in one direction or another; one must remain objective to the scientific (neuropsychological) evidence (data) and have previously communicated this position this to counsel prior to being retained. Despite some pressure from counsel ("Doc I can't get anywhere with him. He says he doesn't remember, and he's always cranky. He seems incompetent to me!) and the examinee's brother, ("Doc, he's a great guy – never tried to steal a dime – he used it to help the poor sick kids – on my mother's grave …"), you stuck to your objective, neutral position and maintained your scientific and ethical principles.

Geriatric neuropsychological assessment requires a set of competencies that a psychologist may not have obtained in pursuing a doctoral degree, state licensure, or recognition by their profession or community (Tuokko & Hadjistavropoulos, 1998). This is so regardless of demonstrated competence in other areas of professional psychology, e.g., general clinical psychology. The examinee was a 78-year-old man in poor health. Neuropsychologists in such situations must be competent in geriatric assessment, familiar with appropriate test procedures, age-education-ethnicity-appropriate norms, and have had supervision in geriatric assessment and diagnoses to competently participate in this evaluation (Standards 2.01, Boundaries of Competence; 2.03, Maintaining Competence; 9.01, Bases of Assessment; & 9.06, Interpreting Assessment Results). Further, the neuropsychologist is obliged to obtain informed consent from the examinee (Standard 9.03, Informed Consent in Assessments).

Case Resolution

In the end the defendant went to trial. The judge read and appreciated your report and applauded your neutrality. Because the judge agreed that the defendant was somewhat compromised, the defendant's ultimate sentence was lessened.

---

[1] The Competency Test: "The test must be whether the defendant has sufficient present ability to consult with his attorney with a reasonable degree of rational understanding and a rational as well as factual understanding of the proceedings against him." See *Dusky v. United States* 362 U.S. 407 (960).

Conclusions/Recommendations

Individuals in the geriatric population often have sensory, motor, cognitive, emotional, social and/or behavioral difficulties that must be understood by neuropsychologists examining and/or treating such individuals. Such competence in geriatric neuropsychology requires special education, training, and experience. competence will be reflected in the use of appropriate measures and norms and the integration of appropriate scientific evidence into data analysis and interpretation.

Scenario 2

The patient is a 93-year-old widow. She had been living rather successfully on her own until recently when she suffered a rather debilitating left hemisphere stroke. She has quite a dense right hemiparesis, and almost total loss of the use of her right hand and leg. Her speech is improving, you are told, but she still has quite an expressive aphasia as far as you can tell. Fortunately, she seems to understand what you are saying to her – when she can hear it! She had significant bilateral hearing loss, premorbidly. But thankfully she can read – though cannot write due to hemiparesis.

Her family is placing her in a nursing home and they have contacted you to do a neuropsychological evaluation as part of the admission process. This nursing home appreciates neuropsychology and what it can add to an understanding of a patient's strengths and weaknesses. You set the appointment.

On the day of her appointment, the patient arrives in a wheelchair accompanied by her daughter and son-in-law. "We'd take mom home with us if we had the room ...," they say. You go over her social, educational, and medical history. She is a 93-year-old, right-handed, widowed female, currently 6 weeks s/p left CVA. Seems the patient was a nurse, not just your basic RN, though, the patient had a Ph.D. in Nursing (Yale,

1930!) and was Dean of the College of Nursing of one of New York's most prestigious universities, a job she held for more than twenty years prior to retirement at age 66 (27 years ago). "She was born and raised in New England and completed her Bachelor's degree and RN from the University of Vermont prior to Yale. Wow," you think, "... pretty impressive credentials." Her family tells you that she was an accomplished woman, had been married to a physician (deceased eleven years ago) and had raised two daughters. You obtain informed consent from the family and proceed with testing – er, assessment.

Well, here are the facts: She cannot hear. She had hearing aides but they were lost, and new ones have not arrived yet. Besides, the audiologist's report indicates that even with hearing aides she will still have 90+% hearing loss, bilaterally. Her children communicate with her by writing and she seems to be able to read okay. She appears to understand and attempts to speak – but she's very Broca-ish and it's very hard to discern what she is trying to say with her paraphasias and staccato speech. She can't write, either, since she's a hemi. You think, "How am I going to do this?" Luckily enough she obviously has vision. Her left hand is unaffected, and she has barely discernable speech. This won't be easy.

Choosing a 'Battery'

You think of what are the best tests to determine if or how much cognitive decline might be present. You know memory testing is critical and you realize that formal tests will be difficult – all but perhaps visual perceptual and recognition memory tests. Fluency is out. But you think you will try the Boston Naming Test (BNT). You decide to administer an "adapted" Dementia Rating Scale (DRS; Mattis, 1973). Here's how you adapt the test: *You write out all the instructions and have her read them, subtest-by-subtest.* You ask her to do the motor part only with her left hand. Any pointing is also done with the left hand. Instead of testing auditory verbal memory, you test *visual* verbal memory. You attempt to discern her responses as best you can. You decide you need more memory testing, so you decide to use a completely visual verbal and non-verbal memory test, the Recognition Memory Test (Warrington, 1984) – but the problem is – the norms only go up to age 70, but she's 93! Can you really use those norms? You use it anyway. You also decide to use the WAIS-III for some areas, such as verbal abstraction (after all, Similarities mostly requires a one or two word answer – she can manage that, you think). But the WAIS-III only goes up to age 89. After a little research, you decide to use the WAIS-R with the Mayo norms supplement (Ivnik et al., 1992).

You collect the data. So okay, you've got what you *think* are "legitimate scores" on the WAIS-R and possibly the BNT. But the "adapted" DRS? The norms on the Warrington? You're not sure how Kosher it was to use them. You decide that the best way to handle the Warrington is to first check with colleagues to see if anyone has developed norms for that age group, even unpublished ones (you think that had you had more time or thought about it earlier, you could have done this in advance for other tests as well, instead of scrambling at the last minute). You even call around and e-mail some senior colleagues and editors of leading journals. But no luck. You think maybe you'll have to throw the data out. Then it dawns on you, why not calculate what the scores for that age group might be based upon the norms for the other age groups, a predicted normative table? You do exactly that. You even check with some senior folks who are far better at statistics, and they tell you that this is a good approach.

Interpreting Cautiously

With it all, you interpret your scores with a great deal of caution. You give caveats about the limitations of these tests and ultimately the validity of the interpretations/conclusions. Since she had a high premorbid level of education, it is clear to you that she was bright, likely very bright. After

deliberating with colleagues, seeking supervision and saying a few prayers, you are ready to announce to the family that you think the patient has only minimal decline; that her aphasia and hemiparesis and a little depression make it appear worse than it actually is. The family, patient, and nursing home are pleased.

Ethical Considerations

The major ethical concern of this case dealt with assessment issues and the appropriateness of tailoring assessment instruments to meet the individual needs of patients in unusual situations, but within the spirit of the Ethics Code. Above all, neuropsychologists must be cognizant of these issues and take every measure to do no harm to their clients (Standard 3.04, Do No Harm). An incorrect diagnosis is very damaging to the patient, their family, and ultimately to the profession. Neuropsychologists make every effort to make correct diagnoses, even if it requires going to great pains to do so.

Neuropsychologists must base their conclusions on established scientific knowledge and procedures (Standard 2.04, Bases of Scientific and Professional Judgments). But what if there are no *established* procedures? As in the case example, one must ensure that all possible stones have been uncovered, seek out supervision by senior colleagues and peers, and adapt instruments with care and caution.

It is crucial that psychologists state the limitations of their conclusions when their methods and procedures have not been scientifically validated. Standard 9.02 (Use of Assessments) informs that we must use instruments that have passed scientific scrutiny (9.02a), that have been validated with members of the population being tested (9.02b), and that psychologists use methods appropriate to a person's language preferences (9.02c). Neuropsychologists make further effort to interpret their test data taking into account many factors and individual differences

(Standard 9.06, Interpreting Assessment Results). This would certainly include age and physical limitations, as in the present case. Limitations of the interpretations in this case were properly noted.

As a final thought, one might argue that the use of the WAIS-R was inappropriate, in consideration of Standard 9.08 (Obsolete Tests and Outdated Test Results). But the utility of the WAIS-R with the Mayo Norms would seem to give less concern about the possible violation of that standard. In fact, this was the logical thing to do, given the age range of the WAIS-III standardization sample. Similarly, one might argue that the use of Warrington Recognition Memory Test was inappropriate since the norms only go up to age 70 and you must attempt to calculate an extension, whereas the norms for the WMS-III Faces subtest goes to 90. But you have carefully considered the characteristics of both measures, have considered the advantages and limitations of both, and have made a decision that you feel you would be on solid ground defending.

Case Resolution

Ultimately, with conservative interpretation, your conclusions seemed to be fairly accurate. With continued speech therapy, the patient regained much of her expressive abilities and indeed, as her speech improved, it became easier to see that she was functioning quite well. In fact, she was one of the highest functioning residents of the nursing home, despite being among the oldest!

Conclusions and Recommendations

Ever have to evaluate a patient who had multi-system sensory-motor loss? What can you do when you'd like to administer the Rey Auditory Verbal Learning Test or CVLT (or any auditory-verbal memory test) – but your patient can't hear at all? How about motor speed tests – Finger

Tapping – in an older person with such profound bilateral arthritis that her hands remain in a rigid knurled position? So much for construction/assembly tasks, too. But you say, "Hey, they never taught me about being this flexible in graduate school, internship, or my post-doc! Is it okay to modify; if so, how much? How do I know what the scores mean?" How do you know, indeed?

Adapting our formal tests and procedures to accommodate the ill and elderly (and any special population) is sometimes necessary in the ethical practice of clinical neuropsychology. The present case is just one example of many encountered on a daily basis.

"A competent, well-trained neuropsychologist should be able to assess anyone at any time, even without formal tests. Imagine for a moment if Wolfgang Kohler had been a neuropsychologist on the island of Tenerife … and the apes had been brain injured humans …" (Harold Goodglass, Ph.D., ABPP, Personal Communication, 1999).

References

Ivnik, R.J., Malec, J.F., Smith, G.E., Tangalos, E.G., Petersen, R.C., Kikmen, E., & Kurkland, L.T. (1992). Mayo's older Americans normative studies: WAIS-R norms for ages 56-97. *The Clinical Neuropsychologist, 6* (Suppl), 1-30.

Kaplan, E., Goodglass, H., & Weintraub, S. (1983). *Boston Naming Test.* Philadelphia: Lee and Fibger.

Mattis, S. (1973). *Dementia Rating Scale professional manual.* Odessa, FL: Psychological Assessment Resources.

Tuokko, H., & Hadjistavropoulos, T. (1998). *An assessment guide to geriatric neuropsychology.* Mahwah, NJ: Lawrence Erlbaum.

Warrington, E. (1984). *Recognition Memory Test.* Berkshire, UK: NFER-Nelson Publishing Co., Ltd.

Section 9

ETHICAL CHALLENGES WITH ETHNICALLY AND CULTURALLY DIVERSE POPULATIONS IN NEUROPSYCHOLOGY

Introduction

Ethical challenges in the consideration of racial, ethnic and cultural diversity pose considerable difficulty for neuropsychologists, as they cut across practice settings, age ranges, and neuropathological conditions. These challenges are faced not only by neuropsychologists representing dominant U.S. demographics but also by those neuropsychologists who are members of the minority groups with whom they work, as many of the measures used were not developed with such groups, and many of the studies relied upon for interpretation of test data did not adequately include such groups. In addition, some of the abilities commonly assessed by neuropsychologists may not be those that are important to members of different cultures, and the expression of certain abilities may differ (Iverson & Slick, 2003; Manly & Jacobs, 2002).

Neuropsychological functioning is dependent upon one's sociocultural background. Yet, despite commonalties that exist among members of the same races, ethnic backgrounds, and cultures, considerable intragroup heterogeneity also exists (Manly & Jacobs, 2002). Therefore, the neuropsychological evaluation must include a thorough clinical interview of the examinee's unique racial and ethnic identity and cultural background. Failure to consider factors such as race, nationality, place of birth, immigration status, the level at which the culture of origin is maintained, and perception of health care institutions and professionals will result in an increased likelihood of misdiagnosis. In addition, failure by examiners to consider their own feelings toward, and understanding of, members of different groups may contribute to misunderstanding of patients' neuropsychological functioning.

The use of interpreters poses unique challenges in neuropsychological assessment. Questions regarding when interpreters are necessary and who should serve as interpreters are difficult to answer in a universal and definitive manner. Although some generalization can be offered, questions about appropriate use of interpreters must often be answered on a case by case basis.

Many of the psychometric challenges faced in the assessment of racial or ethnic minorities are potentially insurmountable (Iverson & Slick, 2003). Ethical Standard 9.06 (Interpreting Assessment Results) requires psychologists to "take into account" the various factors that may affect the accuracy of their interpretations. However, due to the number of potentially invalidating factors, "in some situations, it is impossible to determine if the interpretations made by psychologists under these circumstances could be valid" (Iverson & Slick, 2003; p. 2078). When the neuropsychological assessment procedures are modified due to linguistic needs or the data used for interpretation do not adequately represent the sociocultural background of the examinee, the neuropsychologist must describe *explicitly* the limitations of the reliability and validity of the test results and the conclusions drawn (Iverson & Slick, 2003). Description of such limitations must go beyond the statement that "caution" was used in the interpretation and state clearly that the test results likely underrepresent the examinee's true level of neuropsychological functioning.

The challenges faced by neuropsychologists attempting to conduct valid assessments of diverse individuals may seem prohibitive, but they are not. With appropriate consideration of the issues examined in the following cases, neuropsychologists can continue to provide a valuable service to those in need. Although the APA Ethics Code offers guidance, as Harris (2002) pointed out, "The Ethics Code itself will not definitively instruct neuropsychologists on the course of action to take with ethnically, culturally, or linguistically diverse individuals" (p. 236). The neuropsychologist will best serve such individuals through personal acculturation, development of expertise, and support of the expansion of the empirical knowledge base related to specific languages, races, ethnic backgrounds, and cultures.

References

Harris, J. (2002). Ethical decision-making with individuals of diverse ethnic, cultural, and linguistic backgrounds. In S.S. Bush & M.L. Drexler (Eds.), *Ethical issues in clinical neuropsychology*, 87-101. Lisse, NL: Swets & Zeitlinger Publishers.

Iverson, G.L., & Slick, D.J. (2003). Ethical issues associated with psychological and neuropsychological assessment of persons from different cultural and linguistic backgrounds. In I.Z. Schultz & D.O. Brady (Eds.), *Psychological injuries at trial*, 2066-2087. Chicago: American Bar Association.

Manly, J.J., & Jacobs, D.M. (2002). Future directions in neuropsychological assessment with African Americans. In F.R. Ferraro (Ed.), *Minority and cross-cultural aspects of neuropsychological assessment*, 79-96. Lisse, NL: Swets & Zeitlinger Publishers.

Chapter 18

ETHICAL CHALLENGES WITH ETHNICALLY AND CULTURALLY DIVERSE POPULATIONS IN NEUROPSYCHOLOGY, PART I

Duane E. Dede

Scenario 1

A 57-year-old African-American woman is referred for neuropsychological testing after a one-year history of memory and attention problems. Her daughter became concerned about her level of functioning after the patient had difficulty recalling the names of family members during her visit over the holidays. Her daughter also stated that the patient had trouble coordinating the timings on the holiday meal and was unable to find her car in the parking lot during a visit to a local mall.

The patient lives alone, having become a widow nine months before. She lives in the southern United States. She has three adult children, the youngest living locally, and two small grandchildren. Her middle child has multiple sclerosis, and the patient is involved in her care periodically. She is recently retired from her work as a teaching assistant at a local elementary school. The patient completed the tenth grade in a small southern school before stopping school to care for her ailing mother at the time. She later obtained her GED but was unable to go on to college because she started raising her family.

The patient denies any history of abuse of alcohol or illicit substances. She does not smoke or use an excessive amount of caffeine. Further medical history is significant for hypothyroidism and mild obesity. She has no history of head injury or neurological disorder, nor is she taking any medications. She denied a family history of neurological disorders. Her appetite is within normal limits, but her sleep is occasionally marked by early and middle insomnia. Neuroimaging had not been ordered.

After being referred by her internist, the patient was seen for a neuropsychological evaluation by a European-American clinical psychologist who had some general training in neuropsychology but no formal education or training in cross-cultural issues. The patient's daughter came into town to accompany the patient to the appointment. Testing consisted of an interview with both women and a four-hour testing battery with the patient. She was cooperative with interview questions and most aspects of testing, save a few complaints about how long it was taking and "why are you asking all of these personal questions." She would occasionally say "I don't know" to the more difficult items.

She was oriented to person, place and time. Speech was fluent and free of evidence of thought disorder. Affect was of full range and congruent with the various subject matter.

Testing began with a Mini-Mental State Exam to establish baseline mental status. The patient earned a score of 28, missing two memory items. Her WAIS-III Full Scale IQ was in the lower end of the Average range, with only a slight PIQ > VIQ difference. Verbal Fluency (COWA) was intact, although she scored a little low (50) on the Boston Naming Test.

Psychomotor slowing was noted on the Trail-making Test, Part A, where she scored in the Mildly Impaired range. Yet, her Trails B score was in the Low Average range. Finger tapping speed was mildly impaired bilaterally, although dexterity (Grooved Pegboard test) was intact bilaterally.

The greatest relative difficulty was seen in the area of memory, where the patient scored in the Mild to Moderate Impairment range with the initial and delayed recall on the Wechsler Memory Scale-III stories. Interestingly, she only lost one bit of information of the limited amount she initially recalled on the story that was presented once, and she improved slightly following repeated exposure to the story that was repeated. Visual memory was in the Average range for both immediate and delayed recall. Further difficulty with verbal memory was seen on the California Verbal Learning Test, 2nd edition. Both List1 and Total Trial recall were in the Mildly Impaired range. Short delayed free recall was mildly impaired, but she did manifest a slight benefit from cueing. Recognition memory was perfect.

Assessment of emotional state consisted of an interview, observations, and her performance on the Beck Depression Inventory (BDI). In the interview, she acknowledged occasional periods of sadness and loneliness. Sleep was marked by early insomnia and she had lost twelve pounds since the death of her husband. The patient's score on the BDI was in the mildly depressed range. Symptoms included insomnia, decreased appetite, depressed mood, and increased problems with physical concerns.

The report concluded that the patient was suffering from the beginning stages of Dementia of the Alzheimer's Type. Evidence offered to support this diagnosis included the low memory scores, slowed processing speed, and naming difficulty. The psychologist concluded that the emotional issues were "diagnostically mild and reactive to her declines." The psychologist continued to note that grief was not likely a primary issue given the time since her husband had passed away. His recommendations included a referral to a neurologist for a trial of Aricept and talking with the family about planning for placement in the future. The family did not agree with the findings and asked a second psychologist to review the report to determine if there were grounds for a repeat evaluation.

Relevant Ethical Issues

Competence

Professional competence appears relevant in that the psychologist did not have the necessary neuropsychological or cross-cultural training to reach the conclusions he did in his report (Standard 2.01, Boundaries of Competence). The psychologist's diagnoses did not follow the convention of the collective knowledge base (Standard 2.04, Bases for Scientific and Professional Judgments). Several of the conclusions appear premature and appear to neglect some of the contextual issues in this case. The examiner did not appear to fully appreciate the contribution of culture and educational background to scores in this case. He also appeared to give short shrift to the impact of grieving and caregiving in this patient. The result is inappropriately attributing low test scores to a neurodegenerative process. The psychologist has a further responsibility to stay current with standards of practice and emerging knowledge through ongoing education (Standard 2.03, Maintaining Competence).

Assessment

The psychologist in the case example did not appear to fully appreciate the limitations of some of the measures in this case (Standard 9.02, Use of Assessments). For example, the Boston Naming Test has been found to yield false positives in individuals with limited formal education or in African American subjects (Lichtenberg, Ross, & Christensen, 1994). While a GED is a high school equivalency certificate, neuropsychological studies have found that individuals perform closer to the point that they discontinued their formal education than to that of a high school graduate. So, attributing impairment to a score of 50 on the Boston Naming Test seems inappropriate in this instance given her educational history and cultural status. In addition, a potential contributor to test performance in this case is the construct of stereotype threat (Stelle & Aronson, 1995). This construct has demonstrated that older African-American subjects often underperform on cognitive tests because of perceived demand characteristics of the test. Her good memory savings and her ability to profit from the cueing strategy on the California Verbal Learning Test offer further evidence of her relatively good memory functioning. The conclusions did not appear to fully appreciate the contribution of medical factors (hypothyroidism), cultural reasons for less than optimal effort, or emotional factors on her test scores. The patient's expression of emotional factors may have also been muted for cultural reasons. The BDI, for example is a face valid measure of depression and is open to response bias. Possible reasons for the patient to respond in a biased fashion are limited exposure or mistrust of mental health professionals. This subsection of the 2002 Code would call for the psychologist to qualify the limitations of his findings, which he failed to do.

Individual Differences

The psychologist did not appear to adequately consider the individual characteristics of this patient (Standard 9.06, Interpreting Assessment Results, 9.06). It is unlikely that in a one-hour interview he was able to determine her psychosocial history, medical history, current neuropsychological difficulties and their history, and her unique racial and cultural identity and experiences. As Manly and Jacobs (2002) explained, cognition is always embedded in the context of one's cultural. Factors such as level of acculturation, comfort with the medical/mental health system should be addressed. There may be many personal or historical reasons for these issues to be more salient.

Although her memory scores were somewhat low, they may be within expectations for someone of limited formal education who is likely depressed and whose scores have been compared to norms that were likely established on individuals who are culturally quite different from oneself.

Case Resolution

The second psychologist, with considerable experience assessing and treating African-Americans, contacted the first psychologist and explained his involvement in the case. He requested, with patient release, copies of the test data. Based on a review of the data, on interviews of the patient and her family, and on limited additional testing, different conclusions were drawn. The second psychologist then contacted the first psychologist again and discussed his concerns about the original evaluation and report. The first psychologist was somewhat receptive to the feedback. Although he refused to stop performing neuropsychological evaluations on ethnic minorities, he did offer assurance that he would seek consultation on such cases in the future.

Conclusions and Recommendations

The psychologist who performed the evaluation clearly drew some erroneous conclusions from the data he was able to gather. More extensive testing may have been useful, had it been performed by a competent clinician. Although the inaccurate interpretation was not done in a malicious manner, the consequences for the patient and her family could be quite serious. If the psychologist were practicing in a rural area where he is the only service provider, then consultation with qualified colleagues via telephone or e-mail would be indicated. In addition, referral to professionals from other disciplines would be indicated for further diagnostic studies. The psychologist who performed the evaluation clearly drew some erroneous conclusions from the data he was able to gather.

Even in the best of circumstances with appropriate neuropsychological training and racial and cultural awareness and sensitivity, the current state of psychological and neuropsychological testing is fraught with racial, ethnic, and cultural limitations (Manly & Jacobs, 2002). For example, (a) the tests may not assess the same abilities in individuals from different cultures, (b) the normative data may not be representative of the individual being evaluated; (c) the skills that are important within a given culture may not be adequately tapped by existing tests; (d) individuals perceive and approach health care institutions and professionals differently, some with distrust; (e) it may be extremely difficult to account for the tremendous diversity *within* racial and ethnic groups and cultures; and (f) examiners may vary in their investment and demeanor when assessing individuals from different backgrounds. Many of these issues represent significant challenges within the field. For the individual psychologist, the primary point to consider is that the test data obtained from racial or ethnic minority patients may have a strong likelihood of under-representing their true abilities.

Unfortunately, the scenario described above is more common than it should be. The Code's guidelines are quite clear and helpful on the standards a psychologist must uphold, and these should guide the decision-making process. If the first psychologist in this case were less receptive to feedback, for whatever reason, stronger

sanctions would appear to be indicated. Such sanctions might force the psychologist to change his/her course of action and take the appropriate steps to eliminate the potential for future violations. Repeat cognitive testing, home assessment, and interviewing other family members besides her daughter (who only saw a "sample" of behavior over the holidays) seem indicated.

Great sources of cross-cultural education are the Guidelines on Multicultural Education, Training, Research, Practice, and Organizational Change for Psychologists (American Psychological Association, 2002) and, for African Americans specifically, Manly and Jacobs (2002). These documents and contemporary readings on multicultural topics are essential for neuropsychologists as we work in an increasingly diverse society. Guidelines for handling such issues as appropriate versus inappropriate interpretation of race in reduced test performance and race-specific norms are discussed. Finally, as the Code indicates in the General Principles, consultation with peers is a very useful first step when there are any questions.

Scenario 2

A neuropsychologist seeks consultation from a colleague about a neuropsychological evaluation that a postdoctoral student working under her license recently performed. The patient was a 24-year-old Hispanic gentleman who presented for neuropsychological evaluation two years status-post an apparent mild traumatic brain injury. He was a restrained driver in a motor vehicle accident that occurred as he was leaving a bar late one night. His friend who was driving behind him (and the accident report) stated that he rear-ended a stalled semi truck. The patient did not experience any alteration in consciousness. A CT in the ER and a later MRI were both unremarkable. Blood alcohol levels taken at the hospital revealed that he was intoxicated at the time of the accident. The examiners later learned that the patient had two previous DUIs. He and his family stated that the young man has not used alcohol since the MVA. He was able to recall events prior to and after the accident accurately.

The patient had recently moved to the United States from Columbia, where he was working as a waiter at the time of the accident. He was educated in a small school system in a rural Columbian city. He stopped attending school in the ninth grade to work in his father's clothing business. He started learning English his last year of school and had become fluent over the past year. Medical history is unremarkable.

The patient was accompanied to the interview by his parents, with whom he now lives. He was cooperative with all aspects of the evaluation, stating that he just wanted to improve. He has not worked since the accident. His parents stated that he has been very irritable and impatient since coming home from the hospital. The patient and his parents also acknowledged dysnomia, disinhibition, and variable memory. The patient denied any other substantive changes in his activity, but, when queried, reported that he had actually lost interest in several activities. He had recently started working on the computer at his home and spent a lot of time in Internet chat rooms. He also did some basic computer repairs for members of his family. He was never married and broke up with his girlfriend three months after the MVA.

The patient had a previous neuropsychological evaluation three months after the MVA. It found borderline intellectual functioning, naming difficulties, and very poor memory (verbal memory worse than visual memory). The patient was tested in English, although it was noted that at times he had difficulty with comprehension. Psychomotor processing speed was also mildly compromised bilaterally. Emotional testing was not done in the initial evaluation.

The patient arrived for the evaluation on time, accompanied by of his both parents. The evaluation consisted of a clinical interview of the patient and his parents, as well as five hours of test administration with the patient alone. The neuropsychologist and her postdoctoral fellow conducted the interview jointly. He was fully cooperative with all aspects of the interview and testing. Several items had to be repeated because of apparent comprehension difficulty. Speech was fluent and free of evidence of a thought disorder. There was a mild Spanish accent noticeable. He was oriented to person, place and time. Affect was of full range and congruent with the various subject matter.

Testing began with a MMSE to establish general mental status. His score of 29 was improved from a score of 26 to a score of 29 since the last evaluation. His FSIQ was now 84, up 6 points from the FSIQ 3 months after the MVA. PIQ had improved 8 points, with VIQ only improving a few points and still less than the PIQ. Several subtest scores did not change: Information 6, Vocabulary 7, Picture Arrangement 8, and Picture Completion 8. A few subtest scores improved: Block Design 8 to 9, Digit Symbol 9 to 10, and Object Assembly 8 to 10. Scores on the Boston Naming Test and the Verbal Fluency test remained in the Mildly Impaired range.

Visuoperceptual and psychomotor processing speed were intact bilaterally. Mild difficulty was seen on the total speed of Trailmaking Test B, although the measure was performed accurately. This was essentially equal to the previous testing. His performance on the Booklet Category Test was in the Low Average range, with some difficulty with mental flexibility noted. On the final subtest, he failed to correctly solve items that he had previously missed.

Memory testing was intact for visual stimuli on the Wechsler Memory Scale-III, but difficulties were seen on indices of verbal memory. After the patient scored poorly on the recall of stories, initial and delayed (Moderately Impaired), the postdoctoral fellow felt that the patient's status of having English as a second language was contributing negatively to his performance on verbal subtests. The fellow, who had some facility in Spanish, therefore administered a "Spanish version" of the verbal portion of the Wechsler Memory Scale, California Verbal Learning Test, and another memory measure. Performance on all three measures was essentially in the Mild to Moderately Impaired range. These levels were slightly worse than previous testing, although previous testing was only done in English.

Assessment of mood consisted of interview observations and completion of a Spanish version of the Beck Depression Inventory. This test was used after the patient had noticeable difficulty comprehending the MMPI-2. He did not report a clinically significant level of distress, although he endorsed symptoms of occasional sadness, increased irritability, and physical discomfort.

The fellow's report concluded that the patient continued to have significant memory problems and that they had worsened since the last evaluation. It was felt that these results represented impairments that were secondary to a mild traumatic brain injury suffered in the MVA two years prior. The conclusion was "strengthened" by the fact that he scored worse on Spanish measures of several of the tests, especially memory tests. The report did not conclude that there was significant emotional distress and only recommended cognitive rehabilitation.

Relevant Ethical Issues

Competence

The neuropsychologist's concerns for the accuracy of her report appear warranted. The postdoctoral fellow, and ultimately the neuropsychologist, did not appear to fully assess the impact of English being a second language and how to evaluate the patient in the most accurate form of Spanish. Therefore, minor problems were inappropriately attributed to brain dysfunction. As in the previous case, by not knowing/applying the most appropriate norms, the neuropsychologist failed to exemplify the competence required in the above case (Standard 2.01, Boundaries of Competence; Standard 2.03, Maintaining Competence). In addition, by falsely interpreting mild TBI as a progressive condition, the

neuropsychologist failed to follow the "collective knowledge base" of her field (Standard 2.04, Bases for Scientific and Professional Judgments). As a supervisor, the neuropsychologist failed to ensure that her fellow perform the necessary services competently (Standard 2.05, Delegation of Work to Others).

Assessment

The Ethics Code mandates that psychologists use assessment measures that have had validity and reliability established for use with members of the population being assessed and that are appropriate given the patient's language preference (Standard 9.02b & c). This was certainly the intent of the postdoctoral fellow in selecting Spanish measures; they were just not the appropriate versions. The neuropsychologist also had responsibility for appropriate interpretation of the test data (Standard 9.09c, Test Score and Interpretation Services) and for describing limitations of her interpretations (Standard 9.06, Interpreting Assessment Results).

Case Resolution

After the report had been sent to the referring physician, a deposition was scheduled. As the neuropsychologist reviewed the data for her deposition, she noticed that the "Spanish versions" of several of the memory and personality tests were actually normed on Cuban and Haitian-American samples. This was of concern on two levels. The first was that there exist several dialects within the Spanish language and, given that the patient is from Columbia and only recently learned English, it is possible that his performance may represent these dialectical differences rather than actual cognitive functioning. The second issue relates to the first concern; that is, since no explicit translations and back-translations were utilized, is not possible to know what the patient "heard" on the various translations. It was at this point, before the deposition, that the supervising neuropsychologist consulted a colleague.

The neuropsychologist who was involved in the evaluation of the patient produced a report that likely drew some erroneous conclusions from the data obtained. The intent, while admirable, resulted in interpretation of measures that were inappropriately administered, given the specific Hispanic background of the patient. The neuropsychologist that was consulted suggested that the appropriate action would to be to produce a corrected report and notify the patient and his counsel about the errors. In that the supervising neuropsychologist ultimately consulted with a colleague, she appeared to recognize that she had handled the case poorly and would likely avoid doing so in the future. Toward that end, additional education on the impact of culture, particularly dialect, on test performance is indicated. The supervising neuropsychologist in this case then has the added responsibility of disseminating this knowledge to her supervisees.

Conclusions and Recommendations

This case represents an unfortunately all too common occurrence. Both the neuropsychologist and her postdoctoral fellow had some knowledge that alternative language forms may have been useful in this case but were not fully aware of the variety of measures available, nor did they look at the standardization data to make an informed decision. As a result, their conclusions were faulty. Based on subsequent re-interpretation of the data, the patient did not appear to have suffered significant brain trauma. It is also unlikely that the patient would *get worse* over time. His overall scores appeared marginal like some patients who are evaluated in their second language. That his language scores continued to be low was evidence of such an effect. That he was able to demonstrate some facility for computer repair speaks to his capacity to learn. The patient

was a young man in a new country who had not been able to find employment. Thus, there may have been more distress than the patient was willing to acknowledge (also possibly for cultural reasons), so this needed to be more thoroughly evaluated. If possible, referral to an appropriate neuropsychologist who could perform an evaluation in the patient's dialect may be helpful. Puente and others discuss these issues thoroughly in the Guidelines on Multicultural Education, Training, Research, Practice, and Organizational Change for Psychologists (APA, 2002).

Both cases illustrate the complexity of these issues in neuropsychological assessment and call for the neuropsychologist to rule out as many other factors as possible before attributing impairment to brain dysfunction. Given the potential for exposure to cultures different from one's own and different from those represented in a given measure's normative samples, professional neuropsychologists must truly be lifelong learners.

References

American Psychological Association (2002). Guidelines on Multicultural Education, Training, Research, Practice, and Organizational Change for Psychologists. www.apa.org/pi/multicultural-guidelines. Retrieved 7/2/03.

Lichtenberg, P. A., Ross, T., & Christensen, B. (1994). Preliminary normative data on the Boston Naming Test for an older urban population. *The Clinical Neuropsychologist, 8*, 109–111.

Manly, J.J., & Jacobs, D.M. (2002). Future directions in neuropsychological assessment with African Americans. In F.R. Ferraro (Ed.), *Minority and cross-cultural aspects of neuropsychological assessment* (pp. 79–96). Lisse, NL: Swets & Zeitlinger Publishers.

Steele, C.M., & Aronson, J. (1995). Stereotype threat and the intellectual test performance of African Americans. *Journal of Social Psychology, 69*, 797–811.

Chapter 19

ETHICAL CHALLENGES WITH ETHNICALLY AND CULTURALLY DIVERSE POPULATIONS IN NEUROPSYCHOLOGY, PART II

Thomas A. Martin

Scenario 1

A 40-year-old Filipino woman with a recent history of marital problems and dysphoric mood began to experience frequent headaches and vocational difficulties. Although considered to be one of her company's most efficient and conscientious bookkeepers, management had noticed a gradual decline in the quality of her work. The patient's employer, through its employee assistance program (EAP), subsequently encouraged her to undergo a neuropsychological evaluation and they provided her with the name of a local clinical psychologist. The patient contacted the psychologist and discussed her history of emotional and vocational difficulties and frequent headaches. She also voiced complaints of attention, memory, and word-finding difficulties. The psychologist was familiar with the patient's employer, as this company had referred many patients to him in the past for vocational assessments and psychotherapy. Although he had received some general training in neuropsychology early in his career, the psychologist had not conducted any neuropsychological evaluations

in many years. Not wanting to offend the patient's employer, and suspecting that her neurological symptoms were related to emotional factors, the psychologist scheduled the patient for an evaluation.

The patient reported for the evaluation with her husband. The psychologist discussed the general purpose of the evaluation and explained the procedures involved in the evaluation. He stated that he would bill her health insurance and that he would provide the patient and her husband with the results of the evaluation in one week. The patient gave consent based on the information discussed.

The clinical interview revealed that the patient was born and raised in the Philippines. She had married a U.S. soldier 21 years earlier, and the couple immigrated to the United States shortly after their marriage. They had no children. The patient indicated that while Tagalog was her first language, she was generally fluent in English. She indicated that she completed high school in Manila and earned an Associate's degree in accounting after moving to the U.S. The patient did not smoke, and she had no history of substance abuse. Her prior medical history was unremarkable, and she was taking no medications.

The patient reported struggling with stress and anxiety over the past twelve months secondary to marital problems and her vocational difficulties. She declined to offer specifics about her marital problems, while reporting that her vocational difficulties were related to her frequent headaches (two to three times per week), diminished attention and memory functioning, and word-finding problems. She also reported increasing difficulty solving arithmetic calculations mentally, reporting that that she occasionally made "silly" arithmetic errors on her reports. While the patient denied experiencing anhedonia, feelings of hopelessness, or changes in her appetite, she reported trouble falling asleep at night. The patient's husband offered very little during the interview, except to say that he had noticed no significant changes in his wife's cognitive functioning or ability to manage their finances.

Following the interview, the patient completed a half-day testing battery that included measures of response validity, intelligence, verbal and visual memory, object naming, executive functions, upper extremity motor speed and dexterity, and mood. The patient was cooperative and she appeared to work to the best of her abilities. She was oriented to person, place, and time, and she demonstrated a mildly anxious affect. While her speech was generally fluent and goal directed, mild word-finding difficulties were noted.

Test results revealed a High Average FSIQ, with no statistically significant difference noted between verbal comprehension and perceptual organization skills. Regarding memory functioning, the patient demonstrated High Average visual memory abilities with Average immediate and delayed verbal recall. Confrontation naming was Low Average. Measures of executive functioning fell in the Average range. Assessment of upper extremity motor functioning suggested High Average left (nondominant) hand finger tapping speed and dexterity, with Low Average right hand (dominant) tapping and dexterity.

Assessment of emotional functioning revealed symptoms consistent with moderate anxiety and mild depression.

The psychologist was aware that some clinicians have attributed difficulties on neuropsychological tests to brain dysfunction when they could be better explained by cultural-linguistic differences, and he did not want to make the same mistake. Therefore, based on the test results and on his previous experience treating a woman of Filipino decent, the psychologist concluded that emotional difficulties were of primary concern and that her neurological symptoms likely represented a physical manifestation of her emotional distress. Recommendations included individual psychotherapy with the examining psychologist and a trial of an SSRI. Wanting to maintain a favorable relationship with the patient's employer, the psychologist sent a copy of his report to her company and called the patient to schedule a feedback session.

Relevant Ethical Issues

Descriptions below of Ethical Standards and Principles refer to the 2002 revision of the APA Ethics Code (APA, 2002), except where the 1992 version of the Ethics Code is specified (American Psychological Association, 1992).

Professional Competence

The psychologist in this case failed to satisfy the requirement to maintain competence in the skills that are required or may be required to perform his professional responsibilities (Standard 2.03). Although he had had some degree of training in neuropsychology, he had not provided neuropsychological services in a number of years and likely had not kept up to date with changes in the field. He also failed to consider the importance of making a referral to a neurologist. Additionally, he likely overstepped the boundaries of his competence by recommending in his report a specific class of medications be prescribed to treat her condition. While many physicians and psychologists have relationships such that specific recommendations may be presented informally, and other psychologists work in contexts in which they hold prescription privileges, the above vignette offered no such information.

In addition, the psychologist's experience treating individuals from the Philippines was limited to one patient, and he relied on that sole experience when making decisions about the current patient. Thus, while attempting to be sensitive to cultural-linguistic factors and their potential impact on test results (Standards 2.01b, Boundaries of Competence & 9.06, Interpreting Assessment Results), he demonstrated the stereotyped thinking that he was attempting to avoid.

Informed Consent

The psychologist did not adequately discuss information required for informed consent (Standards 3.10, Informed Consent, & 9.03, Informed Consent in Assessments). For example, he failed to clarify the employer's role, including any desire by the employer for feedback and any potential implications for her employment (see also Standard 3.11, Psychological Services To or Through Organizations). Individuals from different cultures may have widely varying preconceptions about how the test results will be used, which may affect how they approach the evaluation.

Privacy and Confidentiality

Although the patient was encouraged to have a neuropsychological evaluation by her employer, she was actually self-referred and the psychologist was providing services independent of the employer. By sending a copy of the neuropsychological report to the patient's employer, he violated her right to privacy and confidentiality (Standard 4.01, Maintaining Confidentiality). He should have clarified with the patient her desire to have a copy of the report sent to her employer, as well as the potential uses of this information by her employer (Standard 4.02, Discussing the Limits of Confidentiality). As it

was, the psychologist did not seek authorization to release a copy of the report to the employer, and there was no indication that the employer even sought such information.

Assessment

The psychologist failed to adequately consider alternative explanations for the test results (Standards 2.04, Bases for Scientific and Professional Judgments & 9.06, Interpreting Assessment Results). He went into the evaluation believing that the patient's neurological symptoms were likely the result of emotional factors and, given her performance in the Low Average range or better on all measures, failed to consider the relative weaknesses present with abilities typically subsumed by the left cerebral hemisphere. He also failed to describe limitations of the test results and interpretations due to cultural differences between the patient and the standardization samples of the measures used (Standard 9.02, Use of Assessments).

Case Resolution

During the feedback session, the psychologist provided the patient and her husband with the results of the evaluation and his recommendations. Agreeing that she was anxious and depressed, the patient scheduled her first therapy session for two weeks from the date of the feedback session. In the interim, upon earlier referral from the EAP case manager, the patient was evaluated by a neurologist. The neurologist ordered an MRI of the brain, which revealed a small neoplasm in the left temporal lobe. Surgery was scheduled, and the patient cancelled her psychotherapy appointment. In preparation for surgery, the neurosurgeon ordered a neuropsychological evaluation. Upon meeting her new psychologist, who had significant training in neuropsychology, the patient informed her that she had recently undergone an evaluation. With patient consent, the neuropsychologist contacted the first psychologist and obtained a copy of the report and test scores. Upon review of those materials, she immediately contacted the first psychologist to discuss the ethical implications of his work. An informal resolution was reached.

Conclusions and Recommendations

This case illustrates a series of ethically questionable events that could have resulted in significant harm to the patient. Many of these ethical dilemmas originated from the psychologist's insufficient understanding of cultural issues. For example, the psychologist's preconception that the patient's difficulties were likely related to emotional factors was based in part on his limited experience with a previous patient of Filipino descent. This assumption led the psychologist to believe that he possessed the expertise necessary to conduct the evaluation. In addition to his lack of competency working with Filipino patients, and in conducting neuropsychological evaluations, the psychologist's failure to appreciate alternate etiologies to explain the patient's cognitive dysfunction, contributed to a diagnosis and recommendations that were at best inadequate, and at worst detrimental to the patient's well-being. Additionally, while the psychologist committed no ethical violation by referring the patient to himself for psychotherapy, he had an ethical obligation to appreciate and take steps to minimize the potential for such a self-referral to impair his ability to objectively conceptualize the patient's case, interpret her test performance, and make appropriate recommendations. Lastly, by failing to sufficiently discuss the information required to obtain informed consent and sending a copy of the patient's report to her employer, the psychologist demonstrated disregard for the patient's autonomy and right to confidentiality.

Despite the psychologists well meaning intentions, he made several decisions that were inconsistent with the ethical principles and standards that psychologists should employ to guide their professional work. Neuropsychologists who work with ethnically diverse populations have an obligation to develop and maintain the skills necessary to provide competent services. Pursuing formal continuing education in this regard can help a neuropsychologist develop and maintain these necessary competencies. Moreover, maintaining appropriate familiarity with the Ethics Code, frequently assessing areas of competency, and consulting with peers as needed, are additional safeguards that will help neuropsychologists increase their likelihood of maintaining ethically appropriate behavior.

Scenario 2

The patient is a 45-year-old, right-handed, Chinese-American woman who was emergently hospitalized six weeks ago following a two-day period of progressive cognitive deterioration and eventual loss of consciousness. She was subsequently diagnosed with type II diabetes mellitus and ketoacidosis. Following insulin treatment, the patient regained consciousness, and she was discharged home after four-days of hospitalization. During a follow-up appointment with her primary physician to assess her vocational readiness, the patient reported experiencing memory and receptive language difficulties. Her physician subsequently made a referral for a neuropsychological evaluation with a neuropsychologist who was employed at one of the city's teaching hospitals.

Upon receiving the referral, the neuropsychologist contacted the patient by telephone to schedule her appointment and to obtain background information. During their conversation, the neuropsychologist had some difficulty understanding the patient secondary to her Chinese accent and use of broken English. He was able to determine that she was born and raised in China and that she had immigrated to America with her husband and three children fifteen-years ago. She indicated that while Chinese was her first language, she was comfortable conversing in English. When asked if there was a family member who could accompany her to her evaluation and translate if needed, the patient reported that her children did not live in the area and that her husband would not be available to come with her. Realizing that communication difficulties could compromise her testing performance, the neuropsychologist obtained the patient's agreement to work with an interpreter that he would have available for the evaluation.

Although the neuropsychologist was well trained and experienced with a variety of medical conditions, he had limited experience working with patients of Asian descent. Nonetheless, he felt comfortable accepting the referral because he was aware of a nurse in the hospital who was fluent in Chinese and who had acted as an interpreter for other hospital staff in the past. He subsequently contacted this nurse and broadly discussed the case, stressing the importance of translating his instructions and all of the patient's responses as literally as possible. The nurse subsequently agreed to provide this service.

The patient and the interpreter reported for the evaluation as scheduled. The neuropsychologist made introductions and then proceeded to provide the information necessary for the patient to make an informed decision about her desire to participate in the evaluation. When he concluded, it appeared that the patient was confused, and he instructed the interpreter to translate what had been said. During this translation it became apparent that the interpreter and the patient were also having some difficulty understanding each other. When he inquired about this, the interpreter reported that while she spoke Cantonese, the patient spoke Mandarin, a different dialect. The interpreter reassured the neuropsychologist that this would not be a significant problem, as the dialects were similar and she could figure out what the patient was trying to say.

Convinced that the interpreter would be effective, the neuropsychologist began to conduct a clinical interview. While the patient appeared to understand much of what was being said, the interpreter was utilized when it became clear that the patient was confused or the neuropsychologist had difficulty understanding a response. During the interview, it was determined that the patient had completed the equivalent of a high school education in China. After relocating to America, she maintained employment as a housekeeper for a number of years. However, for the past five years she had worked as a dental assistant for a local dentist who was fluent in Chinese. The patient reported that her responsibilities included preparing the instruments before appointments and assisting the dentist as needed during procedures. She indicated that she was very eager to return to work and resume earning an income. When asked about her current neuropsychological problems, the patient reported experiencing concentration, memory, and receptive language difficulties. She felt that these cognitive inefficiencies were compromising her daily functioning. She also reported experiencing fatigue and occasional light-headedness. She denied experiencing current emotional distress or any history of psychiatric illness. The patient reported that her diabetes and hypertension were currently well controlled with medication, and she denied any other history of significant illness or injury. Regarding behavioral health, the patient acknowledged a remote history of tobacco use, while she denied any history of alcohol or illicit substance use.

Following the interview, the patient completed a full-day of neuropsychological testing that included measures of response validity, intelligence, verbal and visual memory, expressive language, executive functions, upper-extremity motor functioning, and mood. Given the periodic need for the translation of information, testing time was extended by one to two hours. During the evaluation, the patient was found to be oriented to person, place, and time, and she evidenced normal affect. While she was fully cooperative and appeared to work to the best of her abilities, she appeared to have difficulty understanding test instructions that were more complex. She also became somewhat restless and fatigued during the final hours of testing.

Test results revealed variable neuropsychological abilities. While WAIS-III Full Scale I.Q. fell at the higher end of the Low Average range, VIQ was in the Borderline range. Memory scores ranged from Borderline to Low Average. Measures of executive functioning ranged from Impaired to Average. Expressive language abilities fell in the Impaired range. Upper extremity motor functioning was High Average, bilaterally. Assessment of emotional functioning revealed no indication of depression or emotional distress.

Given the variable test results and limited background information available for consideration, the neuropsychologist had significant difficulty estimating the patient's premorbid level of functioning or assessing possible changes in her cognition. Reasoning that the patient's cultural-linguistic differences and fatigue likely resulted in an underestimation of many of her abilities, the neuropsychologist recommended to the physician that the patient be allowed to return to work on a part-time basis with appropriate supervision so that her vocational competencies could be assessed by her employer.

Relevant Ethical Issues

Access to Neuropsychological Services
The neuropsychologist recognized that cultural and/or linguistic factors may interfere with the evaluation process or the validity of the results obtained; however, he believed that performing the evaluation would be more beneficial to the patient than referring her to a psychologist with little or no training in neuropsychology (Principles A, Beneficence and Nonmaleficence, & D, Justice). Additionally, failure to provide appropriate services to the patient in the absence of a more culturally or linguistically qualified neuropsychologists may have been seen as unfair discrimination (Standard 3.01).

Professional Competence
The neuropsychologist had minimal experience working with Chinese-American patients (Standard 2.01, Boundaries of Competence). However, he knew of no neuropsychologists in the city with such experience to whom he could refer the patient. He believed he could make an adequate determination of her neuropsychological status through the use of an interpreter – someone who was also a professional employed by the medical center (Standard 3.09, Cooperation With Other Professionals). However, given the different dialects spoken by the patient and the interpreter, the neuropsychologist may have violated Standard 2.05 (Delegation of Work to Others) by authorizing the interpreter to provide a translation that she was not competent to provide.

Privacy and Confidentiality
Interpreters are considered agents of the neuropsychologist and, as such, should be held to the same standards of confidentiality as the neuropsychologist and any other employees (Standard 9.03c, Informed Consent in Assessments). Confidentiality issues should be clarified for all parties during the informed consent process, and the patient must provide consent for the use of the interpreter.

Assessment
The neuropsychologist did not use measures that were developed for use specifically with individuals born and raised and China. In addition, he used an interpreter during test administration who was not fluent in the patient's dialect. While such situations may be preferable to not providing any services, the neuropsychologist's primary failure was in not emphasizing the limitations of the test results and interpretations (Standards 9.01, Bases for Assessments; 9.02, Use of Assessments; 9.03, Informed Consent in Assessments; 9.06, Interpreting Assessment Results). Also, neuropsychologists have a responsibility to educate interpreters about test security issues (9.03c, Informed Consent in Assessments),

and the extent to which such education was provided in the current case is unclear.

Case Resolution

After several days of feeling uneasy about the recommendations he had made, the neuropsychologist sought consultation with a counseling psychology colleague who had experience working with Asian clients. The colleague discussed the importance of working within the boundaries of ethnic and cultural competence and advised the neuropsychologist to send an addendum to the report to the patient and her physician, discussing the difficulties noted during the evaluation and how these issues may have affected the assessment results and his conclusions. The neuropsychologist agreed with the recommendation.

Conclusions and Recommendations

This case illustrates some of the ethical dilemma's that can confront even well-trained neuropsychologists. For example, while this neuropsychologist anticipated the impact that cultural-linguistic differences could have on testing, and he was careful to secure the services of an interpreter, he did not know enough about the patient's culture to inquire about the specific Chinese dialect that she spoke. Given the neuropsychologist's minimal experience working with Chinese-American patients, he may have considered searching for a local neuropsychologist who was experienced in this area. At a minimum, seeking out consultation/supervision with a peer who had experience working with clients of Asian descent, prior to testing the patient, would likely have prepared him for some of the issues that he faced.

Additionally, this case demonstrates the importance of referring to the Ethics Code when confronted with new or challenging situations. For example, while the neuropsychologist stressed the importance of providing literal translations to the interpreter, he failed to appreciate the fact that the interpreter was his agent and it was his responsibility to clarify with her issues related to confidentiality. Lastly, the neuropsychologist's eventual consultation with a peer highlights the utility of discussing ethical concerns and issues with colleagues. Through this peer consultation, the neuropsychologist gained insight into his professional competencies and limitations, as well as a resolution to minimize any potential harm that his evaluation conclusions and recommendations may have caused.

References

American Psychological Association (1992). Ethical principles of psychologists and code of conduct. *American Psychologist, 47*, 1597-1611.

American Psychological Association (2002). Ethical principles of psychologists and code of conduct. *American Psychologist, 57*, 1060-1073.

Knapp, S., & VandeCreek, L (2003). An overview of the major changes in the 2002 APA Ethics Code. *Professional Psychology: Research and Practice, 34*, 301-308.

Section 10

ETHICAL CHALLENGES WITH THE USE OF INFORMATION TECHNOLOGY AND TELECOMMUNICATIONS IN NEUROPSYCHOLOGY

Introduction

The rapid advances in information technology and telecommunications (ITT) offer exciting opportunities for neuropsychological research and practice. However, the use of such technology with individuals with cognitive, psychological, and/or physical limitations brings with it added responsibility. Due to limitations in the ability to understand or manipulate information technology, neuropsychologically vulnerable patients and research participants are entitled to increased protection from the potential negative effects of ITT use (Bush, Naugle, & Johnson-Greene, 2002). Perhaps more than most emerging areas of professional activity, the development and use of ITT has outpaced the development and implementation of ethical guidelines pertaining to its use. The authors of this chapter take another important step toward reducing that discrepancy. By bringing together the latest neuropsychological applications of ITT and the most recent ethical considerations pertaining to ITT use, the authors provide a valuable resource for negotiating ethical challenges that most neuropsychologists now are at least beginning to face.

Reference

Bush, S., Naugle, R., & Johnson-Greene, D. (2002). Interface of information technology and neuropsychology: Ethical issues and recommendations. *The Clinical Neuropsychologist, 16 (4)*, 536-547.

Chapter 20

ETHICAL CHALLENGES WITH THE USE OF INFORMATION TECHNOLOGY AND TELECOMMUNICATIONS IN NEUROPSYCHOLOGY, PART I

Jeffrey N. Browndyke

Scenario 1

A biotechnology company has approached a neuropsychologist working at a major medical center to determine if he would be interested in joining the company's growing network of cognitive assessment clinics. The company's clinics are centered on the implementation of a Internet-enabled, remote neuropsychological assessment (RNA)[1] screening battery and associated international normative database. The broadly stated goal of the company is to provide cognitive assessment results to third-party interests (e.g., clinical trials; employment screening; physicians interested in gaining rapid access to cognitive assessment results; etc.) via a network of company-approved assessment clinics. The company's proprietary computerized neuropsychological assessment battery would be administered in "real time" within one of the company's approved assessment clinics, while the raw data would be transmitted over the Internet to the biotechnology company for analysis. Fee-for-service cognitive evaluation reports would be generated remotely by the company and returned over the Internet to referring clinics, which, in turn, would then be distributed by the clinic operators to third-party interests. The contractual agreement between the company and neuropsychologist would involve the neuropsychologist's assumption of supervisory control over an assessment clinic franchised by the company and responsibility for implementing the RNA screening battery in accordance with the company's assessment protocol. Under the agreement, the company would collect a flat fee for each participant run through the RNA system, while the total cost of the procedure would be at the discretion of clinic owners. The neuropsychologist is intrigued by the company's efforts and flattered that he would be asked to contribute; however, being uncertain of the ethical and legal ramifications involved in telecommunications-mediated service delivery, he asks for more time to consider the company's proposal.

---

[1]Defined as any computerized assessment measure enabled to allow for task selection, stimuli response and feedback, data aggregation, or analysis via currently available telecommunications technologies (e.g., Internet, wireless networks, telephony, etc.).

Relevant Ethical Issues

To some the scenario above may seem far-fetched or beyond the concerns of current neuropsychological practice. However, telecommunication-mediated RNA techniques have been in existence since the mid-1990s (Ball, Scott, McLaren, & Watson, 1993; Montani et al., 1997). RNA is currently being used for research trials in dementia and sports medicine, and by the time this book is published, there will be no less than three well-funded private companies targeting RNA measures and techniques to a wider market of health professionals. At this point, it is clear that the development and implementation of Internet-mediated assessment techniques is being driven by commerical interests, but as Reed, McLaughlin, and Milholland (2000) so aptly point out, "if the technology drives consumer applications and systems development, rather than the technology being responsive to the needs of its users, the result could be extremely costly and elaborate systems that do not deliver better – or even effective – care" (p. 171). The same "cart before the horse" warning could apply to RNA applications indifferent to the ethical and legal responsibilities of the end user (Buchanan, 2002; Bush, Naugle, & Johnson-Greene, 2002; Schatz & Browndyke, 2002).

The presented scenario presumes the biotechnology company and all concerned parties are based within the United States; an assumption that often cannot be made in a world of overseas test publishers and business globalization. Should the biotechnology company or any third-party recipients of the assessment data be located outside the United States, unresolved ethical and legal issues might come into play (e.g., international electronic transmission of assessment data, varying laws governing security and confidentiality, HIPAA compliance, etc.; Bashur, 1997; Koocher & Morray, 2000), which for the sake of brevity, will not be touched upon in this case scenario review. Two advantages are presented by the biotechnology company's use of networked local assessment clinics. By allowing for participant contact and data collection within the purview of a neuropsychologist's licensed practice, thorny and unresolved legal issues related to interjurisdictional practice and licensure portability may be avoided (Huie, 1996; U.S. Department of Commerce – National Telecommunications and Information Administration, 1997). Additionally, by having clinic participants engage in face-to-face contact and presumably some observation by clinic operators during the execution of the computerized assessment battery, a level of professional control and decision-making is maintained by participating neuropsychologists.

Positive aspects aside, the case scenario is still fraught with ethical issues with which the neuropsychologist will have to contend should he choose to participate in the company's efforts. The most prescient ethical issues raised are within the APA Ethics Code domains of Competence, Human Relations, Privacy and Confidentiality, Record Keeping and Fees, and Assessment. In addition to relevant ethical issues, more intensive legal considerations are raised by the case scenario within the areas of privacy, confidentiality, and record keeping, as dictated by nascent Health Insurance Portability and accountability Act (HIPAA) regulations (Calloway & Venegas, 2002; Gue, n.d.). HIPAA-related issues will be touched upon where appropriate. However, the bulk of the case scenario commentary will be reserved for those APA Ethical Standards applicable to the RNA service delivery model.

Boundaries of Competence (Standards 2.01c and e)

Competence within the content domain or patient population with which a new assessment application will be employed should serve as an initial decision rule, regardless of the application modality. Assuming core competency issues are met, Boundaries of Competence clauses "c" and "e" provide the most direct guidance applicable to new technologies and techniques. It is incumbent upon neuropsychologists to keep abreast of the issues surrounding any RNA application or technique.

Bases for Scientific and Professional Judgments (Standard 2.04)

Consulting representative books, journals or professional practice directives provides the best methods for maintaining awareness of the scientific and ethical issues surrounding RNA or other telecommunication-mediated techniques. At this time, the peer-reviewed journals (*The Clinical Neuropsychologist*; *Professional Psychology: Research and Practice*; and, *Behavior Research Methods, Instruments, and Computers*) serve as the most direct outlets for information involving the juncture of telecommunications, computerized assessment, and neuropsychological practice. At this time, practice directives specific to telecommunications and psychology are relatively non-existent (American Psychological Association Ethics Committee, 1998); however, APA Division 40, National Academy of Neuropsychology (NAN), and International Neuropsychological Society (INS) have all formed technology sub-committees, which may serve as consultative outlets for concerned parties.

Avoiding Harm (Standard 3.04)

Presumed to be ubiquitous to all practice considerations, this APA ethical standard extends to issues unique to telecommunications-mediated technology; namely maintaining test security and patient confidentiality within an inherently transferable electronic medium. Both issues are discussed in greater detail under the Maintaining Confidentiality and Maintaining Test Security ethics standards.

Informed Consent (Standards 3.10a and d)

Given the element of face-to-face contact in the presented case scenario, obtaining informed consent from prospective participants undergoing the biotechnology company's RNA battery would be less problematic than in other purely remote

assessment efforts (i.e., no in-person contact between parties). In the case scenario, informed consent would be carried out in a purely traditional fashion. However, assuming no personal contact was required for a RNA effort, how could informed consent be ascertained when a remote practitioner cannot even be reasonably certain of the identity of the person taking the test? Streaming televideo in conjunction with a RNA procedure may aid in the informed consent process, but this addition still does not provide a completely satisfactory solution. One proposed method for those considering the use of RNA without in-person contact requirements would be the assignment of a unique identification code that could be mailed or phoned to prospective participants. The unique identification codes could be used by participants to reasonably confirm their identity online and serve as electronic signatures for informed consent agreements. An additional benefit of a unique electronic code assignment system will be discussed under the APA Ethical Standard governing patient/subject confidentiality (Standard 4.01). HIPAA security rules compliance would also be enhanced through the institution of a unique electronic code identifier system (Gue, n.d.).

Psychological Services Delivered To or Through Organizations (Standard 3.11a)

In the case scenario, the participating neuropsychologist ultimately is a representative of the biotechnology company and their assessment product. As a result, any informed consent agreements should clearly state this relationship and touch upon the methods through which participant assessment data is collected, transmitted, and analyzed.

Maintaining Confidentiality (Standard 4.01)

Confidentiality concerns are paramount when discussing electronically-mediated data collection, transmission, or storage, particularly when data is transmitted over open computer networks. Neuropsychologists considering RNA should ascertain whether any company involved in the RNA battery or system has implemented a comprehensive data security policy that is compliant with HIPAA security provisions (Calloway & Venegas, 2002). Additionally, a chain of trust partner agreement should be established between any involved parties to protect the integrity and confidentiality of data being exchanged via the Internet (Gue, n.d.). Neuropsychologists would want to inquire about the presence of strong data encryption techniques (e.g., 128-key RSA encryption) at all points along the data collection and electronic transfer routes; the use of unique code identification systems to assist in insuring participant confidentiality; the existence of audit controls to track data security; and any assigned security responsibilities assumed by the end-user of the RNA measure or battery. An additional consideration involves an explicit understanding by neuropsychologists as to which parties involved will retain copies of participant raw data or interpretative reports generated by a RNA system.

Discussing the Limits of Confidentiality (4.02a-c)

Although security of confidential electronic patient/subject records cannot be guaranteed with 100 percent certainty, neuropsychologists employing strong encryption techniques, unique code identifier systems, and secure Internet firewalls, can assure RNA participants that their personal information and assessment data are reasonably secure. Where security holes may be present or unavoidable, these should be explicitly stated to prospective participants during the informed consent process. Materials should also be provided regarding the rights and recourse RNA participants may have under HIPAA guidelines should a security breach occur (Calloway & Venegas, 2002).

Maintenance, Dissemination, and Disposal of Confidential Records of Professional and Scientific Work (Standard 6.02a, b)

This APA ethical standard may be satisfied via the competent use of data encryption and unique code identification systems, as noted in earlier APA standards concerning informed consent and the maintenance of patient/subject confidentiality. For neuropsychologists considering the implementation of a unique code identification system for patient data, security may be enhanced if a separate personal information key database or file is encrypted and stored on a computer not equipped with external connection capabilities (e.g., modem, Internet, etc.). Following a relational database system, neuropsychologists would create a primary assessment database devoid of any personally identifiable information and a separate database for personal information. Individual records would be matched via a unique code variable entered in both databases. Not only does a relational database allow for some degree of confidentiality for select databases, but it also is inherently expandable as long as the unique identifier code is included in additional databases.

In order for a database to be considered de-identified and not subject to HIPAA confidentiality requirements, it can only contain age, general geographical information (e.g., zip code), gender, race, ethnicity, marital status, and education information (Calloway & Venegas, 2002). However, if any database contains personally identifiable information or is matched to confidential information via a unique key code, it would be subject to all pertinent HIPAA security and information dissemination restrictions.

Use of Assessments (Standards 9.02a-c)

Striking at the Achilles heel of most computerized assessment and RNA applications, this ethical standard may be hard to completely meet when employing newly developed assessment measures or techniques. Save for a few well-designed and tested measures, most computerized assessment and RNA applications do not have enough reliability and validity data or published independent investigation to warrant confidence at or above the level with which traditional (i.e., non-computerized) measures are held. Furthermore, analytical methods by which some computerized versions of traditional assessment measures are determined to have equivalence may be inadequate to substantiate that claim. (APA, 1986; Mead & Drasgow, 1993). Even if measurement equivalence is obtained using the most stringent of methodologies, it is important to underscore that any determination of equivalence is strictly limited to those populations tested. Computerized assessment measures or RNA applications determined to be equivalent to an analog measure based upon a normal population, but then applied to an untested clinical population would not meet the *"for use with members of the population tested"* clause noted in this ethics standard. The relative infancy of RNA and computerized assessment, however, should not dissuade their judicious use. As this ethics standard points out, *"when ... validity or reliability has not been established, psychologists describe the strengths and limitations of test results and interpretation."* Accordingly, it will be incumbent upon neuropsychologists to be aware of the pitfalls and limitations specific to any RNA or computerized assessment measure and not to overextend the measure's applicability to all populations (APA, Division 40 – Committee on Professional Standards, & Committee on Psychological Tests and Assessment, 1987). Keeping these issues in mind, neuropsychologists would want to examine the quality and results of any reliability and validity studies carried out by a test development company and the populations used to characterize the measurement properties of any computerized assessment measure or battery.

Interpreting Assessment Results (Standard 9.06)

As an extension of comments from the previous ethical standard, human and environmental factors unique to computerized assessment, such as computer familiarity, computer-related anxiety, and apparatus ergonomics, should be considered when interpreting the results from any computerized assessment measure or battery (Browndyke et al., 2002; Schatz & Browndyke, 2002).

Test Scoring and Interpretation Services (Standards 9.09a-c)

It is clear that the neuropsychologist in the case scenario, while possibly being retained as a franchised assessment clinic owner by the biotechnology company, would still be ultimately responsible for the proper use of the RNA system, including confirmation of the veracity and appropriateness of any interpretative reports returned by the biotechnology company. The ethical considerations discussed under the Use of Assessment standard would apply toward this determination.

Explaining Assessment Results (9.10)

Neuropsychologists should determine at the outset of any potential collaborative or employment agreement with a RNA development company any limitations placed upon the explanation of results generated by the company's system. As is typical of most computerized assessment measures, "boilerplate" interpretations are likely to be generated based upon participants' test results. However, this should not preclude neuropsychologists from developing further explanatory refinements based upon clinical judgment and observation of factors often not accounted for in simple data analysis algorithms (Adams & Heaton, 1985).

Maintaining Test Security (Standard 9.11)

Because the RNA system described in the case scenario is limited to assessment administration within a company-approved clinic under the observation of the neuropsychologist, test security can be assumed to be reasonably secure as long as certain safeguards are put into place (e.g., encrypted password access to start RNA battery, adjust settings, transfer raw data, view interpretative reports, etc.). If the RNA battery were to be administered remotely, then test security concerns would become much more salient. Even with the use of secure firewalls and encryption protections, information transmitted over the Internet is still to some small degree vulnerable to unwanted observation or alteration. A key term used in this standard, however, is *"reasonable effort,"* and it is argued that as long as up-to-date and stringent levels of security are implemented for RNA applications (both local and remote administration types), then a level of test security can be reasonably assumed that meets the spirit of this ethical standard.

Case Resolution

The neuropsychologist chose not to accept the biotechnology company's offer, but for reasons independent of the primary ethical and legal details applicable to the use of RNA. He was unable to gain assurances from the company that other franchised assessment clinics would be run by similarly qualified individuals, and he took his participation in the company's efforts as a tacit endorsement of the unrestricted use of neuropsychological assessment techniques by unqualified persons (see Standard 9.07, Assessment by Unqualified Persons).

Had the company agreed to limit the administration of their RNA battery to psychology professionals and adequate reliability and validity for the assessment battery were demonstrated, the neuropsychologist would have agreed to participate. However, he would have insisted upon a contractual agreement to establish the boundaries of responsibility for the administration, maintenance, databasing, and control of any data

collected by the company's assessment battery before proceeding with the establishment of a clinic franchise. An additional clause in the contractual agreement would have included a caveat allowing the neuropsychologist the freedom to reject or modify any interpretative reports generated by the company, as well as the clinical discretion to decide when participants would not be appropriate for the RNA battery. Mindful of HIPAA regulations governing security and confidentiality of patient information, the neuropsychologist and the biotechnology company would have drawn up a chain of trust partner agreement, and collaboration would have been expected to insure that both the franchise clinic and the remote component of the RNA battery (e.g., data transfer over the Internet to the company for analysis) were HIPAA compliant. An informed consent agreement would have been crafted by the neuropsychologist detailing (1) any limitations to participant confidentiality, (2) the fact that participants' data would be electronically transferred for analysis, (3) alternative assessment options for those wishing not to participate in the RNA battery, and (4) any recourse available to participants in the event of a security breach.

Conclusions and Recommendations

1. *Develop and maintain competency.* Reference any published materials pertinent to the RNA measure or battery being considered; attend conference workshops or symposia dealing with RNA and computerized assessment; and, if possible, establish a route of professional consultation with peers who have already had experience in the use of RNA.

2. *Obtain contractual and explanatory materials from any company licensing or distributing RNA measures or techniques.* HIPAA security rules dictate that policies and procedures should be developed between parties regarding certification of any technical

evaluation required of local and remote data systems security; a contingency plan documenting maintenance of operations continuity and data recovery process; responsibility for auditing procedures and maintenance of records; and chain of trust partner agreements to explicitly disclose the covered entities with which health information is to be shared (for more detailed information regarding HIPAA security compliance requirements, see Gue, n.d.).

3. *Develop informed consent agreement specific to any telecommunication-mediated practice.* Practitioners should explain in plain language the process by which RNA participants' data will be collected, transferred, and stored and the security procedures put into place to reasonably guarantee confidentiality of their personal information.

4. *Determine level of data security and implement safeguards to protect confidentiality and integrity of test data.* Consideration should be given to instituting a unique electronic code identifier system for any primary assessment database, which would be kept separate from another database containing matched personal information. Strong encryption methods should be implemented to limit internal and external access to RNA measures, personal information, raw assessment data, or interpretative reports.

5. *Ascertain the reliability and validity of any RNA measure or technique.* If the reliability and validity of computerized assessment measure is being inferred from the properties of a well-established analog version of the measure, examine the methodological stringency and population characteristics by which measurement equivalence was determined.

6. *Understand limitations specific to assessment modality or participant population applicability.* When considering participant appropriateness or the validity of results derived from computerized assessment measures, idiosyncratic (e.g., lack of computer familiarity,

computer-related anxiety), environmental (e.g., apparatus ergonomics, technological barriers), and measurement (e.g., measure's applicability in participant population) factors should be taken into account.

Scenario 2

A geriatric neuropsychologist is called by a programming representative from a local television station. The station's news division is interested in developing a five-part news series covering Alzheimer's disease and other dementing disorders, and the programming representative is soliciting the aid of local health professionals to contribute material for the news series. The programming representative tells the neuropsychologist that the series producer requests a videotaped demonstration of what prospective patients undergo when referred for neuropsychological assessment, parts of which will be aired during certain segments of the news series. In exchange for the neuropsychologist's participation, the programming representative indicates that television station will air any professional contact information the neuropsychologist may provide, including a World Wide Web (WWW) homepage address, during the news series. Recognizing the opportunity to educate the public about neuropsychological practice, as well as providing a venue for free advertisement for her assessment clinic, the neuropsychologist agrees to participate conditionally and rushes to establish a WWW presence for her assessment clinic before the news series airing date.

Relevant Ethical Issues

This case scenario appears to present two routes of ethical considerations with which neuropsychologists must contend – one involving considerations associated with the proposed televised news series and another for the construction of an assessment practice WWW homepage. However, the two routes are not mutually exclusive, and the majority of the applicable ethical standards are pertinent to both aspects of the case scenario. Shared ethical considerations are subsumed within the ethics domains of advertising and other public statements, privacy and confidentiality, and assessment. The construction of an assessment practice WWW homepage presents an additional and unique challenge within the domain of human relations; specifically, the avoidance of unfair discrimination. Each aspect of the case scenario is discussed in relation to the relevant ethical standards, but particular emphasis is placed upon the ethical difficulties and possible solutions associated with the creation of a private practice presence on the WWW. The case scenario critique, however, is not exhaustive in positing solutions for Ethics Code conformity when considering the construction of presence on the WWW, and interested parties are referred to materials developed by the World Wide Web Consortium (WWWC, 1999); Maheu, Whitten, and Allen (2001); and, Hsiung (2002).

Media Presentations (Standard 5.04)

The APA Ethics Committee's inclusion of the words "internet, and other electronic transmission" to this ethics standard is clearly addressed to those practitioners who may be interested in increasing professional visibility within cyberspace. WWW private practice homepages are an attractive advertising venue for a profession long-relegated to local yellow page advertisements (Koocher, 1994). The start-up costs, overhead, and maintenance of a WWW presence are quite reasonable and allow neuropsychologists to not only announce their presence on a worldwide basis, but to also provide greater explanatory materials regarding their professional expertise and practice. However, this ethical standard makes it clear that the new media technologies are not immune from basic requirements to maintain a professional air of honesty and truthfulness in any public statements. Additionally, the last clause

of this ethics statement (e.g., "do not indicate that a professional relationship has been established with the recipient") would be important to address in some form as part of any disclaimer material written for a WWW private practice homepage, particularly if provisions for e-mail contact are going to be made available. Additional ethical concerns regarding e-mail contact are discussed in detail under Standard 4.02c (Discussing Limits of Confidentiality).

Statements by Others (Standards 5.02a)

Neuropsychologists who are interested in developing a presence on the WWW and employ the services of a webpage construction or hosting company are ultimately responsible for the content transcribed or generated by contracted businesses or individuals. Similarly, media content responsibilities exist for televised presentations, particularly if the publicity effort is designed or scripted by the neuropsychologist. Professional control of media content is much more difficult if conducted by independent parties (e.g., local television news, webpage news article, etc.), with whom contact was not initially engaged or employed by a prospective neuropsychologist. Nevertheless, reasonable efforts to retain some form of editorial control should be requested from media outlets. Doing so at the outset of any relationship will help guard against the public release of inadvertent statements or activities that may breach the APA Ethics Code and insures that a reasonable effort to maintain control of statements made by others was undertaken by the neuropsychologist.

Unfair Discrimination (Standard 3.01)

WWW pages often incorporate images and hypertext markup language (HTML) code that cannot be read by interpreter software for the blind or disabled. As a result, often unintended barriers to accessibility are present, which could be construed by some as being discriminatory to the disabled. Guidelines to assist in webpage accessibility are currently available and should be consulted before the construction of a presence on the WWW (WWWC, 1999). Additional consideration should be given to the overall reading level of a private practice or organization website to allow for access to the widest audience possible.

Discussing the Limits of Confidentiality (Standard 4.02c)

"Psychologist who offer services, products, or information via electronic transmission inform client/patients of the risks to privacy and limits of confidentiality."

With the inclusion of this clause to Standard 4.02, the Ethics Code makes clear that it is the responsibility of neuropsychologists to inform and educate about the limitations to privacy and confidentiality when information is being electronically transmitted to, or about, individuals with whom a professional relationship has already been established. However, the provision fails to make clear whether limitation warnings are required for prospective clientele (e.g., unsolicited requests for professional services sent via e-mail; Widman & Tong, 1997). While a requirement for prospective clientele is not stated in the Ethics Code, neuropsychologists establishing a WWW presence should make efforts to inform both current and prospective clients/patients of the risks inherent in electronic information transfer. In the context of a private practice website, a blanket privacy and confidentiality statement posted near any links allowing for electronic contact between parties would appear to satisfy the spirit of this ethical standard.

Maintaining Test Security (Standard 9.11)

Though more applicable to the televised media presentation aspect of the case scenario, test security considerations have also arisen specific to electronic media and the Internet. Ruiz, Drake, Glass, Marcotte, and van Gorp (2002) highlight the serious threat to test security posed by unwise, if not flagrant, online distribution of test stimuli

and instructions. The reproduction and online distribution of test stimuli is an obvious infraction of this ethical standard, but neuropsychologists should also be mindful to avoid any overly detailed descriptions of test procedures or materials on their WWW practice homepages. The same can be said of any televised media presentation of assessment materials or procedures.

To avoid ethical infractions related to media presentations and test security, neuropsychologists should consider the use of mock assessment stimuli or outdated materials and employ the use of a confederate during the demonstration of assessment procedures. If possible, outdated assessment stimuli and procedures should be significantly altered to obscure any hint of the original measure or procedure. It is suggested that media presentations of mock symptom validity measures or procedures be avoided altogether, given the sensitive nature of this type of evaluation.

Case Resolution

The neuropsychologist, mindful of potential test security and confidentiality issues, planned upon the use of a combination of novel and significantly outdated and altered assessment measures (e.g., novel word-list learning task, altered WMS stimuli and subtests, verbal fluency for the letters D, G, P and sports-activities, etc.) during the mock dementia evaluation videotaping and elicited the help of a confederate to act as a patient. In an effort to insure that the mock evaluation and interview were factually accurate and devoid of ethical difficulties, the neuropsychologist insisted that her participation in the news series was contingent upon being able to view and request edits of her video footage.

Satisfied that the news series producers would honor her wishes regarding any televised video materials, the neuropsychologist turned her attention towards the construction of a WWW presence for her assessment clinic. She contacted a reputable local webpage construction and hosting company to build the clinic website based upon text and graphics that she provided and approved. The company made some valuable suggestions regarding universal access provisions for the website (e.g., text only version of any webpage content) that were quickly approved by the neuropsychologist and included into the overall structure of the clinic's website. To address concerns about online security and confidentiality, the neuropsychologist generated two disclaimers for inclusion into the website. One disclaimer served as a blanket copyright statement for the content and design of the website and a legal disclaimer regarding limited liability for any information provided by the clinic website. The other disclaimer detailed the clinic's policy of not engaging in online contact with established clientele and warned of the limited level of confidentiality inherent to any e-mail requests for services from prospective patients or interested family members. Alternative contact information was provided for those wishing to reach the clinic by traditional means. The webpage construction and hosting company contacted the neuropsychologist and provided a working copy of the assessment clinic website, which was reviewed by the neuropsychologist for content before being returned to the company for hosting on a computer linked to the WWW.

Conclusions and Recommendations

1. *Determine media outlet expectations and final content of materials.* If possible, pre-production agreements should be obtained to gain some control over the content and eventual use of any media materials. Agreements should include a provision for the neuropsychologist to review any media before public distribution in an effort to guard against unintended breaches of test security or patient confidentiality.
2. *Provide universal access provisions for any WWW presence.* At a minimum, private practice or organization WWW homepages should provide a "text only" version of all website materials to increase accessibility for the disabled. Additional universal access guidelines are available online (WWWC, 1999).
3. *Clearly state confidentiality and legal considerations related to WWW presence.* The development and posting of a WWW-specific disclaimer statement is highly recommended. Suggested disclaimer coverage should touch upon the policies and procedures for patient/professional online contact, confidentiality limitations, and liability concerns regarding information gained from webpage links to and from a WWW practice homepage (Grossman, 1998; Harroch, 1998).
4. *Maintain test security.* Neuropsychologists wishing to demonstrate assessment procedures or illustrate stimuli examples for media presentations should use long outdated or obsolete measures. If possible, outdated materials or procedures should be significantly altered as to make them wholly unrecognizable from the originals.

References

Adams, K.M., & Heaton, R.K. (1985). Automated interpretation of neuropsychological test data. *Journal of Consulting and Clinical Psychology, 53*, 790-802.

American Psychological Association (1986). *Guidelines for Computer-based Tests and Interpretations.* Washington, DC: Author.

American Psychological Association, Division 40 – Committee on Professional Standards, & Committee on Psychological Tests and Assessment (1987). Task force report in computer-assisted neuropsychological evaluation. *The Clinical Neuropsychologist, 2*, 161-184.

American Psychological Association Ethics Committee (1998). Services by telephone, teleconferencing, and Internet: A statement by the Ethics Committee of the American Psychological Association. *American Psychologist, 53*, 979.

Bashur, R. (1997). Critical issues in telemedicine. *Telemedicine Journal, 3*, 113-126.

Ball, C., Scott, J., McLaren, P. M., & Watson, J. P. (1993). Preliminary evaluation of a low-cost videoconferencing system for remote cognitive testing of adult psychiatric patients. *British Journal of Clinical Psychology, 32*, 303-307.

Browndyke, J.N., Albert, A.L., Malone, W., Schatz, P., Paul, R.H., Cohen, R.A., Tucker, K.A., & Gouvier, W. D. (2002). Computer-related Anxiety: Examining the Impact of Technology-specific Affect on the Performance of a Computerized Neuropsychological Assessment Measure. *Applied Neuropsychology, 9 (4)*, 256-261.

Buchanan, T. (2002). Online assessment: Desirable or dangerous? *Professional Psychology: Research and Practice, 33 (2)*, 148-154.

Bush, S., Naugle, R., & Johnson-Greene, D. (2002). The interface of information technology and neuropsychology: Ethical issues and recommendations. *The Clinical Neuropsychologist, 16 (4)*, 536-547.

Calloway, S.D., & Venegas, L.M. (2002). The new HIPAA law on privacy and confidentiality. *Nursing Administration Quarterly, 26 (4)*, 40-54.

Grossman, M. (1998, February 2). Watch your links, or you'll get framed. *Legal Times*, 31.

Gue, D.G. (n.d.). *The HIPAA security rule (NPRM): Overview.* Retrieved December 20, 2002, from http://www.hipaadvisory.com/regs/security-overview.htm

Harroch, R.D. (1998, February 2). Agreements, disclaimers and disclosures should be no less formal or thorough on the Web. *National Law Journal*, C7.

Hsiung, R. (2002). *E-Therapy: Case Studies, Guiding Principles, and the Clinical Potential of the Internet.* London: W.W. Norton & Company.

Huie, S. (1996). Facilitating telemedicine: Reconciling national access with state licensing laws. *Hastings Communications and Entertainment Law Journal, 18*, 377-400.

Koocher, G.P. (1994). APA and the FTC: New adventures in consumer protection. *American Psychologist, 49 (4)*, 322-328.

Koocher, G.P., & Morray, E. (2000). Regulation of telepsychology: A survey of state attorneys general. *Professional Psychology: Research and Practice, 31 (5)*, 503-508.

Maheu, M., Whitten, P., & Allen, A. (2001). *E-health, Telehealth & Telemedicine: A Practical Guide to Startup and Success.* New York: Jossey-Bass.

Mead, A.D., & Drasgow, F. (1993). Equivalence of computerized and paper-and-pencil cognitive ability tests: A meta-analysis. *Psychological Bulletin, 114 (3)*, 449-458.

Montani, C., Billaud, N., Tyrrell, J., Fluchaire, I., Malterre, C., Lauvernay, N., Couturier, P., & Franco, A. (1997). Psychological impact of a remote psychometric consultation with hospitalized elderly people. *Journal of Telemedicine and Telecare, 3 (3)*, 140-145.

Reed, G.M., McLaughlin, C.J., & Milholland, K. (2000). Ten interdisciplinary principles for professional practice in telehealth: Implications for psychology. *Professional Psychology: Research and Practice, 31 (2)*, 170-178.

Ruiz, M.A., Drake, E.B., Glass, A., Marcotte, D., & van Gorp, W. G. (2002). Trying to beat the system: Misuse of the Internet to assist in avoiding the detection of psychological symptom dissimulation. *Professional Psychology: Research and Practice, 33 (3)*, 294-299.

Schatz, P., & Browndyke, J.N. (2002). Applications of Computer-based Neuropsychological Assessment. *Journal of Head Trauma Rehabilitation, 17 (5)*, 395-410.

U.S. Department of Commerce – National Telecommunications and Information Administration (1997, January 31). *Telemedicine Report to Congress.* Retrieved December 20, 2002, from http://www.ntia.doc.gov/reports/telemed/index.htm

Widman, L.E., & Tong, D.A. (1997). Requests for medical advice from patients and families to health care providers who publish on the World Wide Web. *Archives of Internal Medicine, 157*, 209-212.

World Wide Web Consortium (1999, May 5). *Web Content Accessibility Guidelines 1.0.* Retrieved December 20, 2002, from http://www.w3.org/TR/WAI-WEBCONTENT/

Chapter 21

ETHICAL CHALLENGES WITH THE USE OF INFORMATION TECHNOLOGY AND TELECOMMUNICATIONS IN NEUROPSYCHOLOGY, PART II

Philip Schatz

Scenario 1

A licensed psychologist has a background in clinical psychology, neuropsychological assessment, and teaches within an undergraduate and Master's program in psychology at a small 1500 student, private University with an NCAA Division I athletic program. The Head Athletic Trainer (ATC) invites the psychologist to a meeting with the Team Physician, an M.D., who oversees and is responsible for all medical decisions related to the varsity athletes' participation in athletics program. This Team MD is essentially a consultant to the University who holds "office hours" two days per week in the school health center, during which he sees students for either scheduled examinations or walk-in visits. The Athletics Program and Head ATC have recently purchased computer-based assessment software and are planning on baseline testing all the varsity athletes as part of a new concussion management program. The Athletics Program is interested in monitoring baseline and post-concussion testing data in an effort to assist or guide return to play following concussions.

The psychologist agrees to participate in the project on a consultative basis, in order to assist the Team MD in evaluating the effects of concussion and determining fitness to return to play. The psychologist, along with the Head ATC, attends a workshop on the use and interpretation of the assessment software, and familiarizes himself with the operation and utilization of the software, as well as the psychometric data available in the literature. The Information Technology Department arranges for the psychologist, the Head ATC, and the Team MD to have password-protected access to the raw data, which is stored on a mainframe computer. Throughout the fall semester, when an athlete is suspected of sustaining a concussion, the ATC administers the computer-based assessment, and the psychologist is called. He accesses the data according to the athlete's name, interprets the raw data in the context of comparing it to baseline pre-season performance, and then advises the Team MD as to any preclusion to continued athletic participation. At times, the psychologist discusses cases with colleagues, either by phone or e-mail, prior to making his recommendations.

During the mid-semester break, the Women's Basketball team was on an extended road trip and participated in an evening game during a nationally televised Holiday tournament. During this game, the star athlete on the team was in a severe collision, in which she fell hard, hit her head on the floor, lost consciousness, and was suspected of having sustained a concussion. The student athlete was not permitted to participate for the remainder of the game, and after the game, the traveling ATC administered the tests on a laptop computer, posted the data on the server, and called to discuss the case with the psychologist. The psychologist analyzed the data, and attempted to contact the Team MD, who was unreachable and left no alternate physician to contact. Since there was a game the next day, it was late in the evening, and a swift decision was required by the traveling ATC. The psychologist contacted a group of colleagues via a neuropsychology e-mail listserv in order to get a "second opinion". The psychologist did not provide any demographic data (i.e., gender, age, race) but emphasized the need for a quick reply to his e-mail. Based on the available test data and the opinion of his colleagues, the psychologist made the determination that the student athlete could return to play the next day.

Relevant Ethical Issues

The above-outlined case exemplifies where the use of technology changed the process by which the psychologist obtained, stored, and accessed client data, as well as the manner in which the psychologist sought professional consultation. The psychologist's involvement in this case implicated several ethical guidelines.

Boundaries of Competence
The psychologist has had little formal training in assessing Mild TBI/post-concussion symptomatology, save for one formal workshop and a literature review. While his role as a consultant to the Team MD may be within the boundaries

of his competence, he is not a trained physician and is not qualified to make decisions regarding return to athletic competition after a head-to-floor collision and subsequent loss of consciousness. Such a decision may involve the integration of multiple contributing medical factors. Although the psychologist did attempt to obtain the opinion of colleagues and peers, through his contacts on the listserv, these peers were not medical doctors and could not provide the information needed for the psychologist to arrive at an informed opinion. As the psychologist's participation in this project was stipulated as a consultant to the Team MD, he has gone beyond his authority and competence (Standard 2.01).

Maintenance, Dissemination, and Disposal of Confidential Records of Professional and Scientific Work
As the psychologist was involved in the development of the concussion management program and had been accessing data through password-protected access, he was not naïve to the fact that student athlete data was being stored along with their names. While the use of names may be appropriate for the psychologist's personal data, this data was also being accessed by the ATCs, who were not trained in the interpretation of raw data. The presence of personal identifiers in the database may be in violation of the student athletes' confidentiality. The psychologist may have inappropriately communicated this case to colleagues, via an e-mail listserv, as discussed in the next section (Standard 6.02).

Consultations
The psychologist discussed the case on a public forum, an e-mail based list-serve without prior consent of the client. While he was careful to remove information which might have identified the athlete, based on the small size of the school, the nationally televised audience, and requested speedy turn-around for e-mail feedback, the members of the list-serve may have easily

determined the identity of the psychologist's client (Standard 4.06).

Bases for Assessments

In his capacity as a consultant, the psychologist provided an opinion on the results of cognitive testing which may implicate an athlete's return to play. However, the psychologist's role was to advise the Team MD, who conducts a more comprehensive evaluation of the student athlete. By acting alone and generating a return-to-play decision in the absence of a comprehensive evaluation, the psychologist had not utilized techniques sufficient to substantiate his findings (Standard 9.01).

Assessment by Unqualified Persons

By having an ATC conduct the post-concussion assessments, the psychologist is relying on potentially untrained personnel to obtain important data (Standard 9.07). Student athletes may present with a variety of symptoms that are not detected by the assessment measure, and may also go unnoticed by the ATC. Traditionally, psychometricians are trained to collect behavioral data such as affect, mood, and overall presentation. Recent position papers on the use of psychometricians have assisted and guided clinical psychologists in this manner (National Academy of Neuropsychology, 2000).

Case Resolution

The psychologist's involvement in this case could have been more "ethically sound" had he acted in the following manners.

Boundaries of Competence, Bases for Assessments

The psychologist had acted responsibly in educating himself regarding the use and interpretation of the computer-based assessment measure. However, he should have provided recommendations only for those student athletes whom he

had either seen personally, or those whose records he had an opportunity to fully review. In the case of the latter, his reports should have included a statement stipulating that he had only reviewed existing records. Any recommendations he made should have focused on psychological factors that might have impacted the athlete's ability to perform in her role as either an individual or team participant. He should also have formally recommended external referrals to proper medical professionals. In this case, he should have referred her for a radiological or medical examination and deferred any return-to-play decision making to medical professionals.

Maintenance, Dissemination, and Disposal of Confidential Records of Professional and Scientific Work

The psychologist should have assisted the Head ATC in creating a master list of pseudonyms for each student athlete. All data maintained in the database should have been listed only under the pseudonyms and not the names of the athletes. The master list should be maintained by the psychologist, along with all his client records and reports.

Consultations

The psychologist should not have consulted with colleagues for feedback on this case via an electronic mail list-serve. In spite of the steps taken to minimize infringement of confidentiality, he was unaware of the training and professional background of the list participants, and could not insure that the basketball player was unable to be identified. He should have limited his consultative request to either telephone or personal communications.

Assessment by Unqualified Persons

The psychologist may be relying on incomplete data obtained by the ATC staff, in that he is attempting to assess psychological and cognitive well being following cerebral concussions. While the ATCs may be trained to administer the actual computer-based measure, the psychologist should have personally trained the staff to conduct behavioral observations and document behavioral data. The psychologist would be best suited to personally evaluate each and every athlete following a concussion.

Conclusions and Recommendations

In spite of the exponential increase in the ownership and use of personal computers over the past several years, there remain very few guidelines regarding their use in the practice of (neuro)psychology with respect to the administration of assessment measures, access to and storage of client records, and communication between professionals. In fact, the term "Internet" appears only twice in the 2002 Ethics Code, "technology" only once, and "electronic" five times. Rather, practicing psychologists are left to extrapolate proper ethical conduct to those areas where use of emergent technologies may affect the means by which they carry out their practice.

The above scenario is one in which technology increased the speed of access to test data, allowed access to test data from a distance, and altered the means by which test data was obtained. The ethical guidelines involved do not directly involve the use of technology, as such guidelines do not exist for the use of computer-based assessment measures, digital data storage and retrieval, and consultation by electronic mail. While benefits, limitations, ethics, and applications of computer-based assessment are documented in the literature (French & Beaumont, 1987; Schatz & Browndyke, 2002; Walker & Cobb-Myrick, 1985; Wilson & McMillan, 1991), few would argue that there remains a paucity in this area. Comparison of survey results from the 1980s (Farrell, 1989) and 1990s (McMinn, Buchanan, Ellens & Ryan, 1999), reveals that computer use by psychologists is ever-increasing, and data from the mid-1990s revealed psychologists who were less technophobic, performed frequent assessments, were younger, and saw a higher percentage of managed care patients were more likely to use and embrace technology in their practice (Rosen & Weil, 1997). More recent surveys have focused solely on the ethical implications of consulting with colleagues via telephone or fax (McMinn et al., 1999), but the 2002 Ethical Code is generally replete with reference to the use of computers in psychological practice. Rather, practicing psychologists considering the use of technology are left with the APA Ethics Committee's "Statement on Services by Telephone, Teleconferencing, and Internet" (APA Ethics Committee, 1997): "review the characteristics of the services, the service delivery method, and the provisions for confidentiality … then consider the relevant ethical standards and other requirements, such as licensure board rules."

Recent publications offer detailed recommendations on the ethical use of information technology and telecommunications in clinical practice (Bush, Naugle & Johnson-Greene, 2002), and outline specific ethical considerations for psychologists participating in on-line discussion groups in a professional capacity (Humphreys, Winzelberg & Klaw, 2000). To this end, it appears to be time for APA to revise their 1997 Statement on Services by Telephone, Teleconferencing, and Internet to more specifically define the types of services offered by psychologists and the means by which they can be carried out using technology. Guidelines should be established for the use of computer-based assessment measures, and the subsequent storage and retrieval of data. These guidelines should include acceptable digital storage media, back-up systems for digital storage, and security of such stored media. As well, more detailed guidelines and recommendations should be provided for communication between professionals using electronic mail and Internet-based message boards, with specific focus on maintaining client confidentiality and obtaining prior informed consent for such communications.

Scenario 2

A recent graduate begins a two-year post-doctoral neuropsychology fellowship in which he splits his time between a hospital-based "rotation" and a clinic-based rotation in which services are provided through the private practice of his supervisor. As part of the private practice rotation, the postdoc is expected to collaborate on research activities within his area of shared interest with the supervisor, ageing, dementia and memory. The supervisor maintains a web site for his practice, on which there is little information posted, other than practice contact information and services provided. During an informal lunch conversation early in the post-doc, the postdoc tells the supervisor that he has experience with web site design and maintenance, and shares his vision of creating an on-line "presence" for neuropsychologists, clients, and researchers seeking information regarding the practice of neuropsychology as well as information about the etiology, symptomatology, and treatment of memory disorders and dementias. The postdoc offers to improve the practice web site and increase the amount of information posted in this manner, and the supervisor agrees that these activities can be considered part of his research activities within his post-doc.

The postdoc takes on the role of "webmaster", and throughout the year works on redesigning and expanding the web site, developing many new pages using referenced text from the voluminous literature review from his dissertation. As the site begins to grow, the postdoc develops and arranges pages according to each memory disorder and dementia, with separate pages for causes, symptoms, treatments, prognosis and links. He places a copyright symbol ("©") and his name within the html "source code" of each web page that he designed ("©2002, the postdoc"). During the next year, the postdoc registers the domain name "MemoryLoss.com" and designs a comprehensive web-based resource, external to the supervisor's practice site. The postdoc discusses this new Internet site with the supervisor and tells the supervisor that he wishes to move the "content" pages he developed to his site and place links from the postdoc's practice web page. The supervisor states that the pages in question were developed for his practice, and should remain there. The supervisor further states that he is disappointed in the postdoc's professional conduct and may not be able to recommend him well following his post-doc. The supervisor re-claims the role of "webmaster" and places a copyright ("©2002, the supervisor") on the bottom of each page on the site, but does not notice or alter the postdoc's copyright in the html source code. The postdoc confronts the supervisor and states that this is plagiarism, points out his initial copyright, states that these pages are his "intellectual property," and suggests that if the supervisor does not remove his personal copyright he will be reported to the State Licensing Board's ethics committee.

Relevant Ethical Issues

The above-outlined case exemplifies issues related to potentially exploitive and multiple relationships, assessing student and supervisee performance, and resolution and reporting of ethical violations. With specific respect to the use of technology, this case raises issues related to authorship and publication credit, intellectual property, and copyright law. The psychologist's involvement in this case implicated several ethical guidelines.

Exploitive and Multiple Relationships

Although it appears unintentional, the supervisor appears to have entered into a multiple relationship with the postdoc, in that he simultaneously supervised the postdoc as a postdoctoral fellow and as a hired web designer. Because the supervisor maintained a supervisory position, the postdoc's web design performance could affect the supervisor's objectivity when assessing the postdoc's performance as a postdoctoral fellow. As well, since the position of web designer would most likely be a paid position, incorporating these duties as part of the postdoc's training may be interpreted as exploitive (Standards 3.05a & 3.08).

Assessing Student and Supervisee Performance

The supervisor should not have allowed the interaction regarding the postdoc's desire to claim ownership over the web pages he designed to enter into his evaluation of the postdoc's performance. Had the supervisor previously established a formal process for assessing the postdoc's performance, the risk of having bias from extraneous factors influence the evaluation may have been reduced somewhat, but it still would not have eliminated the potential effects of bias (Standard 7.06).

Plagiarism and Publication Credit

Due to the dynamic nature of the Internet, publication and authorship rights are not clearly defined for individuals who post information on the Internet. However, the postdoc was the primary and substantial contributor to the pages he developed for the supervisor's web site (Standard 8.11). By placing a copyright in the html source code of those web pages, he essentially claimed first authorship for those pages. By later placing his own copyright statement on those same pages, the supervisor was presenting this work as his own (Standard 8.12). Intellectual property rights, and copyright claims, laws and violations are constantly being re-defined and challenged with respect to Internet-based materials. A more comprehensive discussion of copyright laws and intellectual property rights will follow in the "Recommendations" section.

Resolution and Reporting of Ethical Violations

The postdoc attempted to resolve the issue informally by confronting the supervisor (Standard 1.04). He thus acted appropriately when he confronted the supervisor regarding his improper ownership of the materials. The postdoc was acting appropriately and ethically when (after the supervisor failed to change his stance and then threatened actions which might ultimately harm the postdoc) he stated his intention to report the supervisor to the State Licensing Board's ethics committee (Standard 1.05).

Case Resolution

The supervisor's involvement in this case could have been more "ethically sound" had he acted in the following manners:

Multiple and Exploitive Relationships

The supervisor should not have involved the postdoc in any web design activities that could be fulfilled by an outside contractor not trained in psychology. By holding a supervisory relationship, the supervisor was in a position to exploit the postdoc, as well as create a dual relationship of post-doc supervisor and web site owner. The supervisor should have invited the postdoc to lend his expertise and assist in hiring, advising, and supervising an appropriate web design contractor.

Assessing Student and Supervisee Performance

The supervisor should not have allowed the postdoc's performance on the web design project to guide his opinion of the postdoc's performance as a postdoctoral fellow in neuropsychology. The supervisor should have had regularly scheduled meetings during which the postdoc's performance was discussed, as well as during which the supervisor's performance was discussed. If new projects were added to the postdoc's responsibilities, appraisal of the postdoc's performance on these projects should have been discussed within supervision meetings. At no time should the supervisor have used a future letter of recommendation as a "negotiating chip" in an argument.

Plagiarism and Publication Credit

While there is little guidance in the literature on this topic, web-based publications should be treated in a similar manner to journal-based publications. Authorship should be determined prior to commencing the work, and relative contributions should be weighed in determining authorship. Had the supervisor wished to retain copyright of the materials, he should have had the postdoc sign a statement transferring ownership and copyright of the materials developed to the supervisor. However, in the absence of such a document, since the postdoc created the content for these Internet pages, and inserted his copyright in the pages, he should be considered first author. By purposely taking control of this work, and inserting his own copyright symbol, the supervisor was essentially plagiarizing the postdoc's work.

Resolution and Reporting of Ethical Violations

The postdoc acted appropriately when he first discussed his feelings with the supervisor, and then stated he would refer the matter to the State Licensing Board's ethics committee. The supervisor should have consulted with a colleague or an ethics committee to guide his thinking and actions in what became an emotional and territorial matter.

Conclusions and Recommendations

As described above, there exist very few ethical guidelines to inform psychologists regarding their role in determining Internet-based professional publication credits, intellectual property rights, or copyright ownership. While psychologists can extrapolate proper ethical conduct from the 2002 Ethical Code, they must look beyond the published psychology literature for guidance.

According to the U.S. Copyright Act (2001), a copyright gives the owner the exclusive right to reproduce, distribute, perform, display, or license his work, as well as the exclusive right to produce or license derivatives of the work. To be covered by copyright, a work must be original and in a concrete "medium of expression," and, under current law, works are covered whether or not a copyright notice is attached and whether or not the work is registered. The essential goal of copyright protection is to secure the interests of the owner/publisher of the information, such as ensuring any income from intellectual work or protecting personal information (Norderhaug & Oberding, 1995). Thus, the owner of a copyright has *exclusive* rights to reproduce their work, prepared derivatives, distribute copies, or display the work publicly.

Use of Internet technology creates an inherently paradoxical arrangement in which the mechanism for viewing content (i.e., the web browser) may actually store the document in memory or in a cache file, or facilitate the creation of copies of source material by the user by allowing them to: save the material as source, print a rendered version of the material, or select, copy and paste the material into a word document program (Norderhaug & Oberding, 1995). By placing a copyright statement in either the code or the content ("©Year, Creator") the developer or creator is able to ensure that any individual accessing or copying their material is aware of its source and ownership. O'Mahoney (2002) suggests that individuals who post materials on the web should either place a copyright symbol on each item developed, much like book publishers or movie producers list transferred copyright for each and every image, graphic, song, or work displayed. As well, much like journal publishers, for those materials created by employees, contractors, or contributors, there should be a mechanism to transfer copyright from those individuals who created the materials. Individuals who place a copyright statement on their web-based work are encouraged to register that work with the

Library of Congress, prior to arguing a copyright claim relative to that information. While the cost of registering a copyright is in the range of thirty dollars, the cost of emergent, expedited registration can be in the range of several hundred dollars.

While specific APA guidelines for Internet-based publications would assist psychologists, when preparing Internet-based materials, psychologists should follow existing ethical procedures for publishing print-based materials, and familiarize themselves with U.S. Copyright Law. Psychologists should always discuss authorship at the commencement of a multiple-author project, consider the contribution of multiple authors, and weigh whether or not the work is based on a student author's thesis or dissertation.

References

American Psychological Association Ethics Committee. (1997). *Statement on Services by Telephone, Teleconferencing, and Internet* [Web Page]. URL http://www.apa.org/ethics/stmnt01.html [2002, December].

Bush, S., Naugle, R., & Johnson-Greene, D. (2002). The interface of information technology and neuropsychology: Ethical issues and recommendations. *The Clinical Neuropsychologist, 16(4)*, 536-547.

Farrell, A. (1989). Impact of Computers on Professional Practice: A Survey of Current Practices and Attitudes. *Professional Psychology: Research and Practice, 20(3)*, 172-178.

French, C.C., & Beaumont, J.G. (1987). The reaction of psychiatric patients to computerized assessment. *British Journal of Clinical Psychology, 26*, 267-277.

Humphreys, K., Winzelberg, A., & Klaw, E. (2000). Psychologists' ethical responsibilities in Internet-based groups; Issues, Strategies, and a call for dialogue. *Professional Psychology: Research and Practice, 31(5)*, 493-496.

McMinn, M.R., Buchanan, T., Ellens, B.M., & Ryan, M.K. (1999). Technology, Professional Practice, and Ethics: Survey Findings and Implications. *Professional Psychology: Research and Practice, 30(2)*, 165-172.

National Academy of Neuropsychology. (2000). The use of Neuropsychology Test Technicians in Clinical Practice: Official Statement of the National Academy of Neuropsychology. *Archives of Clinical Neuropsychology, 15(5)*, 381-382.

Norderhaug, T., & Oberding, J.M. (1995). Designing a Web of Intellectual Property. *Conference proceedings of The Third International World-Wide Web Conference, Computer Networks and ISDN Systems, 27(6)*, 1037-1046.

O'Mahoney, B. (2002). Protecting your website: Ownership, notice, registration. *Copyright Website LLC.* Retrieved from: http://www.benedict.com/digital/webProtect/webProtect.asp

Rosen, L. D., & Weil, M. M. (1997). Psychologists and Technology: A look at the future. *Professional Psychology: Research and Practice, 27(6)*, 635-638.

Schatz, P., & Browndyke, J.N. (2002). Applications of Computer-based neuropsychological assessment. *Journal of Head Trauma Rehabilitation, 17(5)*, 395-410.

U.S. Copyright Office. (2001). *Copyright Law of the United States of America.* Library of Congress: Washington, DC. (Available on-line: http://www.copyright.gov/title17/).

Walker, N.W., & Cobb-Myrick, C. (1985). Ethical considerations in the use of computers in psychological testing and assessment. *Journal of School Psychology, 23*, 51-57.

Wilson, S.L., & McMillan, T.M. (1991). Microcomputers in psychometric and neuropsychological assessment. In A. Ager (Editor), *Microcomputers and Clinical Psychology: Issues, Applications and Future Developments*. (pp. 79-94). Chichester: England: John Wiley and Sons, Ltd.

Section 11

ETHICAL CHALLENGES IN NEUROPSYCHOLOGICAL RESEARCH

Introduction

Neuropsychological researchers often confront ethical challenges that are similar to those found in other areas of psychology but have the additional aspect of involving participants that are cognitively impaired. Educating the administration and support staff of the institutions through which such research is performed about the unique issues involved with having participants that have cognitive impairments is a priority but can be quite challenging. In addition, pressures from a variety of sources to prematurely apply a participant's research findings to his or her clinical situation may result in conflicts with co-workers or the participant's family members and must be handled in a manner that is sensitive to these competing needs and yet consistent with ethical guidelines. The authors of this chapter provide a representative sampling of such cases and illustrate ways of negotiating the difficulties encountered.

Chapter 22

ETHICAL CHALLENGES IN NEUROPSYCHOLOGICAL RESEARCH, PART I

Laetitia L. Thompson

Scenario 1

A neuropsychologist conducts a study of the neurocognitive functioning of patients as they go through detoxification from alcohol or opiates. He relies upon the clinical staff at the Detoxification Program to inform him when the patient-participant is able to give informed consent. He then goes to the program to meet the potential participant and to obtain consent. After that he or his research assistant (RA) administers a neuropsychological battery that lasts for about three hours. Sometimes, the participants complain of fatigue or feeling ill and want to quit, but the neuropsychologist strongly encourages participants at these times to continue on, because it is very important that he obtain complete data. When this happens, he also reminds them of the monetary incentive that is to be given to them at the end of the testing session. In almost all cases, the neuropsychologist is able to convince the participant to stay for the duration of the study.

The program counselors sometimes intimate to potential participants that they will be able to get information about their brain functioning by participating in the study. The participant then presents this query to the neuropsychologist when going over the consent form. Another program counselor is very excited about the project and thinks that all of her patients should participate. She tends to refer potential participants, even if they are still in withdrawal or reluctant to volunteer.

Sometimes after the testing is completed, the participant's clinical counselor comes to the neuropsychologist, asking about the test results and how the "patient" did. The counselor is also interested in discussing the participant's demeanor and behavior during the research testing session. The neuropsychologist is eager to accommodate the clinical staff at the Center because initially the Center staff had been reluctant to bring this type of research into the clinical program. The neuropsychologist appreciates their collaboration and letting him recruit participants on site. The consent form is vague as to whether or not the neuropsychologist is authorized to release information about the participant to the clinical staff. He explains this to the counselor, who says, "Oh, I know. I just wanted your informal assessment." The neuropsychologist indicates that he is sorry but he thinks it would be violating confidentiality to disclose any information and that this would be unethical. The counselor indicates that he understands, but the neuropsychologist becomes concerned, because after this, this particular counselor seems less interested in directing potential participants his way. The neuropsychologist is concerned not only because it affects the number of participants, but also that it might bias the participant sample, because this counselor sees most of the older patients.

The neuropsychologist employs one RA who scores the results and enters them into the computer for data management and analysis, and a second RA who checks the entries to be sure they are accurate. He is conscientious about this until one of the RAs becomes ill and has to take six weeks of sick leave. Feeling some pressure to analyze the data for publication, he relaxes his standards and has the one RA enter the data, with no further checking. This RA also has some background in statistics and data analysis and she volunteers some novel ideas about how to present the data. She and the neuropsychologist work together on a presentation to be given at a national meeting and a paper that will be submitted for publication. The RA contributes several comments and writes much of the Results section of the paper. The neuropsychologist views her work as being of high quality, and she seems very precise and responsible in her work. He makes her a coauthor, given her hard work and contribution to the study. During the initial presentation of the results at a national conference, several colleagues ask some questions, causing the neuropsychologist to realize that a few numbers in one of the Tables could not be right. He has already submitted the manuscript for publication.

Relevant Ethical Issues

Several of the aspirational General Principles are relevant to one or more aspects of this scenario. The researcher should consider the principles of Beneficence and Nonmaleficence (Principle A) and Respect for People's Rights and Dignity (Principle E) in determining how to treat the study participants. His subject selection process and coercive "encouragement" are likely to result in short-term, and possibly long-term, physical and/or psychological discomfort or distress and may result in data that do not accurately reflect the neuropsychological constructs being assessed. He has an obligation to respect the participants' rights to discontinue testing upon request, without pressure. In addition, given the nature of the patient population involved in the study, the researcher should probably have anticipated the potential for fatigue and illness and designed the study to have briefer testing sessions. The researcher also needs to consider the principles of Fidelity and Responsibility (Principle B) and Integrity (Principle C) in his professional behavior and in his commitment to the accuracy and honesty of the data obtained in the study.

Specific Standards that apply are:

Delegation of Work to Others (2.05)
The neuropsychologist has delegated several research tasks to his RA but has not maintained the necessary oversight to ensure the accuracy of the work performed by the RA. In addition, he delegated to the Center staff the authority to determine when patients are ready for participation in the study. However, based on the patients referred, it does not appear that the Center staff were adequately trained in inclusion and exclusion criteria.

Maintaining Confidentiality (4.01)
The neuropsychologist wants to maintain appropriate confidentiality of the research information, but he appears not to have outlined the confidentiality requirements with the Center staff prior to beginning the study. Similarly, he failed to provide clarity on this issue in his informed consent with study participants. The researcher also appears willing to consider sharing more information about participants with their counselors in order to maintain and increase referrals from certain counselors.

Informed Consent to Research (8.02)

Potential participants need to be competent and fully informed before signing consent. In this case, the consent form was vague, the participants undergoing detoxification may not have been able to fully understand the study parameters and implications, and the researcher did not appear to take the necessary steps to rectify these problems.

Client/Patient, Student, and Subordinate Research Participants (8.04)

These participants are also clinical patients in a treatment program. Furthermore, they are being tested at the Clinical Program, potentially causing confusion as to their research status and making them more vulnerable to subtle coercion. Such factors may have negative effects on both their effort in the study and their investment in their treatment program.

Reporting Research Results (8.10)

It is the responsibility of the neuropsychologist to ensure that research results are reported accurately. In this case, the researcher relied on the work of his RA without checking the accuracy of the results prior to presenting them at a conference and submitting them for publication.

Publication Credit (8.12)

The neuropsychologist, as the principle investigator, has the responsibility of granting authorship to individuals who have made significant scientific or professional contributions to the project. Acknowledgement in a footnote or introductory statement would be appropriate in situations in which an assistant's contribution is not at a level consistent with co-authorship.

Use of Assessments (9.02)

The neuropsychologist needs to be clear that the tools he is using in the research study are experimental tasks for which there are no norms, and clinical interpretation is inappropriate. Such

information should have been explained clearly to Center staff before the study began and to potential participants during the subject selection and informed consent processes.

Case Resolution

While the study is underway, the neuropsychologist becomes aware that the treatment counselors have made assumptions about the research project, some of which are not accurate. One of these assumptions is that the research protocol is like a clinical evaluation in terms of tests administered and information available to the patient-participant. The neuropsychologist does not want to offend any of the counselors because they are helping him with the study, but he does not want potential participants to be misled about receiving their individual test results. He is happy to provide general information about the study results, but since the evaluation includes experimental tasks rather than clinical tests, it is not appropriate to give participants feedback about their individual results. A second assumption is that the neuropsychologist is free to talk about the participant with the clinical staff. This is not the case, but the clinical staff does not fully perceive the difference in status when the patients are participating in a research study. A third problem occurs because one of the counselors is too enthusiastic about the study and does not use good judgment in deciding if and when a patient is ready and able to give informed consent to participate. This makes the neuropsychologist's job more difficult because he has to carefully screen out individuals who appear too ill or confused to consent, and he has to protect the participant from subtle coercion to participate.

The neuropsychologist decides that it is necessary to convene a meeting of the clinical staff to discuss some of these issues. With the consent and attendance of the program director, the neuropsychologist meets with the counselors to openly discuss the issues, and how the goals of research are different from those in the clinical setting. They discuss privacy, confidentiality, the importance of respecting participants' rights and dignity, and the appropriate use of different kinds of assessment information. After considerable discussion, the parties are able to identify the potential conflicts between research and clinical service, and are able to settle on procedures that will ensure ethical work.

In his enthusiasm for collecting as much data as possible, the neuropsychologist loses sight of his responsibility to respect the rights of participants to freely withdraw from the study. He oversteps his bounds in strongly urging participants to continue when they wish to withdraw, and it is inappropriate to bring up the financial incentive at this time. He lets his desire to obtain complete data on participants get in the way of his regard for the autonomy and well being of participants. This is compounded because these participants are clinical patients in a treatment program. Although they are informed that they are participating in a research study, the fact that their counselors refer them for participation and the fact that the testing takes place on the clinical premises may make these individuals more vulnerable to coercion.

The neuropsychologist delegates some of the work to his research assistants, but he remains responsible for the quality and integrity of the data. He should more closely supervise the data entry and analysis, and he should not relax his standards when it becomes inconvenient to double check data entry. He becomes aware of this when being asked questions at a conference that show some problems with the data. After the meeting, he returns to his offices and spends some time with the RA going over the tables, the results, and the actual raw data. He realizes that while overall she did an excellent job, she made a few errors in data entry and misunderstood a couple of things that led to errors in the analyses. The neuropsychologist is relieved that this came to light before the manuscript is published. He contacts the journal editor to whom he has submitted the paper and requests that it be returned to him before any further review because he has found some errors. He realizes that he should have monitored the RA more carefully in her work.

Conclusions and Recommendations

This scenario highlights the many "small" ethical challenges that may be encountered on a frequent basis in doing research. All individuals involved in research must keep in mind the inherent conflict between the goals of research and clinical treatment, and it is incumbent upon the researcher to inform and educate clinical staff with whom he or she is collaborating.

Research often is done under time lines that place some pressure on the psychologist to proceed quickly (e.g., before funding runs out, in time to present at an upcoming meeting, pending loss of an employee or student working on the project). Ethical guidelines should never be sacrificed for expediency, however, no matter how innocent or trivial the infraction may seem.

Maintaining adequate supervision of employees and students can be difficult but is vital for maintaining fidelity and responsibility to the science and for maintaining participants' rights and privacy.

Scenario 2

A young neuropsychologist who had just completed a postdoctoral fellowship obtains a highly desirable, competitive academic position at a large medical school. She will be spending part of her time working with a large research team that focuses on the study of Alzheimer's disease and other dementias. The head of the team is an internationally known expert with considerable grant support, and he is funding part of her salary from one of his grants. Initially, the neuropsychologist thinks that this is going to be a wonderful opportunity. Team meetings are intellectually stimulating, and her input is welcomed. The group is doing some cognitive testing with some of the research participants, and they want the help of a neuropsychologist to enhance their studies.

As she settles in, she begins to explore in detail the measures and methods that are in current use. She observes the research assistants who are doing the testing and is surprised to find that they have received very little training or supervision and, as a result, are fairly dissimilar in their testing practices. Standardized test administration is not followed consistently, and there appears to be low reliability among scoring procedures. When the neuropsychologist approaches the senior scientist about this, he is receptive although not overly concerned. He gives her the authority to hold a few group training sessions, and then to observe the individual testing of each research assistant. When she approaches the RAs directly, she meets with a variety of reactions. Two of the RAs are quite interested in getting more training in order to increase the reliability and validity of what they are doing. One of the RAs who has worked with the research group for many years is polite, but dismissive, that anything needs to be done. She gives the neuropsychologist the impression that she will "go along" and humor her but does not regard any changes in procedures as truly necessary. The fourth RA is overtly resistant to change and to being observed. She feels as though it is a criticism of her work and that it demeans her position. In fact, she complains to the director of the research program, arguing that she has been doing this for years and does not need a new, young faculty member looking over her shoulder. The director, who has worked with this RA for a number of years, tells her to go along with the training, but "winks" at her as he does so.

The training proceeds, and the neuropsychologist thinks it is going well for three of the four testers. The fourth RA either will not (or cannot) adapt to the more rigorous rules for standardized administration, and the more the neuropsychologist learns of her work, the more concerned she becomes. The neuropsychologist discovers that the RA is not very supportive or encouraging of participants as they encounter difficult items on the tests; in fact it appeared that she encourages participants to give up because it shortens the testing session. Moreover, the neuropsychologist becomes concerned about this RA's method of obtaining consent from the participants. Expediency seemed to be the priority, so it is not clear whether or not participants are giving "informed consent." This was not always an easy determination in these individuals with progressive dementing disorders. In the training sessions, the RA initially improves her performance on the first two tests, but when she learns the third test, her previous mistakes on the first two tests reappear, so that she always seems to be improving on some parts and relapsing on others.

The neuropsychologist also becomes aware that test protocols with participant identifiers are left lying around in several offices to which a number of different people have access. The neuropsychologist becomes very frustrated and worried. The group is running several studies of experimental medications, and the behavioral test results are among the primary outcome measures. Participant testing occurs on a frequent basis so, as she tries to work with training, the RAs are collecting more data. The research is on a tight timeline, and the neuropsychologist knows there is pressure to collect data rapidly. Also, she is being encouraged to assume the responsibility for analyzing some of the test measures for inclusion in a manuscript being written by one of her colleagues.

Relevant Ethical Issues

Most of the General Principles are relevant for this scenario. The neuropsychologist must consider the Principles of Beneficence and Nonmaleficence and Respect for the Rights and Dignity of Others in training the RAs to interact with the research participants in a standardized and respectful manner. As part of generating research data, she must also consider the Principles of Fidelity and Responsibility as well as Integrity. Specific standards that apply are:

Conflicts between Ethics and Organizational Demands (1.03)

The neuropsychologist has to deal with the conflicts between her ethics and the methods and procedures that have been followed by the research team. She acted appropriately by bringing her concerns to the attention of the senior scientist in the beginning; however, it appears necessary for her approach him again to inform him of the status of the RA training and to work with him or obtain his approval to establish measurable and enforceable training standards.

Delegation of Work to Others (2.05)

The neuropsychologist has to deal with the ethics of working with subordinates in an area of her scientific expertise and to define her role and responsibility in that regard. In order to help the RAs develop the skills necessary to obtain reliable and valid data, the neuropsychologist needs to elicit their cooperation and their investment in the training program and their work. However, she cannot achieve her goals without the full support of the senior researcher. She must work to establish working relationships with all parties so that everyone is clear about what is required and what will happen if such requirements are not met.

Avoiding Harm (3.04)

The neuropsychologist has to take steps to avoid any harm that might accrue to the research participants because of the deficient work of the RAs. In addition, the implications for greater harm based on publication of faulty results must be considered. Future studies, research funding, and individual treatment decisions may all be influenced by the quality of the research team's

work, including the RAs and the young neuropsychologist.

Maintaining Confidentiality (4.01)

Carelessness in the treatment of test protocols with participant identifiers may result in violations of confidentiality and is inconsistent with ethical conduct.

Maintenance, Dissemination, and Disposal of Confidential Records of Professional and Scientific Work (6.02)

The current practice of record keeping is inadequate in keeping the records confidential. The neuropsychologist has become aware of the carelessness and is ethically obligated to reminding others of the necessity of safeguarding records and ensuring participant confidentiality. If friendly reminders are insufficient, additional steps would need to be taken.

Assessing Student and Supervisee Performance (7.06)

The young neuropsychologist did not initially establish a clear process for training and feedback, partly because of the initial ambiguity of her role. She found herself in the awkward position of coming into the study midway and needing to disrupt the established patterns of behavior. Once she determined what changes needed to be made, it became her responsibility to ensure that they occurred. Establishing training protocols and assessing the performance of the RAs was one of her roles on the research team.

Informed Consent to Research (8.02)

In supervising the RAs, it is imperative that the neuropsychologist ensure that consent procedures are thorough and complete. Information necessary for informed consent that seemed to have been neglected include (a) the participants' right to decline to participate and to withdraw from the research once participation has begun, (b) reasonably foreseeable risks that may influence their willingness to participate, potential limits of confidentiality, and (c) whom to contact for questions about the research and research participants' rights. In addition, since the research participants are patients, the neuropsychologist has a responsibility to protect the prospective participants from adverse consequences of declining or withdrawing from participation (Ethical Standard 8.04) and to ensure that financial incentives were not used in a coercive manner (Ethical Standard 8.06). In addition, some of the prospective participants seem to present with questionable cognitive capacity to make informed decisions regarding participation.

Reporting Research Results (8.10)

The neuropsychologist is confronted with errors in data due to poor testing practices, and yet she is not the one in charge of those data. She is obligated to "take reasonable steps to correct such errors."

Assessment by Unqualified Persons (9.07)

The neuropsychologist must not promote the continuation of testing by unqualified persons. She has taken steps to train all of the RAs. Following completion of training, she must make a determination regarding who is qualified and who is not and only allow those who are qualified to continue administering tests. The support of the senior researcher is required in order to execute her plans.

Case Resolution

Like many real-life situations, this scenario depicts a complex array of relationships and issues.

Prior to accepting the position, the neuropsychologist does not obtain information about how research testing has been conducted, and she does not negotiate who formally supervises the research assistants who serve as testing examiners. As a result, she ends up in a position where she feels responsible, but the "chain of command" is not clear. Thus, when she introduces new training and guidelines to the research assistants, her role and authority are not clear. One of the research assistants has worked for the institution for many years and has worked with the program director for a long time. She resents the intrusion of the new faculty member into her domain. Her resistance is fostered by the program director giving her "mixed messages" about how seriously she needs to treat the new procedures.

The neuropsychologist belatedly realizes that she is in an untenable situation. She consults with fellow psychology faculty members about how to proceed and then goes to the program director with her concerns. Although feeling somewhat intimidated, she informs him of her most basic concerns about enrolling participants who might not be competent to give informed consent and the unreliability and invalidity of the data being obtained. She asserts that the testing has to be supervised in order to obtain useful data, and she suggests that as the neuropsychologist on the team, she was the most qualified to do that supervision. The program director is not so concerned, but he recognizes her intensity about the issue, so he revises the organizational structure to make the roles clear.

The program director is not very receptive to the neuropsychologist's assertion that the data that has been obtained thus far are not valid and should not be relied upon. He thinks that in her youthful enthusiasm, she is reacting too strongly. She indicates that she would be interested in analyzing any future data and participating in publications of it, but she does not wish to get involved with the data that has already been collected.

The neuropsychologist is distressed about the lax way the records are kept. Confidentiality is not ensured, and the records are kept so haphazardly, there is a significant chance that some of the data will become lost or misplaced. When she approaches the program director about this issue, he is appalled. He has emphasized careful and confidential storage of research data in locked facilities. He quickly sends out a memo to all of the research staff regarding appropriate storage of data, urging all to comply and to let him know immediately if appropriate facilities are not available.

The neuropsychologist attempts to work with all four research assistants in establishing reliable procedures and methods, but the recalcitrant RA remains deficient. It seems as though she learns one thing, implements it for a while, and then forgets it after learning something else. Neither party is happy with the situation, and it is making the whole training process difficult. Finally, the program director agrees to "transfer" that RA to a different position where she will not be engaged in testing. The neuropsychologist thinks this is probably the best solution available. She carefully documents her training sessions and the results, in the event that questions should arise later.

Conclusions and Recommendations

This scenario highlights some of the issues that can arise when a neuropsychologist first enters an organization. It is difficult to know all of the important questions to be asked and issues to be negotiated when considering a new job, but it is important to determine how the organization functions and what the "ethical culture" is. In this situation, the neuropsychologist and her research program director both thought they were ethical, but they had somewhat different perspectives. She thought she was doing the minimum to be ethical, and he thought she was rather compulsive about small details. In this situation, the two parties were still able to negotiate procedures that both found acceptable.

This scenario also highlights the difficulties that may arise when a junior member of an organization thinks it is necessary to confront a more senior investigator about ethical issues. This is especially challenging when the senior person is the junior neuropsychologist's supervisor. Such situations are not, of course, restricted to research situations, but it is important to remember that ethical issues are as important in research as in clinical treatment. Although it may be intimidating to approach a supervisor about an ethical issue with which he or she is involved, certain occasions call for this. In many situations where the psychologist is dealing with difficult or uncomfortable ethical issues, it can be helpful to consult with trusted colleagues about how to proceed.

References

American Psychological Association (1992) Ethical principles of psychologists and code of conduct. *American Psychologist, 47,* 1597-1611.

American Psychological Association (2002). Ethical principles of psychologists and code of conduct. *American Psychologist, 57,* 1060-1073.

Chapter 23

ETHICAL CHALLENGES IN NEURO-PSYCHOLOGICAL RESEARCH, PART II

Wilfred G. van Gorp

Scenario 1

A neuropsychologist is conducting a research study investigating the relationship among performance on a battery of neuropsychological tests, performance on newly devised tests of "real world" functions, and success or failure in finding employment in a cohort of HIV+ individuals looking for work. An individual study participant found employment during the course of the study but maintained her employment for only eight months before being terminated from the job. Three months later, the participant's treating psychologist (i.e., her psychotherapist) called the research neuropsychologist conducting the study and asked him to write a letter to the social security administration in support of the participant's disability due to HIV-related dementia. The treating psychologist asked the neuropsychologist to especially highlight the participant's scores on the tasks of functional ability devised in the research study to measure "real world" abilities, to use in support of the proposed disability.

The research neuropsychologist offered to write a brief summary of the test findings from the clinical neuropsychological tests and give this to the participant, but did not agree to include interpretation of the experimentally devised functional ("real world") tests, citing the lack of data on the validity and reliability of the experimentally devised functional tasks as well as the lack of data using the clinical neuropsychological tasks to predict work ability. The researcher explained that the functional tests had been devised in his laboratory, and were not yet validated.

The treating psychologist responded with considerable umbrage, and in the course of their conversation, proffered a threat to encourage the participant to file a complaint with the institutional IRB, citing the failure of the researcher to be mindful of the participant's best interests in supporting her claim for disability. When the research neuropsychologist noted the lack of data between performance on "real world" functional tasks and actual work ability, the participant's clinician commented, "Oh, don't get so technical. You know you could write it if you wanted to – just pretend it's a grant application. Besides, I already told the SSD people you have great data relating work ability to your functional measures."

In an effort to obtain independent consultation regarding this thorny matter, the research neuropsychologist consulted a colleague psychologist researcher doing research in HIV and psychosis at his institution regarding this matter. As he described the participant and her background, the colleague recognized the participant, and replied, "Oh, I know her – she's in my studies too. She's a professional research participant; she is working full time for money 'off the books' doing accounting for a wealthy individual and earning quite a bit of money doing it – and doing it well, I might add."

Relevant Ethical Issues

This case raises a host of ethical issues. They can be perhaps grouped into several arenas.

Bases for Assessment (Standard 9.01) and Use of Assessments (Standard 9.02)
A key issue is that the treating psychologist is asking the researcher to base an opinion in part upon experimental tests not yet validated for clinical use. The Ethics Code specifically indicates that opinions from the assessment are based upon "techniques sufficient to substantiate their findings." In the absence of independent data validating these functional assessments and work ability or disability, there seems no solid basis on which to base an opinion. The ethical standards do indicate that when sufficient validity or reliability has not been established, the psychologist can describe the strengths and limitations of test results and interpretation (9.02b), a possible approach the researcher could take. In refusing to reach definitive conclusions based upon the experimental functional tests, the research neuropsychologist is fulfilling the guidelines of Principle C (Integrity) of the Ethics Code.

There are other ethical issues raised by this scenario. Among them:

Misuse of Psychologist's Work (Standard 1.01)
The standard states that psychologists take reasonable steps to correct or minimize the misuse of their work. The participant's psychotherapist has misrepresented the neuropsychologist's work

in talking to the SSD people, stating that the researcher has "*great* data relating work ability to your functional measures."

Informal Resolution of Ethical Violations (Standard 1.04)
If the psychotherapist-psychologist believed the neuropsychologist had violated an ethical principle or standard, s/he is advised by the Ethics Code to attempt an informal resolution of the matter. Instead, the treater is threatening to encourage his patient to file a complaint with the IRB, which may be judged to be improper. Standard 1.07 (Improper Complaints) indicates that psychologists do not file or encourage the filing of complaints that are filed with reckless disregard for facts which would disprove the allegation. The psychotherapist-psychologist appears to utilize the threat of an ethics complaint as a weapon in a tactic to obtain certain statements from the neuropsychologist which the neuropsychologist believes are unwarranted or not based upon valid information.

Maintaining Confidentiality (Standard 4.01 and Standard 4.06)
The research neuropsychologist has properly indicated he will release an interpretive summary of the findings to the participant, to share with whomever (or no one) as she wishes. This properly maintains confidentiality of the information. Nevertheless, the other psychologist researcher (who knows the participant from her own studies of HIV and psychosis) has failed to maintain confidentiality and has improperly divulged information.

Case Resolution

In this instance, the research neuropsychologist provided an interpretive summary of the participant's findings on the neuropsychological tests to the participant, who shared this with the treating psychologist. The treater then asked if the researcher could additionally describe the functional tests in the report and whether or not the participant could complete them successfully. The researcher agreed, provided he indicates they were not yet validated and conclusions could not be drawn upon as yet unvalidated techniques. The participant and clinician agreed. No complaint was ever filed. The neuropsychologist researcher informally met with his colleague conducting research on HIV and psychosis and expressed distress at her sharing of confidential information. The researcher colleague agreed it was improper and ill advised and promised not to do so again.

Conclusions and Recommendations

In this case, a research participant's treating psychotherapist attempted to persuade a neuropsychologist researcher to base opinions of an assessment upon unvalidated techniques, and to skew the interpretation accordingly. He also threatened to file an ethics complaint in an attempt to intimidate the researcher. Finally, the researcher's colleague improperly divulged information about the participant to the research neuropsychologist. After a number of informal discussions, all parties informally resolved the issues. It is recommended that neuropsychological researchers consider potential ethical challenges unique to their research topic or setting, elicit the experiences of more senior colleagues doing similar research, and prepare responses to some of the more common ethical challenges at the beginning of the study or upon entry to the lab.

Scenario 2

A neuropsychologist is hired to oversee the neuropsychological component of an ongoing longitudinal research study investigating cognitive functioning in older adults who are at risk for dementia. They are deemed at risk as they and/or their significant others have expressed complaints of their exhibiting poor memory functioning without clear-cut signs of dementia as yet. The research protocol includes administration of a longitudinal neuropsychological test battery, laboratory tests including an MRI brain scan and genetic testing for APOE-4 allele, a genetic marker which is present in some individuals who will go on to develop Alzheimer's disease.

The principal investigator (PI) (who has a Ph.D. in experimental psychology with a specialization in statistics) has hired a young neuropsychologist to oversee the neuropsychology component of the research study. The PI requests that, among other things, the neuropsychologist administer the original Wechsler Adult Intelligence Scale (not Revised or the Third Edition), as it has been used in all his other longitudinal research, and he can then compare test results from this instrument to findings in his associated longitudinal studies from years back. He makes similar requests for the Wide Range Achievement Test, and the Wechsler Memory Scale.

Six months into the study, a participant's spouse telephones the neuropsychologist, pressing the neuropsychologist to answer, "Does my husband have Alzheimer's Disease?" The neuropsychologist refers the caller to the PI, and tells the PI the neuropsychological test findings were equivocal in several areas compared to the group of "normal control participants" recruited by the PI, but the results were not conclusively abnormal. When the spouse reaches the PI, he tells the spouse, "Your husband has a positive finding on the APOE-4 allele, and an abnormal neuropsychological examination. The findings indicate Alzheimer's Disease."

Upon learning of this, the neuropsychologist questions the PI's methods and conclusions, citing use of out of date versions of tests, the equivocal nature of the test findings, and ambiguities of the meaning of a positive finding on an APOE-4 allele test in which 50% of positive findings develop Alzheimer's Disease, but 30% of non-demented older adults have positive findings. The PI states, "I told them the truth, and that's that."

Relevant Ethical Issues

Given the ambiguity regarding the meaning of results of APOE-4 allele testing, and the equivocal neuropsychological test results, it appears that the PI may have violated the "do no harm" admonition of the Ethics Code (Principle A, Beneficence and Nonmaleficence; Standard 3.04, Avoiding Harm). Of course, telling a patient and his or her significant other that the patient has Alzheimer's Disease when the diagnosis is not so certain can do considerable harm by creating potentially unnecessary anxiety, pursuit of needless medical evaluations and treatments, etc. It also appears that the PI has misrepresented the findings of the neuropsychological evaluation (Standard 1.01, Misuse of Psychologist's Work) and did not possess the proper base for his conclusions regarding the neuropsychological examination (Standard 9.01, Bases for Assessments).

Although use of earlier versions of psychological and neuropsychological tests may be appropriate in certain situations, the PI has utilized obsolete and out of date tests (the original WAIS, the original Wechsler Memory Scale and the WRAT) to reach a clinical conclusion (Alzheimer's Disease). Because he is relying upon these out of date measures to reach a clinical conclusion, he may be in violation of Standard 9.08 (Obsolete Tests and Outdated Test Results).

Case Resolution

The neuropsychologist requested a meeting with the PI to go over these issues. The neuropsychologist first discussed the issue of the obsolete tests used to reach clinical conclusions, and the PI agreed to stop using these results to reach firm conclusions regarding participant's

clinical status and conditions. The neuropsychologist sought and received approval from the PI to meet with the participant and his wife to discuss the findings in further detail. The neuropsychologist also presented the PI with several articles discussing the limits and ethics of use of the APOE-4 allele, and the PI agreed to stop telling patients with a positive finding that it indicated they would develop Alzheimer's Disease. Though defensive at first, persistence of the neuropsychologist paid off, especially when the various articles were given to the PI, and the matter was informally resolved.

Conclusions and Recommendations

This case illustrates the "Do No Harm" concept, indicating that knowing our limitations is sometimes as or more important than knowing what our science can offer. This case is fortunate that, despite the egregious nature of many of the errors, the PI was ultimately open to modification of his procedures and conclusions in light of limits of the data with which he was working. Consistent with the Ethics Code, the neuropsychologist on the research team has taken steps to correct the misrepresentation of the PI by informing the PI of this error. It was prudent for the neuropsychologist to discuss with the participant and his wife the limits of the diagnostic certainty and the exact nature and meaning of the neuropsychological test findings. In seeking to informally resolve the matter with the PI, the neuropsychologist has followed Standard 1.04 (Informal Resolution of Ethical Violations).

The use of outdated measures may have been of concern to the neuropsychologist upon initial involvement with the study. In such instances, clarification of how results would be used, as described to participants during the informed consent process, and any objections to study procedures should be discussed between the researchers at the outset of their collaboration.

Section 12

ETHICAL CHALLENGES IN NEUROPSYCHOLOGICAL TEST DEVELOPMENT

Introduction

The accuracy of conclusions drawn about brain-behavior relationships depends on the reliability and validity of the assessment procedures utilized. In addition, the accuracy of statements made about the procedures utilized often depends on the competence and integrity of the developer of those procedures. However, even the most competent and honest test developer may inadvertently limit the utility of the test if he or she is unaware of potential ethical pitfalls associated with test development. The authors of this chapter bring their considerable experience with test development to the examination of the ethical issues associated with neuropsychological test development. Through the vignettes and their analyses, the reader is afforded an opportunity to understand and thus avoid common ethical pitfalls associated with neuropsychological test development.

Chapter 24

ETHICAL CHALLENGES IN NEUROPSYCHOLOGICAL TEST DEVELOPMENT, PART I

Charles J. Golden

Scenario 1

A neuropsychologist noticed the need for a high level verbal memory test. He theorized that a list using more complex words would better test memory functions in higher education clients than traditional tests which he saw as too easy. As a faculty member at a large European university, he used his graduate students to construct a test consisting of fifteen words that were repeated four times, followed by an interference list, and then a thirty minute delayed recall of the initial list. He developed the norms on 100 junior, senior, and graduate students who were rated as performing in the top one-quarter of their respective classes, evenly divided between males and females. Norms were developed from this population and compared against the performance of 100 patients with unilateral temporal lobe injuries secondary to stroke, 50 in the left hemisphere and 50 in the right hemisphere. This group was considerably older and less educated than the control group. From the data, he concluded that those with left temporal strokes did much worse than those with right temporal strokes who in turn did worse than the control group. He published the test and made it generally available as a measure of temporal lobe/memory functioning.

Another neuropsychologist read the article (published in an international English language journal) and used this to put together a test to evaluate temporal lobe function in his patients based on the cutoff points suggested by the first neuropsychologist. He used this in several civil and criminal cases to demonstrate the presence of temporal lobe difficulties either as a result of a head injury (in the civil cases) or as a mitigating circumstance (in murder and other criminal cases.)

Relevant Ethical Issues

The APA Ethics Code of 2002 is relatively quiet on the issue of standards for test construction. Standard 9.05 (Test Construction; part of the general section on Assessment) states that "psychologists who develop tests and other assessment techniques use appropriate psychometric procedures and current scientific or professional knowledge for test design, standardization, validation, reduction or elimination of bias, and recommendations for use." This standard gives wide leeway to the user who can augment this with other considerations about test construction published by APA (but not referenced in the ethical code) as well as in the general literature. This standard relies heavily on the judgment of the test developer and, in many cases, the test user, who may employ the test in situations and circumstances not imagined by the test developer.

There are several problems with this scenario that reflect common problems with existing neuropsychological tests. Some of these errors are obvious and seem to speak to the competence of the test developer, the test user, and the journal editor (Ethical Standard 2, Competence): failure to match the normative groups to the patient group for age and education, failure to consider other loci of brain injury before concluding the test measured temporal lobe function, and translating the test article into English without determining English language norms or posting a strong warning cautioning against use in English.

More important, perhaps, are the more subtle general issues. One such issue involves the normative groups that are selected for neuropsychological tests. These are rarely randomly sampled, stratified groups because few tests have been developed in the field with the monetary resources available to do a large and complex sample. Normative groups are most often a sample of convenience which may frequently include college students or university employees, or other samples which are readily available such as the people who live in a local retirement community. In most cases, the samples emphasize healthy individuals with no history of neurological, medical, psychiatric, or behavioral problems.

The difficulty with this is that such groups are not representative of the people who get brain injuries. They will frequently differ in terms of age and education from the original sample. Equally important, patients are often made up of samples of people who not only have a suspected brain injury, but who may also have a history of psychiatric problems, school problems, other medical disorders, and behavioral problems.

Inferences that someone is brain injured by comparing a person with multiple problems against someone with no problems is questionable as it fails to eliminate clear sources of bias, as do the more obvious problems to match to age, education, gender, or culture.

Another issue regards the type of brain injured group used in developmental studies. In this example, the sample consisted exclusively of stroke patients although the test was used to make inference both about head injury cases (in the civil cases) and clients likely injured early in life (in criminal cases), neither of which populations were used to validate the test. The validation also focused only on participants with specific lesions (temporal lobe) to the exclusion of all other lesions, questioning the use and interpretation of the test in any other localized or diffuse injury. Even when groups are not so narrowly selected, the underlying brain injury populations do have unique characteristics in terms of etiology, location, and time of injury, emotional complications, family support, and other related issues that may affect interpretation. In each case, these factors limit the generalizability of the test results or conclusions that can be reached when applying the test to an individual client.

The second neuropsychologist, by using the test with patients not only seen in another country, but also patients with different levels of age, education, and background has created several ethical problems as the user of the test (Ethical Standards 9.02, Use of Assessments, and 9.06, Interpreting Assessment Results). It is often argued that these issues are solely the responsibility of the user, that as long as the original test data is described by the test publisher/developer, the appropriate use of the test must be determined and defended by the user. To some degree, this is true as it would be impossible for any developer to anticipate every use of a test that might occur, especially in a time when many uses are not even a part of the field when the test was developed. However, placing this onus on the user alone is not adequate; the publisher bears some responsibility for misuse of the test if the limitations have not been made immediately clear.

Case Resolution

A neuropsychologist representing the opposing side in a legal case reviewed the evaluation report of the user of the "temporal lobe test". Noting the inadequacies of the measure for the examinee in the case, the reviewing neuropsychologist decided to make a call to her colleague to informally present her concerns. She had no intention of pursuing the matter further while the case was ongoing. The test user was refreshingly open to the information and agreed that the choice of that measure may have been inappropriate. He maintained, however, that results of the other measures in the test battery also supported his original conclusions and that he had no intention of providing an addendum to his report or otherwise modifying his conclusions.

Conclusions and Recommendations

Users come in very different levels of competence and experience. Since psychology does not screen users for level of competence in neuropsychology before allowing one to use a test, it is incumbent upon the publisher to recognize that the test will be used by individuals with the minimal competence required to purchase or use the test (most often simply a license in clinical psychology at the doctoral or the master's level depending on the state.)

In such a case it is therefore incumbent on the publisher / developer to clearly indicate in test manuals or articles what the limits of the test are. This should include information on the level of competence needed to use the test. This should indicate the level of knowledge needed in neuropsychology before using the test at all or limitations on the uses by individuals with different levels of competence. For example, a test manual could warn that general clinical psychologists without specific neuropsychology training should not use a test, or that such individuals should use the test only as a screening device which could be used as a justification for referral to a more highly trained clinician. There may be several levels of use dependent on whether one is a general psychologist, has minimal training in neuropsychology, or advanced training. Interpretive strategies and the knowledge necessary to implement them at each level might be offered as well.

While no test is appropriate to all populations, it is necessary for test publishers to be aware of and discuss the limitations of a test in terms of the background of control participants and the selection of experimental (brain injured clients.) groups. Such information should be specific as to the age and education ranges employed, the number of male and female participants, the language background of the participants (translating tests and using the old norms is not an adequate procedure), the cultural backgrounds, the method in which the control subjects were chosen (which is curiously absent from many manuals), and how and why potential controls were eliminated. Equally importantly, the developer needs to point out what limitations this data imposes on the generalizability of the data and what kind of patients you can use the test with without additional data and considerations. Since the user may be naïve, the information needs to be as specific as possible.

Similarly, the nature of the brain injured group must be discussed to show limitations of generalizing results to other brain injury populations. Data drawn from head injury populations cannot be applied directly to stroke populations or vice versa. These limitations and concerns needed to be spelled out as carefully as possible.

Scenario 2

The publisher of a neuropsychologist's new test on aphasia is very aware of the possible impact of language, culture, age, and education on the results from this new test. As a result, the publisher commits $20,000,000 to selecting a normative test sample. This sample was based on matching all U.S. Census norms for such factors as age, education, profession, state of residence, citizenship status, immigration status, cultural background, race, ethnicity, religion, first language spoken, current dominant language, and income. The sample excluded anyone defined as not normal: anyone with a history of psychiatric treatment, neurological injury or disease, felony convictions, mental health diagnosis, serious medical conditions such as kidney loss, heart disease which limited daily activity, and chronic pulmonary problems. The data was gathered by selecting paid volunteers ($20 per hour for testing) in each region within each state who were given a three day seminar in administering and scoring the test. Each test administration was recorded (audio and visual) so that all scoring and administrative actions and decisions could be later reviewed by the test developer. Each paid volunteer was given a list of ten participants to recruit with specific criteria based on the demographic variables discussed above. Overall, 500 paid volunteers nationwide collected 5000 participants over a 12 month period. Each participant was also paid $20 per hour for their time in taking the test and filling out demographic forms. Norms published were broken down by age, education, and gender. Based on this unprecedented effort, the publisher argued that the test is appropriate for neuropsychological use in any population within the United States.

Relevant Ethical Issues

On the face of it, many would argue that there is no ethical issue here. The neuropsychologist and the publisher had gone well beyond what anyone has ever done before to insure a truly representative stratified random sample that represented the population of the United States in every

possible respect. However, there are several important issues that need to be recognized. The key issue in regards to this vignette is the statement that "developers of tests and other assessment techniques use appropriate psychometric procedures and current scientific or professional knowledge for test design, standardization ..." (Ethical Standard 9.05, Test Construction). Failure to do so may reflect on the professional competence of test developer (Ethical Standard 2.01, Boundaries of Competence), limitations of the test publisher, or other factors.

First, standardization of this aphasia test did not utilize a truly random sample. It is indeed questionable that any study conducted on human testing could ever include a truly random sample, despite the fact that some may contend that they have done so. For a sample to be truly random, all individuals in the population of interest (everyone living in the U.S. who is defined as healthy and unimpaired) must have an equal chance of being included in the sample. By restricting testing to the sites of the 500 volunteers, some people are already eliminated as potential participants since there are far more than 500 sites within a specific state let alone the entire country. By using only volunteer testers willing and able to work for $20 an hour, the sample of testers is being similarly restricted impacting the site selection. In addition, by assigning each tester a specific quota with specific characteristics, the chance of selecting an 18-year-old male Hispanic native Spanish speaker with ten years of education and a job as a middle level manger in Montana is likely less than picking such an individual in South Florida or Texas, as the quotas for each area are generally assigned based on the dominant population in that area rather than randomly. Finally, using self-selected volunteer participants further increases potential sources of bias.

However, while the sample as a whole is not a true stratified random sample, the sheer size of the sample would suggest that the distribution of any errors are likely normal and quite small.

Thus, it is quite likely that the sample as a whole is indeed representative within a small margin of the healthy population of the U.S. and can be assumed to be accurate absent any source of systematic bias that is not evident in the scenario given.

The difficulty arises with the contention that this data can then be fairly applied to all patients within the sample. Thus, while language of origin was considered in the sample, this is not considered in the norms. While the presence of such individuals would influence the norms, general norms would be more influenced by the predominant population (where English is the first language). It is not adequate to simply include the group in the sample; it is necessary to break out specific norms for each group, which has not been done in this case.

When breaking out such norms, however, the sampling issues become more important as the sample sizes will rapidly shrink as we break down data by individuals who spoke Spanish as their first language (but not speak English) by age, education, and gender. As the sample sizes shrink, the influence of biasing issues and the lack of randomness become of greater significance. Applying the general norms to these groups without such a breakdown is psychometrically inappropriate and will lead to bad conclusions in some cases.

Another issue that arises is the exclusion of "unhealthy" people. Neuropsychologists with experience recognize that clients referred for head injuries often have serious prior history of substance abuse, personality problems, school problems, mental health issues, medical problems, and other "unhealthy traits" at a rate far in excess of the normal population. Indeed, the current author surveyed 100 of his own cases and found that over half of them had premorbid histories that would have excluded them from a normative sample. While this percentage may not hold in other practices or samples, such data suggests that our insistence on selecting "healthy people" may yield norms that seriously underestimate

the degree of personality dysfunction which existed prior to an injury or accident. This oversight poses a serious psychometric limitation when the norms are used with brain injured populations. It should be noted that this does not affect other non-neuropsychological uses of such tests, such as when we simply want to know how a person fares against the population as a whole in terms of ability rather than to make a neuropsychological inference.

Given the potential limitations with certain examinees, the test publisher's contention that the test is appropriate for neuropsychological use in any population within the United States is overly ambitious if not blatantly misleading. Although the test publisher may use such language in an attempt to optimize sales, the neuropsychologist that developed the test is ethically obligated to present his work accurately and honestly (Ethical Standard 5/01, Avoidance of False or Deceptive Statements). When the demands of the organizations with which psychologists are affiliated conflict with the Ethics Code, psychologists are responsible for clarifying the conflict, emphasizing their commitment to the Ethics Code, and attempting to resolve the issue in a manner that permits adherence to the Code (Ethical Standard 1.03, Conflicts Between Ethics and Organizational Demands).

Case Resolution

The neuropsychologist was appropriately confident that, despite the limitations inherent in any test development, he had developed a very good measure of language functioning. He realized that the test publisher had overstated the merits of the test; however, he had invested considerable time, energy and emotion into the development of the test and he hoped he would be rewarded with commercial success. He said nothing to the publisher about the wording of its marketing materials. A few of his colleagues mentioned the apparent exaggeration to him, but he sort of shrugged it off in a "what can you do?" manner. The test sold thousands of copies, and no formal ethical problems ever emerged.

Conclusions and Recommendations

This case illustrates the importance of moving away from the tendency to develop monolithic normative samples towards specific and well chosen samples relevant to a specific population. The development of different normative samples aimed at individuals whose initial language was other than English, who only speak Spanish, Black inner-city participants, individuals in Appalachia with less than eight years of education, patients who are in the hospital but not with a brain injury, and so on might allow the field to more appropriately and accurately deal with a wide range of clients in a more appropriate and quantitative fashion rather than make such adjustments in a qualitative, case by case fashion.

In each case, the need to recognize the limitations of the underlying normative samples and the possible presence of biasing and limiting demographic and personal factors must be discussed by the test developer in as much depth as possible. Only in this way can we move the general psychometric data to reflect the needs of the individual clinical client.

Chapter 25

ETHICAL CHALLENGES IN NEUROPSYCHOLOGICAL TEST CONSTRUCTION, PART II

Abigail B. Sivan

Scenario 1

A neuropsychologist, noting limitations with the ecological validity of many neuropsychological tests, utilized advances in computer technology to create a more ecologically valid measure of memory. The neuropsychologist created a series of scenes that people may encounter in their daily lives, such as a grocery store, a post office, a park, and a house. The rich detail of the scenes was brought to the screen with vivid graphics. In addition to the visual component, the neuropsychologist utilized the most advanced sound cards to bring auditory stimuli, such as conversations and everyday noises, to the examinee. The auditory component also had an option for verbal description of the scenes that could be used with those with visual impairments. The neuropsychologist developed a number of options for assessing all of the omponents of memory tapped by commonly used memory measures. The neuropsychologist believed that the Computerized Ecologically Valid Memory Test (CEVMT) could be a valuable measure of auditory and visual memory that could approximate daily memory better than previously developed measures.

Initial validation studies were designed to assess a wide range of demographically diverse healthy individuals, as well as individuals with various neuropathologies. In particular, it was hoped that the CEVMT would help in the diagnosis of various dementing conditions. Initial pilot studies were promising. However, the neuropsychologist's untested impression was that there was an even greater discrepancy in performance related to education than was seen with more traditional measures of memory. The neuropsychologist hypothesized that those with more education had more experience with computers and therefore felt more comfortable with the computerized test administration.

With the CEVMT and results of initial validation studies in hand, the neuropsychologist contacted the Neuropsychological Test Conglomerate (NTC) to see about publishing his groundbreaking test. NTC was very excited to have the opportunity to publish the CEVMT and moved ahead quickly with refinements and additional studies of reliability and validity. The neuropsychologist was very excited with the progress and turned over control for subsequent standardization and marketing to NTC. When the test was published, the neuropsychologist noted that the norms corrected for age but not for education. Based on the results of the observations made during initial pilot studies, the neuropsychologist believed this to be a critical omission and conveyed his opinion to NTC. Since the test had already been published, however, the neuropsychologist turned his attention toward the forthcoming royalty checks.

Relevant Ethical Issues

The primary ethical issue in this case was not inadequate test development on the neuropsychologist's part, but rather inadequate standardization data on the part of the test publisher. As a publisher of neuropsychological tests, NTC should ideally be bound by the same ethical standards for test development as are neuropsychologists who develop and use such tests, including the "reduction or elimination of bias" for those elderly with limited education (Standard 9.05, Test Construction). NTC, however, was not bound by such ethical standards. Hence, it may have been preferred for the neuropsychologist to attempt to resolve the discrepancy between his belief that the CEVMT needed education corrections and NTC's wish to publish the test as quickly as possible (Standard 1.03, Conflicts Between Ethics and Organizational Demands). By attempting to resolve the problem with NTC, the neuropsychologist would clearly be striving to avoid misdiagnoses based on the results of the CEVMT, consistent with Standard 3.04 (Avoiding Harm).

Case Resolution

The initial marketing campaign brought forth questions from the neuropsychology community about the test's standardization and norms. The neuropsychologist reported to colleagues the reservations about use of the measure with elderly with low education. A colleague with

previous tests published by NTC stated firmly that the neuropsychologist needed to impress upon the publisher the need to withhold publication until age corrected norms were available, which the neuropsychologist did. NTC stated that appropriate studies were underway and that supplemental norms would be soon available to those neuropsychologists who have already purchased the CEVMT, for an additional fee. Although content that the needed information would be available, the neuropsychologist wrote a letter to NTC protesting the additional charge but was unable to have it eliminated.

Conclusions and Recommendations

Although there was an adequate and ethical resolution to the neuropsychologist's conflicts with NTC, in the long run it might have better had he specified in his original contract with NTC that before publication of the CEVMT, there would be norms established based on education as well as gender and age. It is recommended that neuropsychologists developing tests try to anticipate the possible problems that may emerge when they relinquish control to, or work within, organizations. While responsibility for appropriate test development resides with the developer, ultimate responsibility for avoiding harm remains with the neuropsychologist in his or her test selection, utilization, and data interpretation. In some instances, it may be prudent to await independent validation or normative studies before using a newly published test with special populations.

Scenario 2

In the course of his clinical practice, a neuropsychologist noticed that many of his head injured patients showed impaired performances on measures that require sustained and careful visual attention. In an effort to shorten his testing battery, the neuropsychologist began to develop his own measure, a measure that would be substantially shorter than the combination of measures he used in the past. After several years of use, the neuropsychologist decides to market his test as a new measure of brain injury using the data he collected in his clinical practice to support the validity of his new measure. He constructed tasteful and informative flyers that he planned to send to colleagues in the U.S. and abroad detailing the merits of his new brain injury measure, with the first set of flyers going to local neuropsychologists.

Relevant Ethical Issues

Both the 1992 and 2002 Ethics Codes require neuropsychologists to follow the established standards of reliability and validity when developing new measures. The neuropsychologist's data may have met established standards for reliability and construct validity. Without demonstration of discriminant validity showing that only the brain damaged clients (and not persons with psychiatric disorders or other conditions that may impair attention) have impairment on this measure, the neuropsychologist's claims for his test are unwarranted. For the neuropsychologist to make the claims he does for this test is unethical (Standard 9.05, Test Construction). This does not mean, however, that his measure does not have clinical utility.

In addition to the sections of the Ethics Code related to test construction, it may appear that the above scenario also reflects a lack of familiarity with, or disregard for, Standard 5.01(a) (Avoidance of False or Deceptive Statements). However, this standard states, "Psychologists do not knowingly make public statements that are false, deceptive, or fraudulent …" In the above case, the neuropsychologist's flyers would be misleading to those not familiar with test construction. However, he did not appear to "knowingly" mislead his readers; rather, the unintended potential deception was the result of his premature determination that his test was ready for wide dissemination and use.

Case Resolution

In the case above, the neuropsychologist was quickly contacted by concerned colleagues in an attempt to resolve the situation informally. The primary concern was the need for replication studies from different neuropsychology laboratories and for additional validation studies, with particular focus on discriminant validity. The neuropsychologist initially defended the merits of his test and his standardization studies to that point but soon realized that his colleagues were right and agreed that marketing his test at that point was premature. One of the neuropsychologists that had contacted him expressed interest in performing initial replication studies her lab, and the neuropsychologist readily accepted her involvement. The neuropsychologist sent follow-up letters to those who had received his flyers to explain the plan for continued standardization of his test, and he recycled the remaining flyers.

Conclusions and Recommendations

For the neuropsychologist interested in test construction, it is important to recognize that the APA Ethics Code as well as the guidelines derived from them, namely the *Standards for Educational and Psychological Testing* (American Educational Research Association, American Psychological Association, & National Council on Measurement in Education 1999), apply to neuropsychological as well as other types of test construction. It is also essential to remember that a neuropsychological test is defined not by its actual content but by its purpose. This is to say that neuropsychological tests do not differ, or at least need not differ, from other behavioral tests in their content or nature, but by the use to which they are put.

For example, the Wechsler scales are measures of "general intelligence". Nevertheless, they can be used for a variety of purposes, although generally they are used as guides for educational and vocational placement. When these measures are used for the purpose of inferring the probability of the presence of brain disease in a patient, they are neuropsychological tests. The manual of the original Wechsler-Bellevue Scales (Wechsler, 1939) included a description of the performance patterns of patients with brain disease and a discussion of the utilization of the measure for evaluating the presence of brain disease in the undiagnosed patient. In this respect, it is worthwhile to note that intelligence test batteries such as the Binet or the Wechsler made use of subtests that were derived from earlier measures devised by physicians for the express purpose of evaluating and differentiating patients with brain disease. In the recent past, the technical manuals of the most recent Wechsler adult tests (The Psychological Corporation, 1997) included norms for special populations, including neurological disorders (e.g., Alzheimer's, Huntington's, and Parkinson's diseases), and a lengthy section on special group studies that examined the performances of persons with other disorders (e.g., alcohol-related conditions, neuropsychiatric, psychoeducational, and developmental disorders or impairments) that may have particular patterns of performance on these measures.

Given the similarities between commonly used psychological tests that provide normative information related to neurologically-impaired performances and neuropsychological tests, how then does construction of these measures differ? The construction of neuropsychological tests is necessarily guided by conceptions of the relationship between brain function and behavior. These brain-behavior relationships are far from fully, or even satisfactorily, understood, despite the significant advances in knowledge made possible by the application of neuro-imaging procedures, such as computerize axial tomography (CAT) magnetic resonance imagery (MRI),

positron emission tomography (PET), and functional magnetic resonance imaging (fMRI). Aided by these procedures, clinical studies have established some association between defective test performances and the presence and localization of lesions in patients with brain disease. Additional normative studies have found activation of some areas of the brain when certain cognitive tasks are performed. Although many of the observed associations between brain function and behavior have proved to be statistically significant, they are not universal. Failure to appreciate the imperfect nature and the complexity of the association between brain function and test performance has sometimes led to extravagant and unwarranted claims and a precision in prediction that does not in fact exist.

Many neuropsychological tests (or perhaps better stated, techniques) are used as an aid in the process of clinical decision-making with clients or patients referred for assessment of specific complaints, such as memory loss, confusion, or disorientation. The nature of these complaints, as well as the compromised status of the patients, requires the procedures used to be brief and specific. Thus, many neuropsychological tests are really clinical maneuvers rather than tests with elaborate norms. The use of these techniques is integral to the work of neuropsychologists. As Lezak (1995) has pointed out:

> ... to do justice to a field of inquiry as complex as brain-behavior relationships in adult human beings requires an adaptable assessment methodology that incorporates the strengths of both quantitative and qualitative approaches. Standardized procedures eliciting behavior that can be measured along empirically defined and scaled dimensions provide objectivity and the potential to make fine distinctions and comparisons that would be unattainable by clinical observation alone. Still, examination cannot be adequately conducted nor can test scores be properly

interpreted in a psychological and social vacuum. The uniqueness of each patient's capacity, disability, needs, and situation calls for discriminating, flexible, and imaginative use of examination techniques (p.4).

The use of these flexible techniques does not excuse neuropsychologists from ethical standards; instead, it shifts the focus from the ethical standards related to test construction to those related to client welfare and the need to recognize both the limited nature of one's judgments and the need to qualify such judgments appropriately.

References

American Educational Research Association, American Psychological Association, National Council on Measurement in Education (1999). *Standards for Educational and Psychological Testing.* Washington, D.C.: American Educational Research Association.

American Psychological Association (1992). Ethical principles of psychologists and code of conduct. *American Psychologist, 47*, 1597-1628.

American Psychological Association (2002). Ethical principles of psychologists and code of conduct. *American Psychologist, 57*, 1060-1073.

Anderson, Jr., R.M., & Palozzi, A.M. (2002). Ethical issues in test construction, selection, and security. In S.S. Bush & M.L. Drexler (Eds.), *Ethical Issues in Clinical Neuropsychology*, (pp. 39-50). Lisse, NL: Swets & Zeitlinger Publishers.

Lezak, M.D. (1995). *Neuropsychological Assessment, 3rd Edition.* New York: Oxford University Press.

The Psychological Corporation (1997). *WAIS-III WMS-III Technical Manual.* San Antonio, TX: Author.

Wechsler, D. (1939). *Wechsler-Bellevue Intelligence Scale.* New York: The Psychological Corporation.

Section 13

ETHICAL CHALLENGES IN THE DETERMINATION OF RESPONSE VALIDITY IN NEUROPSYCHOLOGY

Introduction

The adequate assessment of response validity/bias, after many years of preliminary research, has come to be understood in recent years as a necessary and integral part of the neuropsychological evaluation. Although the context of the evaluation (e.g., setting, patient population) may influence to some degree the nature and extent of validity testing, a quantifiable, standardized assessment of response validity is required in order to make an informed opinion regarding the validity of the results of neuropsychological ability measures regardless of context.

Although the assessment of response validity is a component of the standard of neuropsychological practice, there is as yet no consensus regarding (a) which procedures are to be used, and with which examinees; (b) how many procedures should be used, or indices computed or considered; (c) at what point in a battery they should be administered; and, (d) exactly how they should be interpreted. Each neuropsychologist will need to consider for any given case the appropriate selection and use of indicators of response validity/bias that will allow sufficient confidence to be placed in conclusions about the validity of the evaluation findings. Familiarity with recent literature and dialogue with colleagues are necessary to address this requirement.

Interestingly, in the assessment of examinee response validity or truthfulness, the examiner often employs deception. Many measures of response validity are not what they may appear to the examinee to be. With some measures, their descriptions as outlined in the instructions to the examinee are intentionally, and apparently necessarily, misleading. Although the Ethics Code addresses the use of deception in research (Standard 8.07), it does not specifically address deception in assessment. However, consistent with General Principle C (Integrity), while neuropsychologists generally seek to practice in a truthful manner, there may be instances in which deception may be "ethically justifiable" in order to benefit the consumers of neuropsychological services. Nevertheless, neuropsychologists must be mindful of the possible effects of deception on the sense of trust or the emotional state of the examinee or others involved in the case, and assume responsibility for correcting any harmful effects resulting from such deception. Although deception in this context would seem necessary, neuropsychologists may wish to provide general information related to the inclusion of measures/indices of response validity during the informed consent process and be prepared to negotiate challenges if they arise during or after the informed consent process or the evaluation. Examinees may feel equally justified in their use of deception, as some have indicated following their evaluations while "debriefing" the examiner.

In this chapter, the authors, both experts in the evaluation of response validity, present scenarios with which neuropsychologists may be confronted. They offer reasoned approaches to negotiating such situations at a time when decisions about examinee effort are often more clear-cut or less clear-cut than many neuropsychologists believe.

Chapter 26

ETHICAL CHALLENGES IN THE DETERMINATION OF RESPONSE VALIDITY IN NEUROPSYCHOLOGY, PART I

David R. Cox

Scenario 1

A referral is made to a neuropsychologist by a nurse case manager working with a worker's compensation carrier. The case manager has a reputation in the community as being fair and honest, yet very intent on "catching" examinees in the worker's compensation system that are "milking the system." Because of this, the neuropsychologist is also aware that the case manager will be specifically requesting that the examination address the issue of potential malingering. This is not a problem, as the neuropsychologist is accustomed to doing so routinely as part of examinations, particularly in cases where there may be such clear secondary gain issues.

What the neuropsychologist did not anticipate on initial receipt of the referral, however, was that the case manager now requests administration of *specific* tests for symptom exaggeration or malingering. The request is not merely that such testing be done, but in fact the case manager wants specific tests (Test A and Test B) administered. The neuropsychologist expresses to the case manager that, although there is no problem with testing for response bias, it is the

neuropsychologist's opinion there are better, more appropriate measures available than the ones requested.

Nonetheless, the case manager demands that the neuropsychologist administer the specific tests, Test A and Test B. The case manager indicates that the neuropsychologist may administer other validity measures as desired, but that the time for administration, scoring and reporting of those measures will not be reimbursed. Since the requested measures will be paid for, indicates the case manager, "there is no medical necessity" for the additional measures.

Despite the fact that the neuropsychologist sees the situation as less than ideal, the neuropsychologist agrees to see the examinee. The neuropsychologist makes a determination to administer all measures deemed necessary in order to formulate diagnostic and causality opinions, whether they are paid for or not. That way, the neuropsychologist provides the service that the case manager (the client) wants and also has the data that is considered appropriate and necessary for answering the referral questions.

The examinee presents as a fairly savvy individual who indicates problems after a slip and fall accident in which he injured his knee, back and struck his head on a table in the fall. There was no loss of consciousness, no hospitalization and few, if any, postconcussive symptoms reported early on after the injury. It is now six months post-injury and the examinee indicates that his problems with attention, concentration and memory have worsened. He denies any emotional distress other than "I am frustrated that I can't do what I used to do" and "This whole worker's comp system gets me angry and depressed." He expresses frustration that it takes some time to get his appointments with any new doctors and reports that he feels that none of his doctors really care. "Some of the doctors have even said I could be working, which is obviously crazy," he reports.

While off from work because of his condition, the examinee has been "researching" his symptoms on the internet, has been involved in "chat groups", and has come to know some other examinees that have worked through the same case manager. He has also retained an attorney for legal representation of his case. He indicates that his friends from the chat groups have been helpful and supportive, and have helped him know what to expect. His attorney has apparently instructed him to be cooperative with requested examinations such as this one, but has also reinforced the notion that he should not return to work. The examinee indicates that he has learned that his symptoms often lead to a "disabling condition called fibromyalgia and I think I'm getting that". Notably, he does not complain of symptoms that he specifically relates to the mild head strike in the fall. Rather, he just reports that he cannot concentrate, is more forgetful, and "I'm just not myself anymore".

On testing the examinee, it appears that he is putting forth a reasonable effort. When Test A (one of the requested validity measures) is administered, the examinee indicates "Oh, I've heard about this one." Apparently, other examinees have indicated that they had to go through exams, have talked about the testing, and have learned that the case manager routinely requests

Test A and B. Word is out, and, indeed, the support group has "helped one another". The examinee performs quite well on both Test A and B. As planned, the neuropsychologist proceeds with examination and includes other measures of symptom validity. On those, the examinee does not fare as well. The results suggest symptom exaggeration. Internal consistency checks such as performance on multiple choice portions of standard testing and the like do not indicate gross exaggeration to the point of "flat out malingering", yet the neuropsychologist believes the obtained performance may not represent the examinee's best.

Finally, given the nature of the referral, a request has been made that the report of findings be sent directly to the case manager and workers compensation system without review of the findings with the examinee or his representative. The neuropsychologist sent the report with a cover letter that provided information about recent advances in the assessment of symptom validity. The cover letter included a clear rationale for why the tests required by the case manager were inappropriate and provided specific test recommendations for the case manager to consider adopting for her preferred test battery.

Relevant Ethical Issues

This scenario involves issues relevant to a number of the Ethical Standards. These will be addressed below in an order corresponding to the major areas of the 2002 APA Ethics Code.

Resolving Ethical Issues

The third party is requesting that specific tests be administered, and the neuropsychologist feels there may be a conflict between the organization (workers' compensation as represented by the case manager) and the neuropsychologist (Standard 1.03, Conflicts Between Ethics and Organizational Demands). Although one might argue that you do not *work for* the case manager, it is quite possible (perhaps probable) that you have a contract with the organization that the case manager is representing. By indicating your belief that there are tests better suited for the purpose of this examination, you are indicating the nature of the conflict. By indicating your desire to administer the tests you believe to be best suited, you are making known your commitment to follow the Ethics Code. By administering the requested tests as well as your preferred tests, you are proceeding in a fashion that attempts to resolve the conflict while adhering to the Ethics Code.

Competence

The request by the case manager for one or more specific tests may conflict with the neuropsychologist's opinion in the matter (Standard 2.04, Bases for Scientific and Professional Judgments). The neuropsychologist is obligated to base his or her opinion on knowledge of the discipline, and this includes knowledge of the relative merits of one test versus another when used for particular purposes. Clarification and explanation of the bases of the neuropsychologist's opinion for test selection, as well as rationale for inclusion of any requested tests the neuropsychologist may otherwise not have administered, is in order.

Human Relations

The request for services is made by a third-party (Standard 3.07, Third-Party Requests for Services), a professional with whom the neuropsychologist may need to cooperate (Standard 3.09, Cooperation With Other Professionals). There is a need for informed consent (Standard 3.10, Informed Consent), with additional considerations due to the fact that there are psychological services delivered to or through organizations. (Standard 3.11, Psychological Services Delivered To or Through Organizations).

The neuropsychologist has a duty to the requesting party as client, as well as to the examinee. Clarification of the role of the neuropsychologist needs to be made particularly clear to

the examinee, who may not understand the nuances of these relationship issues without explanation at the outset of services. Relative to this are the limits of confidentiality (see below). At the onset of the examination, the neuropsychologist is required to discuss the role(s) of each party and obtain informed consent for the examination (Section 3.11). The neuropsychologist has a duty to cooperate with the other professionals involved (in this case, the case manager) in serving the client(s) (case manager, worker's compensation carrier) effectively and appropriately. Although this cooperation does not necessitate agreeing to perform the requested specific tests, it may; and in this case the neuropsychologist has agreed to do so in a cooperative fashion. As part of the discussion regarding test selection, the neuropsychologist had an ethical obligation to educate the case manager about the advances in symptom validity assessment that have been made in recent years, information that may result in improved diagnostic accuracy and more appropriate test preferences of the case manager (Ethical Principles A, Beneficence and Nonmaleficence, and B, Fidelity and Responsibility).

Privacy and Confidentiality

The neuropsychologist will need to maintain confidentiality (Standard 4.01, Maintaining Confidentiality), as well as discuss the limits of confidentiality (Standard 4.02, Discussing the Limits of Confidentiality) and disclosures (Standard 4.05, Disclosures) with the individual being examined. These may be both very different than the examinee expects and different from other work that the neuropsychologist does, due to the worker's compensation issue.

The neuropsychologist has an obligation to discuss the limits of confidentiality with the individual being examined at the onset of the examination. This includes those areas directly relevant to the examination (e.g., confidentiality may be limited due to the worker's compensation laws, issues of possible future sworn testimony and responding to questions under oath), as well as other limits (e.g., mandated reporting issues such as child abuse). In this particular situation, the individual being examined potentially has very limited confidentiality in that the neuropsychologist may well be asked to provide sworn testimony that may then become public record. It is imperative that the examinee understand *and agree* to said limitations prior to the neuropsychologist proceeding with examination.

Record Keeping and Fees

The neuropsychologist may have specific documentation requirements regarding professional work and maintenance of records due to the worker's compensation law (Standard 6.01, Documentation of Professional and Scientific Work and Maintenance of Records). These requirements may also involve the maintenance, dissemination, and disposal of confidential records (Standard 6.02a, Maintenance, Dissemination, and Disposal of Confidential Records of Professional and Scientific Work). There is an issue regarding the fees and financial arrangements (Standard 6.04a-d, Fees and Financial Arrangements) due to the non-reimbursed testing the neuropsychologist elected to conduct, and this may require attention to the accuracy in reports to payors and funding sources (Standard 6.06, Accuracy in Reports to Payors and Funding Sources).

The neuropsychologist may well have a duty to report certain types of information to the client (case manager and/or worker's compensation carrier) due to state worker's compensation law. This may or may not mandate *different* information than would otherwise be included; however, the neuropsychologist needs to be aware of the worker's compensation law so that the reporting is in compliance and so that any limits of confidentiality and disclosure are adequately discussed with the individual being examined. Records may need to be disclosed to parties, in compliance with the worker's compensation law, that may or may not have a direct involvement in

the case (e.g., centers that handle the billing for the neuropsychologist and centers that handle payment for the carrier). Again, the examinee needs to be aware of these requirements and limits.

The neuropsychologist is obligated to handle the situation of time spent administering, scoring, interpreting and writing results of the validity testing that was not requested, and specifically identified as not reimbursable, appropriately. Given the discussion with the case manager, it would be unethical to charge for that time unless further discussions ensued in which it was approved. It may be appropriate for the tests that were administered without reimbursement to be identified as such in order to clarify 1) the distinction between tests administered by request of the client (case manager, worker's compensation carrier) and those selected by the neuropsychologist, and 2) the time spent on the reimbursed components of the examination.

Assessment

The neuropsychologist has been asked to conduct testing by a non-psychologist client, in part, for the purposes of rendering an opinion regarding symptom validity, and the neuropsychologist believes the requested tests to be less than ideal (Standard 9.01, Bases for Assessment, and 9.02, Use of Assessments). In order to render the opinion, the neuropsychologist has elected to perform additional testing, despite not being reimbursed for said testing (9.01 and 9.02). Informed consent for assessment is required (Standard 9.03, Informed Consent in Assessments). Some test data may be expected from the referring client (Standard 9.04, Release of Test Data). Due to the request for specific tests that the neuropsychologist feels are less than optimal for this purpose, the neuropsychologist may need to address the issues of obsolete tests (Standard 9.08, Obsolete Tests and Outdated Test Results), among other issues, in the explanation of assessment results (Standard 9.10, Explaining Assessment Results). Additionally, depending on the demands of the worker's compensation law and/or other particulars of this situation, the person being examined may not be entitled to explanation of the testing results by the neuropsychologist, and this needs to be explained at the onset of the relationship (Standard 9.10).

The neuropsychologist has been requested to perform specific testing, albeit in addition to the tests the neuropsychologist personally selects, that may or may not be obsolete. It is clear that the neuropsychologist feels those tests are not appropriate, or are less than ideal, for the situation. The reasons for test selection, use of the tests and interpretation of results are issues that would appropriately be addressed by the neuropsychologist in any report of findings. The neuropsychologist may need to pay particular attention to the release of data in this case, given the significant possibility of such a request if the worker's compensation case becomes litigated. The neuropsychologist should release data to only those appropriate to receive it (e.g., those designated by the individual being examined and/or a licensed psychologist) (Standard 9.04). The examinee in this case may not be entitled to learn of the test results, at least not directly from the neuropsychologist, and this is an issue that needs to be clarified with the referral source prior to examination, as well as discussed with and agreed to by the examinee prior to onset of examination. It would be appropriate for the neuropsychologist to also discuss the possible implications (e.g., on working, driving, etc.) that the results of testing could have, although it would certainly not be within the scope of the neuropsychologist's role to anticipate any and all such implications.

Case Resolution

The neuropsychologist in this case addressed the issues in an acceptable fashion. The resolution of including the requested testing, in addition to the tests deemed more appropriate by the neuropsychologist, provided the information asked for by the client (case manager) as well as deemed necessary by the neuropsychologist to form diagnostic and causality opinions. Reporting of results included the results of the requested testing, with specific mention that they were provided at the request of the referring case manager, and also with clarification that the neuropsychologist's opinion weighed the results of those tests in a fashion appropriate to the situation. Those specific tests were given little or no weight, due to being obsolete/grossly inappropriate to the referral question (a mandate to use only those tests would have led to the neuropsychologist's refusal to conduct the evaluation at all). Appropriate billing procedures were followed, including clarification of time spent on measures that were indicated to be "non-reimbursable". Indication of this matter in the report was made. The examinee decided that the extent of the examination, limits of confidentiality and other issues were fully acceptable *prior to the examination.* If he had not agreed, the neuropsychologist would have declined to perform the examination until such time as appropriate resolution of the examinee's concern had been reached.

Conclusions and Recommendations

Neuropsychologists need to be aware not only of the ethical issues involved in the cases that they take, but also the laws and regulations that govern certain types of cases. Worker's compensation cases, for example, can impose additional requirements on the neuropsychologist as well as the examinee, and can alter limits of confidentiality and other areas that might otherwise be significantly different. Examinations under circumstances such as worker's compensation can, in essence, mandate that the individual being examined waive many rights that otherwise would be intact. A neuropsychologist performing such examinations needs to be fully informed about the variations in practice that arise in such circumstances, and proceed with such examinations only when all involved parties understand, and consent to, any limitations, restrictions and uses of the examination results.

Neuropsychologists must maintain familiarity with the literature on response validity so that appropriate decisions can be made when selecting measures. Issues such as sensitivity and specificity must be considered. In addition, familiarity with the advantages and disadvantages of study design (such as the composition of "malingering" groups) will help the neuropsychologist make an informed choice and may strengthen arguments against those requesting that specific tests be administered.

Neuropsychologists retained by clients other than the examinee may serve their clients well by educating them about advances in neuropsychological practice and the need to periodically update policies based on such advances. Nevertheless, it remains the neuropsychologist's responsibility to use the most appropriate measures, including those addressing symptom validity, to answer the questions at hand. Ultimately, it is the neuropsychologist who will be required to address the rationale for test selection and conclusions reached from administration of tests.

Scenario 2

A neuropsychologist evaluates a 66-year-old, native English-speaking male who has ten years of education. The patient was referred by a neurologist due to apparent cognitive problems and a question of possible brain injury as a result of a motor vehicle accident. The auto insurance carrier is the party expected to pay for the examination. The nature of the accident is in question insofar as the patient's current report is distinctly different from the facts surrounding the accident when it occurred. The patient's report has changed over time from being a relatively minor accident in which he bumped his head to one in which mechanical intervention was necessary to disconnect the two vehicles involved. Review of records indicates that the referring neurologist concluded that the patient suffers from a dementia not related to the accident.

During examination, the patient is noted to present with expressive language difficulties, is not fully oriented and his performance on standard tests is quite low. For example, intelligence testing reveals performance in the mid 60s. Scores on the Dementia Rating Scale suggest that he is performing in the range of the 50th percentile relative to patients with dementia. Response time is noted to be quite slow at times, and rather rapid in an impulsive fashion at others. The patient presents as quite impaired, yet the severity of problem suggests that the deficits could not plausibly have arisen from a mild head trauma. Indeed, the patient's GCS at the scene of the accident was determined to be 15, and there was no complaint of cognitive difficulty for months following the accident. The neuropsychologist tends to believe that the patient may have a cognitive disorder, perhaps a dementia of some type. However, when specific validity/response bias testing is conducted, the patient performs very poorly – well below chance – and is noted to have not responded to a number of items. The computer-administered test scored the items that did not receive a response as "incorrect" responses. The results of this two-choice measure indicate a performance of about 20% accuracy. In order to ascertain the impact that "no-response" had on the final accuracy rating, the neuropsychologist decides to re-score the test discarding the "no-response" items and analyzing only those items to which the patient actually responded. Following this analysis, the resulting accuracy is 24%.

The neuropsychologist is expected to report the results of the examination to the neurologist and the two attorneys involved in the case, as well as to the insurance company paying for the examination. Both analyses are reported in the final written report, and it is indicated that the patient's performance is sub-optimal.

Relevant Ethical Issues

This scenario involves issues relevant to a number of the Ethical Standards. These are addressed below in an order corresponding to the major areas of the 2002 APA Ethics Code.

Human Relations

The patient indicates that there are several "third-parties" involved in his care and case: a neurologist who suggested that the patient come see the neuropsychologist, two attorneys involved in litigation surrounding the alleged brain injury (Standard 3.07, Third-Party Requests for Services), and the insurance carrier. There is a need for cooperation with the neurologist who requested neuropsychological services, and this can likely easily be handled with a standard informed consent and release of information form. There is a need for informed consent also regarding the possible impact of this evaluation on the patient's litigation (Standard 3.10, Informed Consent). As the neuropsychologist has not been retained as an expert witness, but rather consulted as a treating professional, the patient needs to understand that the results of the examination may be subject to subpoena at some point in the future.

The clarification of the role of the neuropsychologist needs to be made clear to the patient, who may not understand the nuances of these relationship issues without explanation at the outset of services. This may, in fact, be an issue that arises only in the midst of a clinical interview when the patient indicates that there is active litigation. It may, however, arise at the onset if the referring neurologist has provided that information in making the referral. Relative to this are the limits of confidentiality (see below). At the onset of the examination, the neuropsychologist is required to discuss the role(s) of each party and obtain informed consent for the examination (Section 3.11). The neuropsychologist has a duty to cooperate with the other professionals involved (in this case, it is initially the neurologist) in serving the patient effectively

and appropriately. Yet the neuropsychologist also has a responsibility to cooperate with the attorneys involved once the patient has signed a release to do so. As such, the neuropsychologist has a duty to the patient to indicate the possibility that the results of the examination may or may not impact positively on the patient's legal case. Because the patient's cognitive status is in question and he already carries a diagnosis of dementia, there may exist a question of whether or not the patient understands the informed consent issues as described by the neuropsychologist. As a result, the neuropsychologist must be certain that such understanding exists before proceeding with the examination. If in doubt, the neuropsychologist should obtain consent from another responsible party, such as the patient's spouse.

Privacy and Confidentiality

The neuropsychologist will need to maintain confidentiality (Standard 4.01, Maintaining Confidentiality), as well as discuss the limits of confidentiality (Standard 4.02, Discussing the Limits of Confidentiality) and disclosures (Standard 4.05, Disclosures) with the individual being examined.

The neuropsychologist has an obligation to discuss the limits of confidentiality with the individual being examined at the onset of the examination. These limits include (1) areas directly relevant to the examination (e.g., standard confidentiality issues and instances in which the law may require the neuropsychologist to notify authorities such as in child abuse), (2) confidentiality as it pertains to communication between the neuropsychologist and neurologist, (3) issues of possible future sworn testimony and responding to questions under oath, and (4) other potential limits (e.g., in this situation, the neuropsychologist may also be required to provide a report of the examination to an insurance company paying for the exam). It is imperative that the patient understand *and agree* to these limitations prior to the neuropsychologist proceeding with examination.

Record Keeping and Fees

The neuropsychologist will have requirements that involve the maintenance, dissemination, and disposal of confidential records (Standard 6.02a, Maintenance, Dissemination, and Disposal of Confidential Records of Professional and Scientific Work). The neuropsychologist's records may be subject to examination by individuals who have access to the report that may or may not have a direct involvement in the case (e.g., centers that handle the billing for the neuropsychologist and personnel in the various offices to which the patient has requested a report be forwarded). Again, the patient needs to be aware of these issues, requirements and limits. In addition, the neuropsychologist should be conducting practice in compliance with HIPAA laws and regulations, education regarding which should be an ongoing part of the neuropsychologist's practice in order to maintain compliance with the HIPAA mandates.

The issue of fees and financial arrangements (Standard 6.04a-d, Fees and Financial Arrangements) may require attention as may accuracy in reports to payors and funding sources (Standard 6.06, Accuracy in Reports to Payors and Funding Sources). It would be appropriate for the neuropsychologist to address with the patient the possible implications of findings of examination. For example, the auto insurance carrier may conclude that coverage does not exist for this situation and therefore leaves the patient responsible for the bill. However, it would certainly not be within the scope of the neuropsychologist's role to anticipate all such implications. Similarly, depending on the confidence placed in the determination of suboptimal effort and the wording used by the neuropsychologist to describe invalid test results, the insurance company also may determine that responsibility for payment rests with the patient.

Assessment

The neuropsychologist has been asked to perform an examination. This may or may not include the use of tests as well as interview procedures. In determining the need for any testing, the neuropsychologist will need to consider the rationale for and against such procedures (Standard 9.01, Bases for Assessment, and 9.02, Use of Assessments). Informed consent for assessment is required (Standard 9.03, Informed Consent in Assessments). The referring neurologist, insurance carrier and/or attorneys involved at the request of the patient may expect release of some or all of the test data (Standard 9.04, Release of Test Data). The neuropsychologist may need to address the decision-making process that was involved in the administration, or lack thereof, of specific tests, including measures of response bias, in the explanation of assessment results (Standard 9.10, Explaining Assessment Results).

The reasons for test selection, use of the tests and interpretation of results are issues that would appropriately be addressed by the neuropsychologist in any report of findings. The neuropsychologist will need to address the rationale for the decision to "re-score" the response bias testing so as to exclude the "no-response" items (Standard 9.09c, Test Scoring and Interpretation Services). As well, discussion of the varying interpretations based on that analysis is appropriate. In this case, the results do not change significantly; however, under different circumstances, they may have required substantial discussion.

The neuropsychologist should release raw data to only those appropriate to receive it. This may include release of raw data to all parties, or it may be much more limited depending on the state laws involved. The neuropsychologist will need to consider the need for a signed release from the individual being examined (should be obtained prior to examination) as well as clarifying whether state law may require release of raw data only to a licensed psychologist, as is true in some jurisdictions (Standard 9.04). It would be appropriate for the neuropsychologist to also discuss the possible implications (e.g., that the litigation is impacted) that the results of testing could have, although it would certainly not be within the scope of the neuropsychologist's role to anticipate all such implications.

Case Resolution

The neuropsychologist in this case addressed the issues in an acceptable fashion. The slowed response time and possible impact on response bias testing raised a concern for the neuropsychologist, as the neuropsychologist did not want to report as "sub-optimal effort" scores that may have been optimal, yet adversely affected by psychomotor slowing. The resolution of the effect of the "no-response" items on response bias testing was dealt with by using standard scoring and analysis as well as "non-standard re-analysis". The results were interpreted as not substantively different. An explanation of the "re-analysis" and its impact on the neuropsychologist's final conclusions/opinions was included in the written report, as is appropriate. Should there have been a substantial difference between the performances as indicated by the two analyses, this aspect of the examination would have necessitated yet additional exploration. The report of the response bias testing was written so as to indicate sub-optimal performance. Given the clinical presentation in interview, however, the neuropsychologist did not opt to rule out the possibility that the patient does in fact have a cognitive disorder.

Conclusions and Recommendations

Neuropsychologists need to appreciate the medical, legal and psychosocial implications of the work that they do as it may impact a patient or others in ways in which a patient may not be aware prior to engaging in a relationship with a neuropsychologist. Limits of confidentiality as well as the future use of information by others (e.g., in this case the attorneys) should be anticipated as best as possible at the onset of the examination. A neuropsychologist performing such examinations needs to be as certain as is possible that all involved parties understand, and consent to, any limitations, restrictions and uses of the examination results. Neuropsychologists must understand not only how to administer tests and interpret them, but also the mechanisms involved in any automated procedures of scoring and/or interpretation used. In this scenario, the "re-analysis" made no significant difference in the outcome of the case. However, there may have been a very significant impact on the case were the "re-analysis" to have indicated that the patient had correctly responded to most all items for which a response was given, and merely scored low on the overall test due to a lack of responding to a number of items. Although the latter may have technically yielded the same results on the test itself (assuming that a "no-response" is indeed intended to be scored as an error), the neuropsychologist may well have reached different conclusions about the overall case (e.g., perhaps the patient was dozing or over-medicated). The neuropsychologist must maintain familiarity with the literature on response validity so that appropriate decisions can be made as to whether or not formal test administration is indicated, how to select such tests, scoring procedures and subsequent interpretation of tests. With the use of scoring services, including those scored locally on one's own computer, the neuropsychologist retains responsibility for appropriate interpretation of the data.

Chapter 27

ETHICAL CHALLENGES IN THE DETERMINATION OF RESPONSE VALIDITY IN NEUROPSYCHOLOGY, PART II

John A. Crouch

Scenario 1

The examinee is a 23-year-old Hungarian-born male who was referred to Neuropsychologist II for a re-evaluation of his cognitive status by an attorney for the respondent (defendant) in a legal case. The attorney states that she suspects the claimant (the examinee) might be exaggerating his claim of disability. She cites evidence from various sources, including videotaped surveillance to support her hypothesis.

The examinee was reportedly injured in a work-related accident approximately three years prior to the referral. The accident reportedly occurred when he tripped and fell off of a five-foot retaining wall while working as a landscaper's assistant. The examinee stated that he "landed on" his head from the fall, but also acknowledged that he fractured his ankle in the incident. Unfortunately, due to limited staffing issues on the day of the accident, no one witnessed the event or its initial effects on the examinee.

The examinee apparently worked the remainder of the day of the accident, going to a nearby "walk-in" emergency clinic that night. Medical personnel who examined the examinee noted that he was "alert, oriented, and in no apparent distress." His Glasgow Coma Scale (GCS) was entirely normal (GCS = 15) at that time. Records indicated that there were no complaints of blow to the head, loss of consciousness, or other neurological issues at that time. Aside from being placed in a cast for his ankle, the examinee declined any additional medical intervention and returned home. According to employment records, the examinee returned to work in two days, reportedly without incident.

Due to a reported decline in his functioning approximately four months subsequent to the incident in question (see below), the examinee and his mother sought legal counsel. The attorney then referred him to a neurologist to provide documentation of his client's disability.

Results from the neurological evaluation were "within normal limits" aside from some confusion during the verbal portions of a cognitive screening (e.g., had difficulty naming objects). Laboratory and neuroradiological (MRI) test results were normal. However, the neurologist, in an effort to obtain clarity regarding the examinee's functioning, referred him to Neuropsychologist I for an evaluation.

The initial neuropsychological evaluation occurred approximately five months subsequent to the incident in question. The assessment included a limited cognitive examination (e.g., dementia screen, etc.) as well as a collateral interview of the examinee's mother. Based on this information, Neuropsychologist I concluded that that the examinee had suffered a mild traumatic brain injury (MTBI) secondary to the accident, was experiencing symptoms of "post-concussion syndrome", and would be unable to work, drive, or live independently in the future. Recommendations for residential care and conservatorship were provided. During a discussion about these issues, Neuropsychologist I reportedly provided the examinee and his mother with brochures from a residential placement that was managed by the neuropsychologist's sister.

The neurologist, considering Neuropsychologist I's findings and recommendations, provided the examinee with documentation for disability compensation. He subsequently stopped working, began living with his mother, and started collecting Worker's Compensation benefits. Rehabilitation and other treatment (e.g., mental health assistance) was neither requested by the examinee nor recommended by his neurologist.

The respondent's attorney reviewed these details with Neuropsychologist II and stated that, in her opinion, the examinee was not disabled and must be "malingering his deficits." Neuropsychologist II asked that the examinee's raw data from the assessment be obtained from Neuropsychologist I. Despite providing Neuropsychologist I with an appropriate signed release, the data were not provided to Neuropsychologist II for approximately eight months, until a court order was obtained.

Neuropsychologist II had concerns regarding several aspects of Neuropsychologist I's evaluation of the examinee. For example, although the examinee had resided in the U.S. for nearly

five years, he reportedly had difficulty understanding instructions and verbal test items. A closer review of the examinee's history revealed that English was actually his third language.

Additionally, records indicated that Neuropsychologist I's evaluation included administration of a dated measure of effort as well as multiple administrations of a new symptom-validity test. Neuropsychologist II noted that the examinee initially failed the older test of effort, but it was incorrectly interpreted by Neuropsychologist I as representing "valid effort". The symptom validity test was also incorrectly interpreted by Neuropsychologist I as being indicative of "good effort," although the results of the test were clearly below standards of valid effort established by the test developers. Interestingly, Neuropsychologist I's records indicated that the same test was re-administered in a subsequent session, resulting in the examinee demonstrating a truly "normal" pattern of performance. No explanation for this re-administration was provided in the report.

Other portions of Neuropsychologist I's records suggested that the examinee's presentation might be pertinent to the issue of effort. For example, the examinee reportedly was unable to recognize Neuropsychologist I at the time of their second assessment appointment (two days following the initial meeting) and stated that he could not recall his mother's first name. These behaviors were not integrated into Neuropsychologist I's formulation of the case aside from being viewed as "pathogenic" and further "evidence of disability." Neuropsychologist II noted that no collateral information (e.g., records, interviews with others, etc.) was gathered by Neuropsychologist I aside from discussions with the examinee's mother. Finally, it appeared that Neuropsychologist I did not collect, or he avoided collecting, information about the examinee's medical history prior to the incident in question. It was later revealed that Neuropsychologist I had initially included a review of the examinee's medical history (including an account of a motor vehicle accident in which he had been injured), but the examinee and his attorney objected to this information being included stating that it was "irrelevant" to the matter at hand. Moreover, the examinee apparently was confused about Neuropsychologist I's role in his case, believing that information obtained in his interview was "confidential".

Neuropsychologist II proceeded with the re-evaluation. A professional Hungarian interpreter was utilized to assist with the interview and evaluation. The examinee provided a signed consent for the assessment and limits of confidentiality. The range of tests was limited primarily to nonverbal (visual) tests, including two current measures of response bias. Findings from the assessment were qualified due to the sociocultural background of the claimant. The examination revealed results that were inconsistent with MTBI due to (a) the examinee's difficulty on numerous tests in manner that was indicative of limited facility with English (e.g., Verbal IQ significantly worse than Performance IQ), (b) differences in the course of the symptoms from those of MTBI patients (e.g., four month delay in development of symptoms, worsening functioning, etc.), (c) collateral information that revealed pre-existing difficulties from a prior brain trauma (e.g., employment records that indicated he had difficulty learning and remembering the operation of new landscaping machinery, re-mowed the front portion of a lawn due to confusion as to whether he had already done so, etc.), and (d) invalid response patterns on several formal tests of effort (e.g., 22/50, 26/50, and 21/50 on the TOMM, etc.). Moreover, a number of issues regarding Neuropsychologist I's assessment were revealed that raised questions about its reliability and validity.

Relevant Ethical Issues

This scenario includes several issues that are relevant to the Ethical Standards of Psychologists

and Code of Conduct (APA, 2002). These issues will be addressed in an order corresponding to their appearance in the Code.

Boundaries of Competence (2.01)

Neuropsychologist I's competence to perform the initial neuropsychological evaluation appears questionable due to several factors. For example, his interpretation of the test results appeared to lack appreciation of key aspects of the examinee's background (e.g., non-English speaking status), his medical history, and his presentation (e.g., symptom course, severity of symptoms, etc.). Errors of this type suggest possible limited training in neuropsychology, a factor that was revealed during a review of Neuropsychologist I's curriculum vitae. In particular, he reported no supervised training in clinical neuropsychology at any time in his education. Although definitions of "clinical neuropsychologist" (American Psychological Association, Division of Neuropsychology/ Division 40/, 1989; Hannay, Bieliauskas, Crosson, Hammeke, Hamsher, & Koffler, 1998; National Academy of Neuropsychology, 2001) are debated, basic competency standards include both training and experience in neuropsychology that were clearly not present in this case.

Conflict of Interest (3.06)

Neuropsychologists avoid taking on a professional role when other interests could impair their objectivity or could expose others to harm. At times, this issue can take the form of recommending services that primarily meet the needs of the neuropsychologist. At times, this can take the form of only referring patients to oneself for treatment following an assessment. In this case, Neuropsychologist I recommended placement in a residential facility managed by his sister, clearly raising questions about his objectivity. This issue also raises concerns about possible multiple and exploitative relationships (Ethical Standards 3.05 & 3.08).

Cooperation with Other Professionals (3.09)

Due to the nature of the examinees that clinical neuropsychologists see, they are often asked to re-evaluate individuals who have previously been assessed. It is crucial that professionals who are re-evaluating such patients have information from prior examinations, particularly the tests that were administered, scores of those tests, and the demographics of the patient at the time of the evaluation (e.g., age, educational level, etc.). In legal cases, copies of raw data may also be required so that scoring and administration procedures can be evaluated more closely by the re-assessing neuropsychologist.

Neuropsychologist I was asked by Neuropsychologist II to provide raw data from his evaluation. Repeated attempts to obtain this information through conventional means (e.g., letters, telephone calls, etc.) yielded no response. Eventually, the defense attorney in the case obtained a court order that compelled Neuropsychologist I to provide Neuropsychologist II with the information. Neuropsychologist I's failure to respond in any way to requests for this information until placed under the duress of a court order appears to violate this standard.

Discussing the Limits of Confidentiality (4.02)

Prior to performing a neuropsychological evaluation, it is important for examinees to understand the role of the neuropsychologist. Within this discussion, as in the practice of psychotherapy, it is crucial that the neuropsychologist explain the limits of confidentiality (see discussion regarding "Informed Consent in Assessments" below). This is particularly important in forensic matters in which patients' privacy and confidentiality are often greatly limited. In addition to mentioning limitations of confidentiality in emergencies (e.g., imminent suicide, abuse, etc.), examinees in forensic contexts need to understand that, if information from the evaluation is utilized in the legal case, there are no protections

against others being informed about that information. In fact, records from neuropsychological evaluations are routinely copied and sent to experts for opposing counsel.

Moreover, it is important for examinees to be made aware that all information obtained in the evaluation, if relevant to the assessment, will be revealed and cannot be "taken back." This issue is most likely to arise when conducting an evaluation with a plaintiff (claimant) when historical information is revealed that could have causal significance to his/her case. For example, revealing an examinee's history of prior brain trauma, substance usage, or mental health problems may weaken his/her legal case and will likely draw ire from his/her attorney.

Lastly, examinees should be informed that their effort and accuracy of self-report will be formally evaluated during the evaluation. Again, results from these tests will not remain confidential, regardless of whether they benefit or hurt the examinee's legal case.

Avoidance of False or Deceptive Statements (5.01)

While it is clear that Neuropsychologist I's conclusions were insufficiently supported and at times clearly inaccurate, what is less certain is whether his actions were solely the result of incompetence or were also influence by intentional misrepresentation of the information and data that he obtained (see also Principle C, Integrity).

Bases for Assessments (9.01)

Neuropsychologists are ethically bound to conduct evaluations that are sufficient in content and depth to support their opinions. Although many different assessment approaches exist (e.g., fixed battery approach, flexible battery approach, etc.), standards of practice in neuropsychology demand that the tests chosen are appropriate for the case at hand. In this case, Neuropsychologist I's use of a dementia screening measure in the context of a forensic TBI case appears inappropriate.

Additional issues arise with respect to the assessment of response bias. For example, although different approaches may be taken to assessing effort/honesty, current standards of practice in Independent Medical Examination (IME) referrals specify that (a) at least two measures of effort are administered, and (b) the measures of effort must be recently developed tests (e.g., Test of Memory Malingering [TOMM], Word Memory Test, Validity Indicator Profile [VIP], Computerized Assessment of Response Bias [CARB], etc.). Similarly, indices of response validity within, or based on, ability measures must be considered. Additional recommendations regarding personality tests to assess for accuracy of self-report (e.g., Minnesota Multiphasic Personality Inventory, Second Edition [MMPI-2]) are also often specified. These standards appear to be motivated by a desire for an adequate basis for assessment conclusions from tests within the battery.

Additionally, an adequate basis for assessment of response bias requires that information be obtained beyond formal tests. In this regard, reviewing records, conducting collateral interviews, and examining consistency/inconsistency between test results and daily life functioning provides crucial information. As with other aspects of neuropsychological assessment, a "multi-modal" approach of this type appears necessary. In this case, Neuropsychologist I did not appear to obtain or integrate such information into his conclusions.

Use of Assessments (9.02)

Neuropsychologists are ethically bound to utilize assessment tools and norms appropriate for the population being evaluated. Neuropsychologist I's failure to consider the examinee's sociocultural and language backgrounds in the choice of tests and norms utilized to judge performance appears ethically questionable. Of course, when it appears unlikely that available methods or norms exist for a particular examinee, the neuropsychologist must qualify his/her opinions

about the test results. Neuropsychologist I did not qualify his opinions about this examinee, possibly leading to an inappropriate conclusion about his functioning.

Other issues related to this examinee's presentation could involve the use of an interpreter. Standards related to Delegation of Work to others (2.05), Maintaining Confidentiality (4.01), and Assessment by Unqualified Persons (9.07) may apply under such circumstances.

Informed Consent in Assessments (9.03)

The examinee appeared confused about Neuropsychologist I's role in the first evaluation. He revealed that he believed Neuropsychologist I was "on his side" and, consequently, would not reveal any negative aspects of his history (including a prior injury of relevance). The examinee's attorney further added to confusion on this issue by instructing Neuropsychologist I not to include information about his client that was "prejudicial".

As in any aspect of psychological practice, neuropsychologists are bound to fully inform their examinees about their roles and the limits of confidentiality (see 'Discussing the Limits of Confidentiality' above) in the particular context of that assessment. With litigation matters in particular, examinees must be fully informed and agree to proceed under evidentiary requirements that mandate the potential for full disclosure of all materials obtained during the evaluation.

Moreover, examinees should be informed that their effort and accuracy of report will be evaluated formally. Their informed agreement to participate in the evaluation formalizes their willingness to cooperate fully and put forth their best effort throughout the evaluation.

An open discussion about these issues as well as formal documentation of the examinee's informed consent on these matters is required. Neuropsychologist I did not appear to obtain this consent prior to proceeding with his evaluation of the examinee.

Interpreting Assessment Results (9.06)

Interpretation of neuropsychological evaluation results requires a complex process of reviewing normatively-based test patterns, the patient's history, his/her current circumstances, and collateral information. Through the use of deductive reasoning and the process of "ruling out" alternative explanations for the patient's presentation, a more complete understanding about his/her functioning may be obtained. Neuropsychologist I apparently did not consider the examinee's pre-existing medical history, choosing to focus exclusively on the incident in question. This violates standards of practice parameters for neuropsychological evaluations and suggests that Neuropsychologist I utilized a biased approach in his assessment. In addition, Neuropsychologist I "misinterpreted" the results of the first symptom validity test. Although plaintiff's attorneys often express frustration when the dutiful neuropsychologist identifies pre-existing injuries, substance usage, questionable response validity, or other pertinent issues in their clients, the neuropsychologist is bound to perform the same investigative process during all evaluations, regardless of the "side" that has hired him/her.

Obsolete Tests and Outdated Test Results (9.08)

New and updated versions of tests are constantly being published. Neuropsychologists are required to utilize updated and current versions of tests, whenever possible, and to avoid use of outdated procedures. Neuropsychologist I's use of an older, outmoded test of response bias was inappropriate.

Case Resolution

Consistent with Principle B (Fidelity and Responsibility), Neuropsychologist II was quite

concerned about the apparent ethical misconduct of Neuropsychologist I in his role in this case. After Neuropsychologist II completed the evaluation and sent the report to the retaining attorney, he attempted once again to contact Neuropsychologist I, this time in an attempt to discuss the areas of ethical concern (Standard 1.04, Informal Resolution of Ethical Violations). Consistent with earlier requests for test data, also via certified mail and telephone calls, Neuropsychologist I did not respond. Neuropsychologist II was mindful both of his responsibility to protect the public from further mistreatment by Neuropsychologist I (Principle A, Beneficence and Nonmaleficence; Standard 3.04, Avoiding Harm) and of the potential appearance of an adversarial attack should he file a formal complaint during the course of legal/disability proceedings.

To obtain an objective, outside opinion regarding these issues, Neuropsychologist II contacted the APA Division of Neuropsychology Ethics Committee and presented the case without identifying information. The committee, based on the information provided, supported his decision to pursue the matter formally, following resolution of the case. Neuropsychologist II knew that since Neuropsychologist I was not a member of APA or the state psychological association, any complaint would need to be made to the state psychology board. Following resolution of the case, he filed the complaint.

Conclusions and Recommendations

The need to assess effort is straightforward, yet how to best go about such assessment is less certain. Nevertheless, the acknowledgement that effort testing is critically important to research and clinical assessment makes this an exciting time for those studying and discussing such practices. Neuropsychologists are ethically obligated to stay informed of the advances in this rapidly changing area in order to best serve patients and others who solicit neuropsychological services.

Scenario 2

A neuropsychologist is employed as a consultant in a university-based medical center. A portion of her work involves assessments on a psychiatric unit with both acute and chronic patients. The neuropsychologist received a referral from the psychiatric Unit Chief, requesting that a "VIP patient" be evaluated as soon as possible. Referral questions included clarification of diagnosis, including "the possibility of malingering."

Discussions with the referring psychiatrist revealed that the patient, a 33-year-old male, was the son of a wealthy state government official. He was brought to the inpatient, unit on transfer after he was observed to be confused and agitated near a busy downtown thoroughfare. Law enforcement personnel found the patient standing in the street, yelling angrily at passing vehicles. He was initially taken to the Emergency Department at a large county hospital before being transferred to the medical center where the neuropsychologist is employed. This transfer reportedly occurred following demands from the patient's father, who had been out-of-state at a government convention.

The patient was reported to have a 12-year history of multiple (at least 30) psychiatric and medical admissions. Voluminous records were reviewed by the neuropsychologist and revealed multiple psychiatric diagnoses including Schizophrenia, Bipolar Disorder I, Delusional Disorder, and Amphetamine Abuse. In addition, numerous medical difficulties were identified in the record including chronic low back pain, chronic headaches, and soft tissue discomfort. Legal issues were identified included multiple arrests following attempts to forge prescriptions for pain medications.

Records from three prior neuropsychological evaluations were available for review. Concerns

about the patient's cooperation and effort were expressed by the examiners during each assessment. Results from the patient's most recent evaluation (four months prior to the current assessment) were judged to be "unreliable and invalid," in part, due to his poor performance on a measure of response bias (i.e., Portland Digit Recognition Test [PDRT], 29/72 trials correct).

On the psychiatric unit, the patient was noted to be uncooperative and "difficult" to engage in treatment. He often openly expressed negative views about staff members, criticizing their competency and threatening legal action from his father if he was not treated as a "dignitary". He stated repeatedly that he was "suing" several psychiatric facilities where he has previously been hospitalized and threatened to do so to the current facility if his needs were not adequately met. During staff meetings, clinicians often expressed hostility toward the patient, angrily stating that they were "counting the minutes" until he could be discharged. Multiple staff members labeled the patient a "faker," hoping that the neuropsychologist's results would substantiate a tendency to exaggerate problems.

The neuropsychologist's assessment of the patient proved to be challenging, and issues related to honesty and effort arose early during the interview. For example, the patient provided details about his history that were grossly inaccurate, including his marital status, geographic area in which he grew up, and institution from which he obtained his college degree. However, based on repeated questioning and interviews with family members, there were no apparent pending legal issues or pending claims for disability compensation. Therefore, obvious motivations for the patient to engage in this behavior were not present.

During the interview, the neuropsychologist realized that she had previously met the patient at a political social function for his father approximately two years previously. She discussed this with the patient, sharing her personal recollections of his father's campaign as well as her positive impressions of the patient. He expressed gratitude to the neuropsychologist for her favorable memory of him, promising to have his father reimburse her personally for the evaluation. The patient stated that he was happy the information he provided would be "confidential," as his father would be purchasing her discretion.

With respect to spontaneous behavior, the patient appeared listless, unconcerned about his performance, and responded in a random or haphazard manner on even the most basic test items (e.g., unable to consistently recall two digits forward during Digit Span). Test results from more challenging tests revealed marked inconsistencies. For instance, on a verbal learning test, the patient was unable to correctly recognize a word that he had remembered spontaneously on six previous learning/memory trials (including long delay recall). A forced choice procedure also demonstrated an apparent amnesia for this word. The neuropsychologist repeatedly confronted the patient about these inconsistencies, but he denied exaggeration of his deficit.

Although the neuropsychologist rarely used measures of effort during her clinical evaluations, the patient's test results and presentation prompted a formal administration of such measures. Due to time management issues, the neuropsychologist employed a graduate student from a local college to administer the test. This individual was student in the neuropsychologist's Clinical Neuropsychology class and had expressed interest in obtaining some "real life" experience to round out her background. The neuropsychologist was unavailable for the appointment but instructed the graduate student to contact her via cell phone if any issues arose. The student later reported that the session with the patient went well, although she was unsure whether she should accept his offer for "lunch" once discharged from the unit.

Formal effort testing revealed inconsistencies between test results. That is, the patient functioned below expectations on one measure of effort (i.e., TOMM; 41/50, 44/50, 43/50), but performed well on another symptom validity measure (PDRT; 62/72 correct). Results from the MMPI-2 and VIP were also in the normal range with respect to reliability and validity. The neuropsychologist was unsure how she should report and resolve this discrepancy. She subsequently delayed completing the report until after a staff rounds meeting in which she would ask other staff members about their opinions on this issue.

In addition, the neuropsychologist contacted another neuropsychologist in the same town to obtain a consultation on the response bias issue. During a discussion of the patient's history, the examining neuropsychologist disclosed several key personal facts about the patient (e.g., his father's government job, etc.), resulting in the colleague correctly "guessing" the father's identity. The neuropsychologist, responding in embarrassment, quickly discontinued the conversation, never obtaining an opinion about how to resolve the issue.

The staff rounds meeting included a number of particularly heated exchanges between staff members regarding the patient. The staff appeared divided regarding whether to continue treatment or whether to discharge him due to "malingering". The chief psychiatrist expressed the latter view and solicited the neuropsychologist to provide test-based confirmation of his opinion. The neuropsychologist agreed with the psychiatrist, her supervisor, stating that "unequivocal evidence for malingering" was found. The psychiatrist began discharge proceedings, asking that the neuropsychologist be present at a meeting in which neuropsychological evaluation findings and discharge recommendations would be explained to the patient and his family. The neuropsychologist stated that she would be unavailable to attend this meeting due to a rapidly developing "flu".

Relevant Ethical Issues

This scenario includes several issues that are relevant to the Ethical Standards of Psychologists and Code of Conduct (APA, 2002). These issues will be addressed in an order corresponding to their appearance in the Code.

Delegation of Work to Others (2.05)

The neuropsychologist utilized a graduate student to conduct the response bias portion of the neuropsychological assessment. The student's competence to administer any test appeared questionable given her lack of experience in clinical situations and obvious confusion regarding "boundary issues" with the patient (e.g., considering a social visit following his discharge). Unfortunately, the test data from this portion of the assessment would likely be questionably valid/reliable, causing further concern about interpretation of the evaluation data. Although the neuropsychologist was available by telephone, the student examiner was not adequately supervised in this situation. If such supervision had been present, the neuropsychologist would likely have removed the student from the role of examiner.

Avoiding Harm (3.04)

Psychologists are mandated to avoid harming or to minimize harm towards others in their work, whenever possible. Harm to the patient in this scenario was a possible result of the neuropsychologist's use of pejorative psychiatric labels including "malingerer". Although appropriate at times, such labels have particularly negative connotations within clinical situations. Patients with documented histories of malingering or factitious conditions may be less likely to receive evaluation or treatment services even when warranted.

Within this scenario, the neuropsychologist is faced with conflicting information from multiple tests of effort/honesty. It should be noted, however, that the one failed measure of motivation (TOMM) yielded results that were nearly in the normal range. Although performance below the cutoff score on one measure of response bias may, to some clinicians, be indicative of questionable validity of the overall test results, other clinicians may use different standards to make this determination. For example, the patient's normal performance on a more sensitive measure of effort (i.e., PDRT) could, for some neuropsychologists, raise questions about the meaning of the TOMM results, including whether or not the TOMM results should be accorded less weight in the determination of the validity of performance on the ability measures. (Of course, other factors, such as possible examinee training with, or past exposure to, the PDRT, could have influenced his performance.) Hopefully, future research will assist neuropsychologists in defining more clearly the behavioral presentations and patterns of test performance necessary to confidently establish the examinee's level of effort to do well and his or her likelihood of producing valid test results.

Poor performance on symptom validity tests is insufficient in and of itself for establishing a diagnosis of malingering. In any given case, there may exist a number of reasons for poor performance on symptom validity tests, and such measures alone cannot distinguish between the various potential reasons. The "Slick criteria" serve as an important step toward making such distinctions (Slick, Sherman, & Iverson, 1999). In this patient's case, no obvious external incentives were present that would motivate him to feign deficits. Rather, the possibility of a Factitious Disorder was present, with his psychiatrically-motivated maintenance of a "sick role" within a medical or psychiatric treatment context. Alternatively, the patient's presentation might have been indicative of a "hysterical" disorder, possibly driven by underlying psychiatric issues that were displayed via neuropsychiatric symptomatology. Finally, the possibility exists that the patient was willfully uncooperative with the neuropsychologist for no obvious external or intrapsychic reason. Such patients, particularly bright individuals in forensic or long-term psychiatric settings, may engage in this type of behavior for "fun" to "pass the time" or to augment their sense of "power" within a setting in which they feel otherwise inadequate. Each of these possible alternative causal scenarios must be considered and ruled out before the neuropsychologist provides the label of "malingerer". In this case, the neuropsychologist appeared to respond to the treatment team's needs to punish the patient rather than the objective assessment data and presentation.

Multiple Relationships (3.05)

The neuropsychologist's pre-existing social relationship with the patient raised the possibility of bias within her interpretation of the evaluation findings. She appeared to exacerbate this situation by engaging the patient in a gratuitous conversation about the prior contact, likely leading to an expectation of "special treatment" by the neuropsychologist. Similar to other clinical situations, discovery of potential multiple relationships should be addressed immediately with the patient. In this case, transferring the referral to another neuropsychologist within the hospital system would have been most appropriate.

Psychological Services Delivered to or Through Organizations (3.11)

Neuropsychologists who conduct evaluations through facilities or organizations are required to fully inform patients regarding their roles and how information will be disseminated. A key issue involves confidentiality of information provided during assessments. The patient clearly had a misperception regarding the "confidentiality" of the information he provided to the neuropsychologist during the assessment. This misunderstanding could lead to surprise and anger if/when the patient learns that, in fact, the neuropsychologist was providing information about him to the treatment team throughout the evaluation process.

Disclosures (4.05)

Neuropsychologists are allowed to disclose confidential information if they obtain appropriately informed consent or if the information is legally required (e.g., child abuse reporting). Issues around this topic often arise when work is performed in an organization or facility (see section on Psychological Services Delivered to or Through Organization above) when multiple parties have access to the information. In this case, the neuropsychologist did not obtain an appropriately informed consent from the patient to disclose information from the assessment to members of the treatment staff. This error justifiably raises the neuropsychologist's exposure to an ethical complaint from the patient.

Consultations (4.06)

Neuropsychologists often seek consultation with other professionals when they are confused by a particular aspect of a case or when they simply need a "second opinion" on an issue. The neuropsychologist appropriately sought out a consultation in relation to conflicting results on measures of response bias. However, in conflict with ethical requirements, she provided the consultant with personal information about the patient that allowed him to determine the patient's father's identity. Consultants may be informed about details of the case but should not be provided with information that would lead to their ability to identify the individual (or others to whom he is related in some manner). Unfortunately, following realization of her mistake, the neuropsychologist impulsively ended the conversation with the consultant and, consequently, never obtained the opinion she sought.

Fees and Financial Arrangements (6.04)

The neuropsychologist is required to inform patients or other responsible parties about financial arrangements for his/her services before services are provided. In this case, the patient's statement that his father would pay the neuropsychologist personally (i.e., "under the table") for the assessment requires clarification prior to the start of the assessment. Accepting money in this manner would likely violate policies of the facility in which the neuropsychologist works and would increase the potential for bias and a lack of objectivity in her work.

Bases for Assessments (9.01)

Following completion of the testing portion of the assessment, the neuropsychologist was confused about how to interpret the test findings. Specifically, inconsistencies between measures of response bias could not be resolved. An additional factor involved pressures from the treatment team and, in particular, the chief psychiatrist on the case who viewed the patient as a manipulative malingerer.

Although the neuropsychologist appeared hesitant regarding the "malingering" label, pressure from the chief psychiatrist apparently led to her kowtowing to his opinion. Basing one's conclusions on those of others likely reduces conflict in team dynamics but is ethically inappropriate when the neuropsychological evaluation data do not provide objective support for the opinion.

Explaining Assessment Results (9.10)

Neuropsychological assessment results are multi-faceted and complex, requiring a broad range of expertise that is unique compared to most other medical or psychological specialists. Neuropsychologists are personally obligated to provide examinees or concerned others with information about the examinee's test findings and their interpretation. This activity varies greatly across practitioners but could include a face-to-face meeting, telephone conference, or written summary. The neuropsychologist's refusal to attend a conference in which the test results and their implications could be discussed appears professionally and ethically inappropriate.

Case Resolution

The neuropsychologist reconsidered her attendance at the family meeting, realizing that she must attend. However, she did not want the patient to be blindsided by the team's conclusion (accusation of malingering), which was based in large part on her report. Therefore, hours prior to the family meeting, she met individually with the patient to prepare him for what he would hear in the meeting. Using her counseling skills, she rather delicately presented the fact that, on at least certain portions of the testing, the patient did not appear to put forth full effort. Somewhat surprisingly, and much to the relief of the neuropsychologist, the patient acknowledged that he saw the mental healthcare system, including its professionals, as "a farce", to be manipulated, and not be taken seriously. He informed the neuropsychologist that he actually "got into" some of the tests but completely "zoned out" or even intentionally misrepresented his ability on others. He said he had no problem admitting that fact in front of his parents and the rest of the treatment team, and that was exactly what happened at the meeting.

Conclusions and Recommendations

The scenarios in this section highlight the range of ethical dilemmas that can arise within the context of symptom validity testing in neuropsychological assessment. Issues related to response bias assessment are different than those associated with traditional cognitive ability assessment in that they challenge the tendency of clinicians to trust the accuracy of what patients say and the behaviors they exhibit, and they challenge the traditional tendency of examiners to rely on their subject impressions of response validity. At this point, assessment of cognitive ability must also include formal assessment of response validity. As neuropsychologists become more skilled at assessing symptom validity in their evaluations, so too must they remain mindful of their ethical responsibilities.

References

American Psychological Association, Division of Neuropsychology (Division 40) (1989). Definition of a clinical neuropsychologist. *The clinical neuropsychologist, 3 (1)*, 22.

Hannay, H.J., Bieliauskas, L.A., Crosson, B.A., Hammeke, T.A., Hamsher, K.deS., & Koffler, S. (Eds.) (1998). Proceedings of the Houston Conference on Specialty Education and Training in Neuropsychology: Policy statement. *Archives of clinical neuropsychology, 13*, 160-166.

National Academy of Neuropsychology (2001). *NAN definition of a clinical neuropsychologist.* Retrieved on December 23, 2003 from http://www.nanonline.org/downloads/paio/Position/NANPositionDefNeuro.pdf.

Slick, D.J., Sherman, E.M.S., & Iverson, G.L. (1999). Diagnostic criteria for malingered neurocognitive dysfunction: Proposed standards for clinical practice and research. *The clinical neuropsychologist, 13*, 545-561.

Appendix A

ETHICAL PRINCIPLES OF PSYCHOLOGISTS AND CODE OF CONDUCT

Effective date June 1, 2003.

Introduction and Applicability

The American Psychological Association's (APA's) Ethical Principles of Psychologists and Code of Conduct (hereinafter referred to as the Ethics Code) consists of an Introduction, a Preamble, five General Principles (A-E), and specific Ethical Standards. The Introduction discusses the intent, organization, procedural considerations, and scope of application of the Ethics Code. The Preamble and General Principles are aspirational goals to guide psychologists toward the highest ideals of psychology. Although the Preamble and General Principles are not themselves enforceable rules, they should be considered by psychologists in arriving at an ethical course of action. The Ethical Standards set forth enforceable rules for conduct as psychologists. Most of the Ethical Standards are written broadly, in order to apply to psychologists in varied roles, although the application of an Ethical Standard may vary depending on the context. The Ethical Standards are not exhaustive. The fact that a given conduct is not specifically addressed by an Ethical Standard does not mean that it is necessarily either ethical or unethical.

This Ethics Code applies only to psychologists' activities that are part of their scientific, educational, or professional roles as psychologists. Areas covered include but are not limited to the clinical, counseling, and school practice of psychology; research; teaching; supervision of trainees; public service; policy development; social intervention; development of assessment instruments; conducting assessments; educational counseling; organizational consulting; forensic activities; program design and evaluation; and administration. This Ethics Code applies to these activities across a variety of contexts, such as in person, postal, telephone, internet, and other electronic transmissions. These activities shall be distinguished from the purely private conduct of psychologists, which is not within the purview of the Ethics Code.

Membership in the APA commits members and student affiliates to comply with the standards of the APA Ethics Code and to the rules and procedures used to enforce them. Lack of awareness or misunderstanding of an Ethical Standard is not itself a defense to a charge of unethical conduct.

The procedures for filing, investigating, and resolving complaints of unethical conduct are described in the current Rules and Procedures of the APA Ethics Committee. APA may impose sanctions on its members for violations of the standards of the Ethics Code, including termination of APA membership, and may notify other bodies and individuals of its actions. Actions that violate the standards of the Ethics Code may also lead to the imposition of sanctions on psychologists or students whether or not they are APA members by bodies other than APA, including state psychological associations, other professional groups, psychology boards, other state or federal agencies, and payors for health services. In addition, APA may take action against a member after his or her conviction of a felony, expulsion or suspension from an affiliated state psychological association, or suspension or loss of licensure. When the sanction to be imposed by APA is less than expulsion, the 2001 Rules and Procedures do not guarantee an opportunity for an in-person hearing, but generally provide that complaints will be resolved only on the basis of a submitted record.

The Ethics Code is intended to provide guidance for psychologists and standards of professional conduct that can be applied by the APA and by other bodies that choose to adopt them. The Ethics Code is not intended to be a basis of civil liability. Whether a psychologist has violated the Ethics Code standards does not by itself determine whether the psychologist is legally liable in a court action, whether a contract is enforceable, or whether other legal consequences occur.

The modifiers used in some of the standards of this Ethics Code (e.g., *reasonably, appropriate, potentially*) are included in the standards when they would (1) allow professional judgment on the part of psychologists, (2) eliminate injustice or inequality that would occur without the modifier, (3) ensure applicability across the broad range of activities conducted by psychologists, or (4) guard against a set of rigid rules that might be quickly outdated. As used in this Ethics Code, the term *reasonable* means the prevailing professional judgment of psychologists engaged in similar activities in similar circumstances, given the knowledge the psychologist had or should have had at the time.

In the process of making decisions regarding their professional behavior, psychologists must consider this Ethics Code in addition to applicable laws and psychology board regulations. In applying the Ethics Code to their professional work, psychologists may consider other materials and guidelines that have been adopted or endorsed by scientific and professional psychological organizations and the dictates of their own conscience, as well as consult with others within the field. If this Ethics Code establishes a higher standard of conduct than is required by law, psychologists must meet the higher ethical standard. If psychologists' ethical responsibilities conflict with law, regulations, or other governing legal authority, psychologists make known their commitment to this Ethics Code and take steps to resolve the conflict in a responsible manner. If the conflict is unresolvable via such means, psychologists may adhere to the requirements of the law, regulations, or other governing authority in keeping with basic principles of human rights.

Preamble

Psychologists are committed to increasing scientific and professional knowledge of behavior and people's understanding of themselves and others and to the use of such knowledge to improve the condition of individuals, organizations, and society. Psychologists respect and

protect civil and human rights and the central importance of freedom of inquiry and expression in research, teaching, and publication. They strive to help the public in developing informed judgments and choices concerning human behavior. In doing so, they perform many roles, such as researcher, educator, diagnostician, therapist, supervisor, consultant, administrator, social interventionist, and expert witness. This Ethics Code provides a common set of principles and standards upon which psychologists build their professional and scientific work.

This Ethics Code is intended to provide specific standards to cover most situations encountered by psychologists. It has as its goals the welfare and protection of the individuals and groups with whom psychologists work and the education of members, students, and the public regarding ethical standards of the discipline.

The development of a dynamic set of ethical standards for psychologists' work-related conduct requires a personal commitment and lifelong effort to act ethically; to encourage ethical behavior by students, supervisees, employees, and colleagues; and to consult with others concerning ethical problems.

General Principles

This section consists of General Principles. General Principles, as opposed to Ethical Standards, are aspirational in nature. Their intent is to guide and inspire psychologists toward the very highest ethical ideals of the profession. General Principles, in contrast to Ethical Standards, do not represent obligations and should not form the basis for imposing sanctions. Relying upon General Principles for either of these reasons distorts both their meaning and purpose.

Principle A: Beneficence and Nonmaleficence

Psychologists strive to benefit those with whom they work and take care to do no harm. In their professional actions, psychologists seek to safeguard the welfare and rights of those with whom they interact professionally and other affected persons, and the welfare of animal subjects of research. When conflicts occur among psychologists' obligations or concerns, they attempt to resolve these conflicts in a responsible fashion that avoids or minimizes harm. Because psychologists' scientific and professional judgments and actions may affect the lives of others, they are alert to and guard against personal, financial, social, organizational, or political factors that might lead to misuse of their influence. Psychologists strive to be aware of the possible effect of their own physical and mental health on their ability to help those with whom they work.

Principle B: Fidelity and Responsibility

Psychologists establish relationships of trust with those with whom they work. They are aware of their professional and scientific responsibilities to society and to the specific communities in which they work. Psychologists uphold professional standards of conduct, clarify their-professional roles and obligations, accept appropriate responsibility for their behavior, and seek to manage conflicts of interest that could lead to exploitation or harm. Psychologists consult with, refer to, or cooperate with other professionals and institutions to the extent needed to serve the best interests of those with whom they work. They are concerned about the ethical compliance of their colleagues' scientific and professional conduct. Psychologists strive to contribute a portion of their professional time for little or no compensation or personal advantage.

Principle C: Integrity

Psychologists seek to promote accuracy, honesty, and truthfulness in the science, teaching, and practice of psychology. In these activities psychologists do not steal, cheat, or engage in fraud, subterfuge, or intentional misrepresentation of fact. Psychologists strive to keep their promises and to avoid unwise or unclear commitments. In situations in which deception may be ethically justifiable to maximize benefits and minimize harm, psychologists have a serious obligation to consider the need for, the possible consequences of, and their responsibility to correct any resulting mistrust or other harmful effects that arise from the use of such techniques.

Principle D: Justice

Psychologists recognize that fairness and justice entitle all persons to access to and benefit from the contributions of psychology and to equal quality in the processes, procedures, and services being conducted by psychologists. Psychologists exercise reasonable judgment and take precautions to ensure that their potential biases, the boundaries of their competence, and the limitations of their expertise do not lead to or condone unjust practices.

Principle E: Respect for People's Rights and Dignity

Psychologists respect the dignity and worth of all people, and the rights of individuals to privacy, confidentiality, and self-determination. Psychologists are aware that special safeguards may be necessary to protect the rights and welfare of persons or communities whose vulnerabilities impair autonomous decision making. Psychologists are aware of and respect cultural, individual, and role differences, including those based on age, gender, gender identity, race, ethnicity, culture, national origin, religion, sexual orientation, disability, language, and socioeconomic status and consider these factors when working with members of such groups. Psychologists try to eliminate the effect on their work of biases based on those factors, and they do not knowingly participate in or condone activities of others based upon such prejudices.

Ethical Standards

Resolving Ethical Issues

Misuse of Psychologists' Work
If psychologists learn of misuse or misrepresentation of their work, they take reasonable steps to correct or minimize the misuse or misrepresentation.

Conflicts Between Ethics and Law, Regulations, or Other Governing Legal Authority
If psychologists' ethical responsibilities conflict with law, regulations, or other governing legal authority, psychologists make known their commitment to the Ethics Code and take steps to resolve the conflict. If the conflict is unresolvable via such means, psychologists may adhere to the requirements of the law, regulations, or other governing legal authority.

Conflicts Between Ethics and Organizational Demands
If the demands of an organization with which psychologists are affiliated or for whom they are working conflict with this Ethics Code, psychologists clarify the nature of the conflict, make known their commitment to the Ethics Code, and to the extent feasible, resolve the conflict in a way that permits adherence to the Ethics Code.

Informal Resolution of Ethical Violations
When psychologists believe that there may have been an ethical violation by another psychologist, they attempt to resolve the issue by bringing it to the attention of that individual, if an informal resolution appears appropriate and the intervention does not violate any confidentiality rights that may be involved. (See also Standards 1.02, Conflicts Between Ethics and Law, Regulations, or Other Governing Legal Authority, and 1.03, Conflicts Between Ethics and Organizational Demands.)

Reporting Ethical Violations
If an apparent ethical violation has substantially harmed or is likely to substantially harm a person or organization and is not appropriate for informal resolution under Standard 1.04, Informal Resolution of Ethical Violations, or is not resolved properly in that fashion, psychologists take further action appropriate to the situation. Such action might include referral to state or national committees on professional ethics, to state licensing boards, or to the appropriate institutional authorities. This standard does not apply when an intervention would violate confidentiality rights or when psychologists have been retained to review the work of another psychologist whose professional conduct is in question. (See also Standard 1.02, Conflicts Between Ethics and Law, Regulations, or Other Governing Legal Authority.)

Cooperating with Ethics Committees
Psychologists cooperate in ethics investigations, proceedings, and resulting requirements of the APA or any affiliated state psychological association to which they belong. In doing so, they address any confidentiality issues. Failure to cooperate is itself an ethics violation. However, making a request for deferment of adjudication of an ethics complaint pending the outcome of litigation does not alone constitute noncooperation.

Improper Complaints
Psychologists do not file or encourage the filing of ethics complaints that are made with reckless disregard for or willful ignorance of facts that would disprove the allegation.

Unfair Discrimination Against Complainants and Respondents
Psychologists do not deny persons employment, advancement, admissions to academic or other programs, tenure, or promotion, based solely

upon their having made or their being the subject of an ethics complaint. This does not preclude taking action based upon the outcome of such proceedings or considering other appropriate information.

Competence
Boundaries of Competence
(a) Psychologists provide services, teach, and conduct research with populations and in areas only within the boundaries of their competence, based on their education, training, supervised experience, consultation, study, or professional experience.
(b) Where scientific or professional knowledge in the discipline of psychology establishes that an understanding of factors associated with age, gender, gender identity, race, ethnicity, culture, national origin, religion, sexual orientation, disability, language, or socioeconomic status is essential for effective implementation of their services or research, psychologists have or obtain the training, experience, consultation, or supervision necessary to ensure the competence of their services, or they make appropriate referrals, except as provided in Standard 2.02, Providing Services in Emergencies.
(c) Psychologists planning to provide services, teach, or conduct research involving populations, areas, techniques, or technologies new to them undertake relevant education, training, supervised experience, consultation, or study.
(d) When psychologists are asked to provide services to individuals for whom appropriate mental health services are not available and for which psychologists have not obtained the competence necessary, psychologists with closely related prior training or experience may provide such services in order to ensure that services are not denied if they make a reasonable effort to obtain the competence required by using relevant research, training, consultation, or study.
(e) In those emerging areas in which generally recognized standards for preparatory training do not yet exist, psychologists nevertheless take reasonable steps to ensure the competence of their work and to protect clients/patients, students, supervisees, research participants, organizational clients, and others from harm.
(f) When assuming forensic roles, psychologists are or become reasonably familiar with the judicial or administrative rules governing their roles.

Providing Services in Emergencies
In emergencies, when psychologists provide services to individuals for whom other mental health services are not available and for which psychologists have not obtained the necessary training, psychologists may provide such services in order to ensure that services are not denied. The services are discontinued as soon as the emergency has ended or appropriate services are available.

Maintaining Competence
Psychologists undertake ongoing efforts to develop and maintain their competence.

Bases for Scientific and Professional Judgments
Psychologists' work is based upon established scientific and professional knowledge of the discipline. (See also Standards 2.01e, Boundaries of Competence, and 10.01b, Informed Consent to Therapy.)

Delegation of Work to Others
Psychologists who delegate work to employees, supervisees, or research or teaching assistants or who use the services of others, such as interpreters, take reasonable steps to (1) avoid delegating such work to persons who have a multiple relationship with those being served that would likely lead to exploitation or loss of objectivity; (2) authorize only those responsibilities that such persons can be expected to perform competently

on the basis of their education, training, or experience, either independently or with the level of supervision being provided; and (3) see that such persons perform these services competently. (See also Standards 2.02, Providing Services in Emergencies; 3.05, Multiple Relationships; 4.01, Maintaining Confidentiality; 9.01, Bases for Assessments; 9.02, Use of assessments; 9.03, Informed Consent in Assessments; and 9.07, Assessment by Unqualified Persons.)

Personal Problems and Conflicts

(a) Psychologists refrain from initiating an activity when they know or should know that there is a substantial likelihood that their personal problems will prevent them from performing their work-related activities in a competent manner.

(b) When psychologists become aware of personal problems that may interfere with their performing work-related duties adequately, they take appropriate measures, such as obtaining professional consultation or assistance, and determine whether they should limit, suspend, or terminate their work-related duties. (See also Standard 10.10, Terminating Therapy.)

Human Relations

Unfair Discrimination

In their work-related activities, psychologists do not engage in unfair discrimination based on age, gender, gender identity, race, ethnicity, culture, national origin, religion, sexual orientation, disability, socioeconomic status, or any basis proscribed by law.

Sexual Harassment

Psychologists do not engage in sexual harassment. Sexual harassment is sexual solicitation, physical advances, or verbal or nonverbal conduct that is sexual in nature, that occurs in connection with the psychologist's activities or roles as a psychologist, and that either (1) is unwelcome, is offensive, or creates a hostile workplace or educational environment, and the psychologist knows or is told this or (2) is sufficiently severe or intense to be abusive to a reasonable person in the context. Sexual harassment can consist of a single intense or severe act or of multiple persistent or pervasive acts. (See also Standard 1.08, Unfair Discrimination Against Complainants and Respondents.)

Other Harassment

Psychologists do not knowingly engage in behavior that is harassing or demeaning to persons with whom they interact in their work based on factors such as those persons' age, gender, gender identity, race, ethnicity, culture, national origin, religion, sexual orientation, disability, language, or socioeconomic status.

Avoiding Harm

Psychologists take reasonable steps to avoid harming their clients/patients, students, supervisees, research participants, organizational clients, and others with whom they work, and to minimize harm where it is foreseeable and unavoidable.

Multiple Relationships

(a) A multiple relationship occurs when a psychologist is in a professional role with a person and (1) at the same time is in another role with the same person, (2) at the same time is in a relationship with a person closely associated with or related to the person with whom the psychologist has the professional relationship, or (3) promises to enter into another relationship in the future with the person or a person closely associated with or related to the person.

A psychologist refrains from entering into a multiple relationship if the multiple relationship could reasonably be expected to impair the psychologist's objectivity, competence, or effectiveness in performing his or her functions as a psychologist, or otherwise risks exploitation or harm to the person with whom the professional relationship exists.

Multiple relationships that would not reasonably be expected to cause impairment or risk exploitation or harm are not unethical.

(b) If a psychologist finds that, due to unforeseen factors, a potentially harmful multiple relationship has arisen, the psychologist takes reasonable steps to resolve it with due regard for the best interests of the affected person and maximal compliance with the Ethics Code.

(c) When psychologists are required by law, institutional policy, or extraordinary circumstances to serve in more than one role in judicial or administrative proceedings, at the outset they clarify role expectations and the extent of confidentiality and thereafter as changes occur. (See also Standards 3.04, Avoiding Harm, and 3.07, Third-Party Requests for Services.)

Conflict of Interest

Psychologists refrain from taking on a professional role when personal, scientific, professional, legal, financial, or other interests or relationships could reasonably be expected to (1) impair their objectivity, competence, or effectiveness in performing their functions as psychologists or (2) expose the person or organization with whom the professional relationship exists to harm or exploitation.

Third-Party Requests for Services

When psychologists agree to provide services to a person or entity at the request of a third party, psychologists attempt to clarify at the outset of the service the nature of the relationship with all individuals or organizations involved. This clarification includes the role of the psychologist (e.g., therapist, consultant, diagnostician, or expert witness), an identification of who is the client, the probable uses of the services provided or the information obtained, and the fact that there may be limits to confidentiality. (See also

Standards 3.05, Multiple Relationships, and 4.02, Discussing the Limits of Confidentiality.)

Exploitative Relationships

Psychologists do not exploit persons over whom they have supervisory, evaluative, or other authority such as clients/patients, students, supervisees, research participants, and employees. (See also Standards 3.05, Multiple Relationships; 6.04, Fees and Financial Arrangements; 6.05, Barter With Clients/Patients; 7.07, Sexual Relationships With Students and Supervisees; 10.05, Sexual Intimacies With Current Therapy Clients/Patients; 10.06, Sexual Intimacies With Relatives or Significant Others of Current Therapy Clients/Patients; 10.07, Therapy With Former Sexual Partners; and 10.08, Sexual Intimacies With Former Therapy Clients/Patients.)

Cooperation With Other Professionals

When indicated and professionally appropriate, psychologists cooperate with other professionals in order to serve their clients/patients effectively and appropriately. (See also Standard 4.05, Disclosures.)

Informed Consent

(a) When psychologists conduct research or provide assessment, therapy, counseling, or consulting services in person or via electronic transmission or other forms of communication, they obtain the informed consent of the individual or individuals using language that is reasonably understandable to that person or persons except when conducting such activities without consent is mandated by law or governmental regulation or as otherwise provided in this Ethics Code. (See also Standards 8.02, Informed Consent to Research; 9.03, Informed Consent in Assessments; and 10.01, Informed Consent to Therapy.)

(b) For persons who are legally incapable of giving informed consent, psychologists nevertheless (1) provide an appropriate explanation, (2) seek the individual's assent, (3) consider such persons' preferences and best interests, and (4) obtain appropriate permission from a legally authorized person, if such substitute consent is permitted or required by law. When consent by a legally authorized person is not permitted or required by law, psychologists take reasonable steps to protect the individual's rights and welfare.

(c) When psychological services are court ordered or otherwise mandated, psychologists inform the individual of the nature of the anticipated services, including whether the services are court ordered or mandated and any limits of confidentiality, before proceeding.

(d) Psychologists appropriately document written or oral consent, permission, and assent. (See also Standards 8.02, Informed Consent to Research; 9.03, Informed Consent in Assessments; and 10.01, Informed Consent to Therapy.)

Psychological Services Delivered To or Through Organizations

(a) Psychologists delivering services to or through organizations provide information beforehand to clients and when appropriate those directly affected by the services about (1) the nature and objectives of the services, (2) the intended recipients, (3) which of the individuals are clients, (4) the relationship the psychologist will have with each person and the organization, (5) the probable uses of services provided and information obtained, (6) who will have access to the information, and (7) limits of confidentiality. As soon as feasible, they provide information about the results and conclusions of such services to appropriate persons.

(b) If psychologists will be precluded by law or by organizational roles from providing such information to particular individuals or groups, they so inform those individuals or groups at the outset of the service.

Interruption of Psychological Services

Unless otherwise covered by contract, psychologists make reasonable efforts to plan for facilitating services in the event that psychological services are interrupted by factors such as the psychologist's illness, death, unavailability, relocation, or retirement or by the client's/patient's relocation or financial limitations. (See also Standard 6.02c, Maintenance, Dissemination, and Disposal of Confidential Records of Professional and Scientific Work.)

Privacy and Confidentiality

Maintaining Confidentiality

Psychologists have a primary obligation and take reasonable precautions to protect confidential information obtained through or stored in any medium, recognizing that the extent and limits of confidentiality may be regulated by law or established by institutional rules or professional or scientific relationship. (See also Standard 2.05, Delegation of Work to Others.)

Discussing the Limits of Confidentiality

(a) Psychologists discuss with persons (including, to the extent feasible, persons who are legally incapable of giving informed consent and their legal representatives) and organizations with whom they establish a scientific or professional relationship (1) the relevant limits of confidentiality and (2) the foreseeable uses of the information generated through their psychological activities. (See also Standard 3.10, Informed Consent.)

(b) Unless it is not feasible or is contraindicated, the discussion of confidentiality occurs at the outset of the relationship and thereafter as new circumstances may warrant.

(c) Psychologists who offer services, products, or information via electronic transmission inform clients/patients of the risks to privacy and limits of confidentiality.

Recording

Before recording the voices or images of individuals to whom they provide services, psychologists obtain permission from all such persons or their legal representatives. (See also Standards 8.03, Informed Consent for Recording Voices and Images in Research; 8.05, Dispensing With Informed Consent for Research; and 8.07, Deception in Research.)

Minimizing Intrusions on Privacy

(a) Psychologists include in written and oral reports and consultations, only information germane to the purpose for which the communication is made.

(b) Psychologists discuss confidential information obtained in their work only for appropriate scientific or professional purposes and only with persons clearly concerned with such matters.

Disclosures

(a) Psychologists may disclose confidential information with the appropriate consent of the organizational client, the individual client/patient, or another legally authorized person on behalf of the client/patient unless prohibited by law.

(b) Psychologists disclose confidential information without the consent of the individual only as mandated by law, or where permitted by law for a valid purpose such as to (1) provide needed professional services; (2) obtain appropriate professional consultations; (3) protect the client/patient, psychologist, or others from harm; or (4) obtain payment for services from a client/patient, in which instance disclosure is limited to the minimum that is necessary to achieve the purpose. (See also Standard 6.04e, Fees and Financial Arrangements.)

Consultations

When consulting with colleagues, (1) psychologists do not disclose confidential information that reasonably could lead to the identification of a client/patient, research participant, or other person or organization with whom they have a confidential relationship unless they have obtained the prior consent of the person or organization or the disclosure cannot be avoided, and (2) they disclose information only to the extent necessary to achieve the purposes of the consultation. (See also Standard 4.01, Maintaining Confidentiality.)

Use of Confidential Information for Didactic or Other Purposes

Psychologists do not disclose in their writings, lectures, or other public media, confidential, personally identifiable information concerning their clients/patients, students, research participants, organizational clients, or other recipients of their services that they obtained during the course of their work, unless (1) they take reasonable steps to disguise the person or organization, (2) the person or organization has consented in writing, or (3) there is legal authorization for doing so.

Advertising and Other Public Statements

Avoidance of False or Deceptive Statements

(a) Public statements include but are not limited to paid or unpaid advertising, product endorsements, grant applications, licensing applications, other credentialing applications, brochures, printed matter, directory listings, personal resumes or curricula vitae, or comments for use in media such as print or electronic transmission, statements in legal proceedings, lectures and public oral presentations, and published materials. Psychologists do not knowingly make public statements that are false, deceptive, or fraudulent concerning their research, practice, or other work activities or those of persons or organizations with which they are affiliated.

(b) Psychologists do not make false, deceptive, or fraudulent statements concerning (1) their training, experience, or competence; (2) their academic degrees; (3) their credentials; (4) their institutional or association affiliations; (5) their services; (6) the scientific or clinical basis for, or results or degree of success of, their services; (7) their fees; or (8) their publications or research findings.

(c) Psychologists claim degrees as credentials for their health services only if those degrees (1) were earned from a regionally accredited educational institution or (2) were the basis for psychology licensure by the state in which they practice.

Statements by Others

(a) Psychologists who engage others to create or place public statements that promote their professional practice, products, or activities retain professional responsibility for such statements.

(b) Psychologists do not compensate employees of press, radio, television, or other communication media in return for publicity in a news item. (See also Standard 1.01, Misuse of Psychologists' Work.)

(c) A paid advertisement relating to psychologists' activities must be identified or clearly recognizable as such.

Descriptions of Workshops and Non-Degree-Granting Educational Programs

To the degree to which they exercise control, psychologists responsible for announcements, catalogs, brochures, or advertisements describing workshops, seminars, or other non-degree-granting educational programs ensure that they accurately describe the audience for which the program is intended, the educational objectives, the presenters, and the fees involved.

Media Presentations

When psychologists provide public advice or comment via print, internet, or other electronic transmission, they take precautions to ensure that statements (1) are based on their professional knowledge, training, or experience in accord with appropriate psychological literature and practice; (2) are otherwise consistent with this Ethics Code; and (3) do not indicate that a professional relationship has been established with the recipient. (See also Standard 2.04, Bases for Scientific and Professional Judgments.)

Testimonials

Psychologists do not solicit testimonials from current therapy clients/patients or other persons who because of their particular circumstances are vulnerable to undue influence.

In-Person Solicitation

Psychologists do not engage, directly or through agents, in uninvited in-person solicitation of business from actual or potential therapy clients/patients or other persons who because of their particular circumstances are vulnerable to undue influence. However, this prohibition does not preclude (1) attempting to implement appropriate collateral contacts for the purpose of benefiting an already engaged therapy client/patient or (2) providing disaster or community outreach services.

Record Keeping and Fees

Documentation of Professional and Scientific Work and Maintenance of Records

Psychologists create, and to the extent the records are under their control, maintain, disseminate, store, retain, and dispose of records and data relating to their professional and scientific work in order to (1) facilitate provision of services later by them or by other professionals, (2) allow for replication of research design and analyses, (3) meet institutional requirements, (4) ensure accuracy of billing and payments, and (5) ensure compliance with law. (See also Standard 4.01, Maintaining Confidentiality.)

Maintenance, Dissemination, and Disposal of Confidential Records of Professional and Scientific Work

(a) Psychologists maintain confidentiality in creating, storing, accessing, transferring, and disposing of records under their control, whether these are written, automated, or in any other medium. (See also Standards 4.01, Maintaining Confidentiality, and 6.01, Documentation of Professional and Scientific Work and Maintenance of Records.)

(b) If confidential information concerning recipients of psychological services is entered into databases or systems of records available to persons whose access has not been consented to by the recipient, psychologists use coding or other techniques to avoid the inclusion of personal identifiers.

(c) Psychologists make plans in advance to facilitate the appropriate transfer and to protect the confidentiality of records and data in the event of psychologists' withdrawal from positions or practice. (See also Standards 3.12, Interruption of Psychological Services, and 10.09, Interruption of Therapy.)

Withholding Records for Nonpayment

Psychologists may not withhold records under their control that are requested and needed for a client's/patient's emergency treatment solely because payment has not been received.

Fees and Financial Arrangements

(a) As early as is feasible in a professional or scientific relationship, psychologists and recipients of psychological services reach an agreement specifying compensation and billing arrangements.

(b) Psychologists' fee practices are consistent with law.

(c) Psychologists do not misrepresent their fees.

(d) If limitations to services can be anticipated because of limitations in financing, this is discussed with the recipient of services as early as is feasible. (See also Standards 10.09, Interruption of Therapy, and 10.10, Terminating Therapy.)

(e) If the recipient of services does not pay for services as agreed, and if psychologists intend to use collection agencies or legal measures to collect the fees, psychologists first inform the person that such measures will be taken and provide that person an opportunity to make prompt payment. (See also Standards 4.05, Disclosures; 6.03, Withholding Records for Nonpayment; and 10.01, Informed Consent to Therapy.)

Barter With Clients/Patients

Barter is the acceptance of goods, services, or other nonmonetary remuneration from clients/patients in return for psychological services. Psychologists may barter only if (1) it is not clinically contraindicated, and (2) the resulting arrangement is not exploitative. (See also Standards 3.05, Multiple Relationships, and 6.04, Fees and Financial Arrangements.)

Accuracy in Reports to Payors and Funding Sources

In their reports to payors for services or sources of research funding, psychologists take reasonable steps to ensure the accurate reporting of the nature of the service provided or research conducted, the fees, charges, or payments, and where applicable, the identity of the provider, the findings, and the diagnosis. (See also Standards 4.01, Maintaining Confidentiality; 4.04, Minimizing Intrusions on Privacy; and 4.05, Disclosures.)

Referrals and Fees

When psychologists pay, receive payment from, or divide fees with another professional, other than in an employer-employee relationship, the payment to each is based on the services provided (clinical, consultative, administrative, or other) and is not based on the referral itself. (See also Standard 3.09, Cooperation With Other Professionals.)

Education and Training

Design of Education and Training Programs

Psychologists responsible for education and training programs take reasonable steps to ensure that the programs are designed to provide the appropriate knowledge and proper experiences, and to meet the requirements for licensure, certification, or other goals for which claims are made by the program. (See also Standard 5.03, Descriptions of Workshops and Non-Degree-Granting Educational Programs.)

Descriptions of Education and Training Programs

Psychologists responsible for education and training programs take reasonable steps to ensure that there is a current and accurate description of the program content (including participation in required course- or program-related counseling, psychotherapy, experiential groups, consulting projects, or community service), training goals and objectives, stipends and benefits, and requirements that must be met for satisfactory completion of the program. This information must be made readily available to all interested parties.

Accuracy in Teaching

(a) Psychologists take reasonable steps to ensure that course syllabi are accurate regarding the subject matter to be covered, bases for evaluating progress, and the nature of course experiences. This standard does not preclude an instructor from modifying course content or requirements when the instructor considers it pedagogically necessary or desirable, so long as students are made aware of these modifications in a manner that enables them to fulfill course requirements. (See also Standard 5.01, Avoidance of False or Deceptive Statements.)

(b) When engaged in teaching or training, psychologists present psychological information accurately. (See also Standard 2.03, Maintaining Competence.)

Student Disclosure of Personal Information

Psychologists do not require students or supervisees to disclose personal information in course- or program-related activities, either orally or in writing, regarding sexual history, history of abuse and neglect, psychological treatment, and relationships with parents, peers, and spouses or significant others except if (1) the program or training facility has clearly identified this requirement in its admissions and program materials or (2) the information is necessary to evaluate or obtain assistance for students whose personal problems could reasonably be judged to be preventing them from performing their training- or professionally related activities in a competent manner or posing a threat to the students or others.

Mandatory Individual or Group Therapy

(a) When individual or group therapy is a program or course requirement, psychologists responsible for that program allow students in undergraduate and graduate programs the option of selecting such therapy from practitioners unaffiliated with the program. (See also Standard 7.02, Descriptions of Education and Training Programs.)

(b) Faculty who are or are likely to be responsible for evaluating students' academic performance do not themselves provide that therapy. (See also Standard 3.05, Multiple Relationships.)

Assessing Student and Supervisee Performance

(a) In academic and supervisory relationships, psychologists establish a timely and specific process for providing feedback to students and supervisees. Information regarding the process is provided to the student at the beginning of supervision.

(b) Psychologists evaluate students and supervisees on the basis of their actual performance on relevant and established program requirements.

Sexual Relationships with Students and Supervisees

Psychologists do not engage in sexual relationships with students or supervisees who are in their department, agency, or training center or over whom psychologists have or are likely to have evaluative authority. (See also Standard 3.05, Multiple Relationships.)

Research and Publication

Institutional Approval

When institutional approval is required, psychologists provide accurate information about their research proposals and obtain approval prior to conducting the research. They conduct the research in accordance with the approved research protocol.

Informed Consent to Research

(a) When obtaining informed consent as required in Standard 3.10, Informed Consent, psychologists inform participants about (1) the purpose of the research, expected duration, and procedures; (2) their right to decline to participate and to withdraw from the research once participation has begun; (3) the foreseeable consequences of declining or withdrawing; (4) reasonably foreseeable factors that may be expected to influence their willingness to participate such as potential risks, discomfort, or adverse effects; (5) any prospective research benefits; (6) limits of confidentiality; (7) incentives for participation; and (8) whom to contact for questions about the research and research participants' rights. They provide opportunity for the prospective participants to ask questions and receive answers. (See also Standards 8.03, Informed Consent for Recording Voices and Images in Research; 8.05, Dispensing With Informed Consent for Research; and 8.07, Deception in Research.)

(b) Psychologists conducting intervention research involving the use of experimental treatments clarify to participants at the outset of the research (1) the experimental nature of the treatment; (2) the services that will or will not be available to the control group(s) if appropriate; (3) the means by which assignment to treatment and control groups will be made; (4) available treatment alternatives if an individual does not wish to participate in the research or wishes to withdraw once a study has begun; and (5) compensation for or monetary costs of participating including, if appropriate, whether reimbursement from the participant or a third-party payor will be sought. (See also Standard 8.02a, Informed Consent to Research.)

Informed Consent for Recording Voices and Images in Research

Psychologists obtain informed consent from research participants prior to recording their voices or images for data collection unless (1) the research consists solely of naturalistic observations in public places, and it is not anticipated that the recording will be used in a manner that could cause personal identification or harm, or (2) the research design includes deception, and consent for the use of the recording is obtained during debriefing. (See also Standard 8.07, Deception in Research.)

Client/Patient, Student, and Subordinate Research Participants

(a) When psychologists conduct research with clients/patients, students, or subordinates as participants, psychologists take steps to protect the prospective participants from adverse consequences of declining or withdrawing from participation.

(b) When research participation is a course requirement or an opportunity for extra credit, the prospective participant is given the choice of equitable alternative activities.

Dispensing with Informed Consent for Research

Psychologists may dispense with informed consent only (1) where research would not reasonably be assumed to create distress or harm and involves (a) the study of normal educational practices, curricula, or classroom management methods conducted in educational settings; (b) only anonymous questionnaires, naturalistic observations, or archival research for which disclosure of responses would not place participants at risk of criminal or civil liability or damage their financial standing, employability, or reputation, and confidentiality is protected; or (c) the study of factors related to job or organization effectiveness conducted in organizational settings for which there is no risk to participants' employability, and confidentiality is protected or (2) where otherwise permitted by law or federal or institutional regulations.

Offering Inducements for Research Participation

(a) Psychologists make reasonable efforts to avoid offering excessive or inappropriate financial or other inducements for research participation when such inducements are likely to coerce participation.
(b) When offering professional services as an inducement for research participation, psychologists clarify the nature of the services, as well as the risks, obligations, and limitations. (See also Standard 6.05, Barter With Clients/Patients.)

Deception in Research

(a) Psychologists do not conduct a study involving deception unless they have determined that the use of deceptive techniques is justified by the study's significant prospective scientific, educational, or applied value and that effective nondeceptive alternative procedures are not feasible.
(b) Psychologists do not deceive prospective participants about research that is reasonably expected to cause physical pain or severe emotional distress.
(c) Psychologists explain any deception that is an integral feature of the design and conduct of an experiment to participants as early as is feasible, preferably at the conclusion of their participation, but no later than at the conclusion of the data collection, and permit participants to withdraw their data. (See also Standard 8.08, Debriefing.)

Debriefing

(a) Psychologists provide a prompt opportunity for participants to obtain appropriate information about the nature, results, and conclusions of the research, and they take reasonable steps to correct any misconceptions that participants may have of which the psychologists are aware.
(b) If scientific or humane values justify delaying or withholding this information, psychologists take reasonable measures to reduce the risk of harm.
(c) When psychologists become aware that research procedures have harmed a participant, they take reasonable steps to minimize the harm.

Humane Care and Use of Animals in Research

(a) Psychologists acquire, care for, use, and dispose of animals in compliance with current federal, state, and local laws and regulations, and with professional standards.
(b) Psychologists trained in research methods and experienced in the care of laboratory animals supervise all procedures involving animals and are responsible for ensuring appropriate consideration of their comfort, health, and humane treatment.

(c) Psychologists ensure that all individuals under their supervision who are using animals have received instruction in research methods and in the care, maintenance, and handling of the species being used, to the extent appropriate to their role. (See also Standard 2.05, Delegation of Work to Others.)

(d) Psychologists make reasonable efforts to minimize the discomfort, infection, illness, and pain of animal subjects.

(e) Psychologists use a procedure subjecting animals to pain, stress, or privation only when an alternative procedure is unavailable and the goal is justified by its prospective scientific, educational, or applied value.

(f) Psychologists perform surgical procedures under appropriate anesthesia and follow techniques to avoid infection and minimize pain during and after surgery.

(g) When it is appropriate that an animal's life be terminated, psychologists proceed rapidly, with an effort to minimize pain and in accordance with accepted procedures.

Reporting Research Results

(a) Psychologists do not fabricate data. (See also Standard 5.01a, Avoidance of False or Deceptive Statements.)

(b) If psychologists discover significant errors in their published data, they take reasonable steps to correct such errors in a correction, retraction, erratum, or other appropriate publication means.

Plagiarism

Psychologists do not present portions of another's work or data as their own, even if the other work or data source is cited occasionally.

Publication Credit

(a) Psychologists take responsibility and credit, including authorship credit, only for work they have actually performed or to which they have substantially contributed. (See also Standard 8.12b, Publication Credit.)

(b) Principle authorship and other publication credits accurately reflect the relative scientific or professional contributions of the individuals involved, regardless of their relative status. Mere possession of an institutional position, such as department chair, does not justify authorship credit. Minor contributions to the research or to the writing for publications are acknowledged appropriately, such as in footnotes or in an introductory statement.

(c) Except under exceptional circumstances, a student is listed as principal author on any multiple-authored article that is substantially based on the student's doctoral dissertation. Faculty advisors discuss publication credit with students as early as feasible and throughout the research and publication process as appropriate. (See also Standard 8.12b, Publication Credit.)

Duplicate Publication of Data

Psychologists do not publish, as original data, data that have been previously published. This does not preclude republishing data when they are accompanied by proper acknowledgment.

Sharing Research Data for Verification

(a) After research results are published, psychologists do not withhold the data on which their conclusions are based from other competent professionals who seek to verify the substantive claims through reanalysis and who intend to use such data only for that purpose, provided that the confidentiality of the participants can be protected and unless legal rights concerning proprietary data preclude their release. This does not preclude psychologists from requiring that such individuals or groups be responsible for costs associated with the provision of such information.

(b) Psychologists who request data from other psychologists to verify the substantive claims through reanalysis may use shared data only for the declared purpose. Requesting psychologists obtain prior written agreement for all other uses of the data.

Reviewers

Psychologists who review material submitted for presentation, publication, grant, or research proposal review respect the confidentiality of and the proprietary rights in such information of those who submitted it.

Assesment

Bases for Assessments

(a) Psychologists base the opinions contained in their recommendations, reports, and diagnostic or evaluative statements, including forensic testimony, on information and techniques sufficient to substantiate their findings. (See also Standard 2.04, Bases for Scientific and Professional Judgments.)

(b) Except as noted in 9.01c, psychologists provide opinions of the psychological characteristics of individuals only after they have conducted an examination of the individuals adequate to support their statements or conclusions. When, despite reasonable efforts, such an examination is not practical, psychologists document the efforts they made and the result of those efforts, clarify the probable impact of their limited information on the reliability and validity of their opinions, and appropriately limit the nature and extent of their conclusions or recommendations. (See also Standards 2.01, Boundaries of Competence, and 9.06, Interpreting Assessment Results.)

(c) When psychologists conduct a record review or provide consultation or supervision and an individual examination is not warranted or necessary for the opinion, psychologists explain this and the sources of information on which they based their conclusions and recommendations.

Use of Assessments

(a) Psychologists administer, adapt, score, interpret, or use assessment techniques, interviews, tests, or instruments in a manner and for purposes that are appropriate in light of the research on or evidence of the usefulness and proper application of the techniques.

(b) Psychologists use assessment instruments whose validity and reliability have been established for use with members of the population tested. When such validity or reliability has not been established, psychologists describe the strengths and limitations of test results and interpretation.

(c) Psychologists use assessment methods that are appropriate to an individual's language preference and competence, unless the use of an alternative language is relevant to the assessment issues.

Informed Consent in Assessments

(a) Psychologists obtain informed consent for assessments, evaluations, or diagnostic services, as described in Standard 3.10, Informed Consent, except when (1) testing is mandated by law or governmental regulations; (2) informed consent is implied because testing is conducted as a routine educational, institutional, or organizational activity (e.g., when participants voluntarily agree to assessment when applying for a job); or (3) one purpose of the testing is to evaluate decisional capacity. Informed consent includes an explanation of the nature and purpose of the assessment, fees, involvement of third parties, and limits of confidentiality and sufficient opportunity for the client/patient to ask questions and receive answers.

(b) Psychologists inform persons with questionable capacity to consent or for whom testing is mandated by law or governmental regulations about the nature and purpose of the proposed assessment services, using language that is reasonably understandable to the person being assessed.

(c) Psychologists using the services of an interpreter obtain informed consent from the client/patient to use that interpreter, ensure that confidentiality of test results and test security are maintained, and include in their recommendations, reports, and diagnostic or evaluative statements, including forensic testimony, discussion of any limitations on the data obtained. (See also Standards 2.05, Delegation of Work to Others; 4.01, Maintaining Confidentiality; 9.01, Bases for Assessments; 9.06, Interpreting Assessment Results; and 9.07, Assessment by Unqualified Persons.)

Release of Test Data

(a) The term *test data* refers to raw and scaled scores, client/patient responses to test questions or stimuli, and psychologists' notes and recordings concerning client/patient statements and behavior during an examination. Those portions of test materials that include client/patient responses are included in the definition of *test data*. Pursuant to a client/patient release, psychologists provide test data to the client/patient or other persons identified in the release. Psychologists may refrain from releasing test data to protect a client/patient or others from substantial harm or misuse or misrepresentation of the data or the test, recognizing that in many instances release of confidential information under these circumstances is regulated by law. (See also Standard 9.11, Maintaining Test Security.)

(b) In the absence of a client/patient release, psychologists provide test data only as required by law or court order.

Test Construction

Psychologists who develop tests and other assessment techniques use appropriate psychometric procedures and current scientific or professional knowledge for test design, standardization, validation, reduction or elimination of bias, and recommendations for use.

Interpreting Assessment Results

When interpreting assessment results, including automated interpretations, psychologists take into account the purpose of the assessment as well as the various test factors, test-taking abilities, and other characteristics of the person being assessed, such as situational, personal, linguistic, and cultural differences, that might affect psychologists' judgments or reduce the accuracy of their interpretations. They indicate any significant limitations of their interpretations. (See also Standards 2.01b and c, Boundaries of Competence, and 3.01, Unfair Discrimination.)

Assessment by Unqualified Persons

Psychologists do not promote the use of psychological assessment techniques by unqualified persons, except when such use is conducted for training purposes with appropriate supervision. (See also Standard 2.05, Delegation of Work to Others.)

Obsolete Tests and Outdated Test Results

(a) Psychologists do not base their assessment or intervention decisions or recommendations on data or test results that are outdated for the current purpose.

(b) Psychologists do not base such decisions or recommendations on tests and measures that are obsolete and not useful for the current purpose.

Test Scoring and Interpretation Services

(a) Psychologists who offer assessment or scoring services to other professionals accurately describe the purpose, norms, validity, reliability, and applications of the procedures and any special qualifications applicable to their use.

(b) Psychologists select scoring and interpretation services (including automated services) on the basis of evidence of the validity of the program and procedures as well as on other appropriate considerations. (See also Standard 2.01b and c, Boundaries of Competence.)

(c) Psychologists retain responsibility for the appropriate application, interpretation, and use of assessment instruments, whether they score and interpret such tests themselves or use automated or other services.

Explaining Assessment Results

Regardless of whether the scoring and interpretation are done by psychologists, by employees or assistants, or by automated or other outside services, psychologists take reasonable steps to ensure that explanations of results are given to the individual or designated representative unless the nature of the relationship precludes provision of an explanation of results (such as in some organizational consulting, pre-employment or security screenings, and forensic evaluations), and this fact has been clearly explained to the person being assessed in advance.

Maintaining Test Security

The term *test materials* refers to manuals, instruments, protocols, and test questions or stimuli and does not include *test data* as defined in Standard 9.04, Release of Test Data. Psychologists make reasonable efforts to maintain the integrity and security of test materials and other assessment techniques consistent with law and contractual obligations, and in a manner that permits adherence to this Ethics Code.

Therapy

Informed Consent to Therapy

(a) When obtaining informed consent to therapy as required in Standard 3.10, Informed Consent, psychologists inform clients/patients as early as is feasible in the therapeutic relationship about the nature and anticipated course of therapy, fees, involvement of third parties, and limits of confidentiality

and provide sufficient opportunity for the client/patient to ask questions and receive answers. (See also Standards 4.02, Discussing the Limits of Confidentiality, and 6.04, Fees and Financial Arrangements.)

(b) When obtaining informed consent for treatment for which generally recognized techniques and procedures have not been established, psychologists inform their clients/patients of the developing nature of the treatment, the potential risks involved, alternative treatments that may be available, and the voluntary nature of their participation. (See also Standards 2.01e, Boundaries of Competence, and 3.10, Informed Consent.)

(c) When the therapist is a trainee and the legal responsibility for the treatment provided resides with the supervisor, the client/patient, as part of the informed consent procedure, is informed that the therapist is in training and is being supervised and is given the name of the supervisor.

Therapy Involving Couples or Families

(a) When psychologists agree to provide services to several persons who have a relationship (such as spouses, significant others, or parents and children), they take reasonable steps to clarify at the outset (1) which of the individuals are clients/patients and (2) the relationship the psychologist will have with each person. This clarification includes the psychologist's role and the probable uses of the services provided or the information obtained. (See also Standard 4.02, Discussing the Limits of Confidentiality.)

(b) If it becomes apparent that psychologists may be called on to perform potentially conflicting roles (such as family therapist and then witness for one party in divorce proceedings), psychologists take reasonable steps to clarify and modify, or withdraw from, roles appropriately. (See also Standard 3.05c, Multiple Relationships.)

Group Therapy

When psychologists provide services to several persons in a group setting, they describe at the outset the roles and responsibilities of all parties and the limits of confidentiality.

Providing Therapy to Those Served by Others

In deciding whether to offer or provide services to those already receiving mental health services elsewhere, psychologists carefully consider the treatment issues and the potential client's/patient's welfare. Psychologists discuss these issues with the client/patient or another legally authorized person on behalf of the client/patient in order to minimize the risk of confusion and conflict, consult with the other service providers when appropriate, and proceed with caution and sensitivity to the therapeutic issues.

Sexual Intimacies With Current Therapy Clients/Patients

Psychologists do not engage in sexual intimacies with current therapy clients/patients.

Sexual Intimacies With Relatives or Significant Others of Current Therapy Clients/Patients

Psychologists do not engage in sexual intimacies with individuals they know to be close relatives, guardians, or significant others of current clients/patients. Psychologists do not terminate therapy to circumvent this standard.

Therapy With Former Sexual Partners

Psychologists do not accept as therapy clients/patients persons with whom they have engaged in sexual intimacies.

Sexual Intimacies With Former Therapy Clients/Patients

(a) Psychologists do not engage in sexual intimacies with former clients/patients for at least two years after cessation or termination of therapy.

(b) Psychologists do not engage in sexual intimacies with former clients/patients even after a two-year interval except in the most unusual circumstances. Psychologists who engage in such activity after the two years following cessation or termination of therapy and of having no sexual contact with the former client/patient bear the burden of demonstrating that there has been no exploitation, in light of all relevant factors, including (1) the amount of time that has passed since therapy terminated; (2) the nature, duration, and intensity of the therapy; (3) the circumstances of termination; (4) the client's/patient's personal history; (5) the client's/patient's current mental status; (6) the likelihood of adverse impact on the client/patient; and (7) any statements or actions made by the therapist during the course of therapy suggesting or inviting the possibility of a posttermination sexual or romantic relationship with the client/patient. (See also Standard 3.05, Multiple Relationships.)

Interruption of Therapy

When entering into employment or contractual relationships, psychologists make reasonable efforts to provide for orderly and appropriate resolution of responsibility for client/patient care in the event that the employment or contractual relationship ends, with paramount consideration given to the welfare of the client/patient. (See also Standard 3.12, Interruption of Psychological Services.)

Terminating Therapy

(a) Psychologists terminate therapy when it becomes reasonably clear that the client/patient no longer needs the service, is not likely to benefit, or is being harmed by continued service.

(b) Psychologists may terminate therapy when threatened or otherwise endangered by the client/patient or another person with whom the client/patient has a relationship.

(c) Except where precluded by the actions of clients/patients or third-party payors, prior to termination psychologists provide pretermination counseling and suggest alternative service providers as appropriate.

History and Effective Date Footnote

This version of the APA Ethics Code was adopted by the American Psychological Association's Council of Representatives during its meeting, August 21, 2002, and is effective beginning June 1, 2003. Inquiries concerning the substance or interpretation of the APA Ethics Code should be addressed to the Director, Office of Ethics, American Psychological Association, 750 First Street, NE, Washington, DC 20002-4242. The Ethics Code and information regarding the Code can be found on the APA web site, http://www.apa.org/ethics. The standards in this Ethics Code will be used to adjudicate complaints brought concerning alleged conduct occurring on or after the effective date. Complaints regarding conduct occurring prior to the effective date will be adjudicated on the basis of the version of the Ethics Code that was in effect at the time the conduct occurred.

The APA has previously published its Ethics Code as follows:

American Psychological Association (1953). *Ethical standards of psychologists*. Washington, DC: Author.

American Psychological Association (1959). Ethical standards of psychologists. *American Psychologist, 14*, 279-282.

American Psychological Association (1963). Ethical standards of psychologists. *American Psychologist, 18*, 56-60.

American Psychological Association (1968). Ethical standards of psychologists. *American Psychologist, 23*, 357-361.

American Psychological Association (1977, March). Ethical standards of psychologists. *APA Monitor*, 22-23.

American Psychological Association (1979). *Ethical standards of psychologists*. Washington, DC: Author.

American Psychological Association (1981). Ethical principles of psychologists. *American Psychologist, 36*, 633-638.

American Psychological Association (1990). Ethical principles of psychologists (Amended June 2, 1989). *American Psychologist, 45*, 390-395.

American Psychological Association (1992). Ethical principles of psychologists and code of conduct. *American Psychologist, 47*, 1597-1611.

Request copies of the APA's *Ethical Principles of Psychologists and Code of Conduct* from the APA Order Department, 750 First Street, NE, Washington, DC 20002-4242, or phone (202) 336-5510.

©2002 American Psychological Association.

Appendix B

SPECIALTY GUIDELINES FOR FORENSIC PSYCHOLOGISTS[1]

Committee on Ethical Guidelines for Forensic Psychologists[2]

Law and Human Behavior, Vol. 15 (6), 1991 Reprinted with permission from Kluwer Academic/Plenum Publishers

The Specialty Guidelines for Forensic Psychologists, while informed by the *Ethical Principles of Psychologists* (APA, 1990) and meant to be consistent with them, are designed to provide more specific guidance to forensic psychologists in monitoring their professional conduct when acting in assistance to courts, parties to legal proceedings, correctional and forensic mental health facilities, and legislative agencies. The primary goal of the Guidelines is to improve the quality of forensic psychological services offered to individual clients and the legal system and thereby to enhance forensic psychology as a discipline and profession. The *Specialty Guidelines for Forensic Psychologists* represent a joint statement of the American Psychology-Law Society and Division 41 of the American Psychological Association and are endorsed by the American Academy of Forensic Psychology. The *Guidelines* do not represent an official statement of the American Psychological Association. The Guidelines provide an aspirational model of desirable professional practice by psychologists, within any subdiscipline of psychology (e.g., clinical, developmental, social, experimental), when they are engaged regularly as experts and represent themselves as such, in an activity primarily intended to provide professional psychological expertise to the judicial system. This would include, for example, clinical forensic examiners; psychologists employed by correctional or forensic mental health systems; researchers who offer direct testimony about the relevance of scientific data to a psycholegal issue; trial behavior consultants; psychologists engaged in preparation of *amicus* briefs; or psychologists, appearing as forensic experts, who consult with, or testify before, judicial, legislative, or administrative agencies acting in an adjudicative capacity. Individuals who provide only occasional service to the legal system and who do so without representing themselves as *forensic experts* may find these *Guidelines* helpful, particularly in conjunction with consultation with colleagues who are forensic experts. While the *Guidelines* are concerned with a model of desirable professional practice, to the extent that they may be construed as being applicable to the advertisement of services or the solicitation of clients, they are intended to prevent false or deceptive advertisement or solicitation, and should be construed in a manner consistent with that intent.

1. The *Specialty Guidelines for Forensic Psychologists* were adopted by majority vote of the members of Division *41* and the American Psychology-Law Society. They have also been endorsed by majority vote by the American Academy of Forensic Psychology. The Executive Committee of Division *41* and the American Psychology Law Society formally approved these *Guidelines* on March 9, 1991. The Executive Committee also voted to continue the Committee on Ethical Guidelines in order to disseminate the *Guidelines* and to monitor their implementation and suggestions for revision. Individuals wishing to reprint these *Guidelines* or who have queries about them should contact either Stephen L. Golding, Ph.D., Department of Psychology, University of Utah, Salt Lake City, UT 84 I J. 2,80 1-58 I-8028 (voice) or 80 1-58 I-584 1 (FAX) or other members of the Committee listed below. Reprint requests should be sent to Cathy Oslzly, Department of Psychology, University of Nebraska- Lincoln, Lincoln, NE 68588-0308.

2. These Guidelines were prepared and principally authored by a joint Committee on Ethical Guidelines of Division 41 and the American Academy of Forensic-Psychology (Stephen L. Golding, [Chair], Thomas Grisso, David Shapiro, and Herbert Weissman [Co-chairs]). Other members of the Committee included Robert Fein, Kirk Heiibrun, Judith McKenna, Norman Poythress, and Daniel Schuman. Their hard work and willingness to tackle difficult conceptual and pragmatic issues is gratefully acknowledged. The Committee would also like to acknowledge specifically the assistance

and guidance provided by Dort Bigg, Larry Cowan, Eric Harris, Arthur Lemer, Michael Miller, Russell Newman, Melvin Rudov, and Ray Fowler. Many other individuals also contributed by their thoughtful critique and suggestions for improvement of earlier drafts which were widely circulated.

Purpose and Scope

Purpose

1. While the professional standards for the ethical practice of psychology, as a general discipline, are addressed in the American Psychological Association's *Ethical Principles of Psychologists*, these ethical principles do not relate, in sufficient detail, to current aspirations of desirable professional conduct for forensic psychologists. By design, none of the *Guidelines* contradicts any of the *Ethical Principles of Psychologists*; rather, they amplify those *Principles* in the context of the practice of forensic psychology, as herein defined.

2. The *Guidelines* have been designed to be national in scope and are intended to conform with state and Federal law. In situations where the forensic psychologist believes that the requirements of law are in conflict with the *Guidelines*, attempts to resolve the conflict should be made in accordance with the procedures set forth in these *Guidelines* [IV(G)] and in the *Ethical Principles of Psychologists*.

Scope

1. The *Guidelines* specify the nature of desirable professional practice by forensic psychologists, within any subdiscipline of psychology (e.g., clinical, developmental, social, experimental), when engaged regularly as forensic psychologists.

   a. "Psychologist" means any individual whose professional activities are defined by the American Psychological Association or by regulation of title by state registration or licensure, as the practice of psychology. "Forensic psychology" means all forms of professional psychological conduct when acting, with definable foreknowledge, as a psychological expert on explicitly psycholegal issues, in direct assistance to courts, parties to legal proceedings, correctional and forensic mental health facilities, and administrative, judicial, and legislative agencies acting in an adjudicative capacity. "Forensic psychologist" means psychologists who regularly engage in the practice of forensic psychology.

   b. "Forensic psychology" means all forms of professional conduct when acting with definable foreknowledge, as a psychological expert on explicitly psychological issues, in direct assistance to the courts parties to legal proceedings, correctional and forensic mental health facilities, and administrative, judicial, and legislative agencies acting in an adjudicative capacity.

   c. "Forensic psychologist" means psychologists who regularly engage in the practice of forensic psychology as defined in I(B)(1)(b).

2. The *Guidelines* do not apply to a psychologist who is asked to provide professional psychological services when the psychologist was not informed at the time of delivery of the services that they were to be used as forensic psychological services as defined above. The Guidelines may be helpful, however, in preparing the psychologist for the experience of communicating psychological data in a forensic context.

3. Psychologists who are not forensic psychologists as defined in I(B)(1)(c), but occasionally provide limited forensic psychological services, may find the *Guidelines* useful in the preparation and presentation of their professional services.

Related Standards

1. Forensic psychologists also conduct their professional activities in accord with the *Ethical Principles of Psychologists* and the various other statements of the American Psychological Association that may apply to particular subdisciplines or areas of practice that are relevant to their professional activities.

2. The standards of practice and ethical guidelines of other relevant "expert professional organizations" contain useful guidance and should be consulted even though the present *Guidelines* take precedence for forensic psychologists.

Responsibility

A. Forensic psychologists have an obligation to provide services in a manner consistent with the highest standards of their profession. They are responsible for their own conduct and the conduct of those individuals under their direct supervision.

B. Forensic psychologists make a reasonable effort to ensure that their services and the products of their services are used in a forthright and responsible manner.

Competence

A. Forensic psychologists provide services only in areas of psychology in which they have specialized knowledge, skill, experience, and education.

B. Forensic psychologists have an obligation to present to the court, regarding the specific matters to which they will testify, the boundaries of their competence, the factual bases (knowledge, skill, experience, training, and education) for their qualification as an expert, and the relevance of those factual bases to their qualification as an expert on the specific matters at issue.

C. Forensic psychologists are responsible for a fundamental and reasonable level of knowledge and understanding of the legal and professional standards that govern their participation as experts in legal proceedings.

D. Forensic psychologists have an obligation to understand the civil rights of parties in legal proceedings in which they participate, and manage their professional conduct in a manner that does not diminish or threaten those rights.

E. Forensic psychologists recognize that their own personal values, moral beliefs, or personal and professional relationships with parties to a legal proceeding may interfere with their ability to practice competently. Under such circumstances, forensic psychologists are obligated to decline participation or to limit their assistance in a manner consistent with professional obligations.

Relationships

A. During initial consultation with the legal representative of the party seeking services, forensic psychologists have an obligation to inform the party of factors that might reasonably affect the decision to contract with the forensic psychologist. These factors include, but are not limited to

1. The fee structure for anticipated professional services;

2. Prior and current personal or professional activities, obligations, and relationships that might produce a conflict of interests;

3. Their areas of competence and the limits of their competence; and

4. The known scientific bases and limitations of the methods and procedures that they employ and their qualifications to employ such methods and procedures.

B. Forensic psychologists do not provide professional services to parties to a legal proceeding on the basis of "contingent fees," when those services involve the offering of expert testimony to a court or administrative body, or when they call upon the psychologist to make affirmations or representations intended to be relied upon by third parties.

C. Forensic psychologists who derive a substantial portion of their income from fee-for-service arrangements should offer some portion of their professional services on a pro bono or reduced fee basis where the public interest or the welfare of clients may be inhibited by insufficient financial resources.

D. Forensic psychologists recognize potential conflicts of interest in dual relationships with parties to a legal proceeding, and they seek to minimize their effects.

1. Forensic psychologists avoid providing professional services to parties in a legal proceeding with whom they have personal or professional relationships that are inconsistent with the anticipated relationship.

2. When it is necessary to provide both evaluation and treatment services to a party in a legal proceeding (as may be the case in small forensic hospital settings or small communities), the forensic psychologist takes reasonable steps to minimize the potential negative effects of these circumstances on the rights of the party, confidentiality, and the process of treatment and evaluation.

E. Forensic psychologists have an obligation to ensure that prospective clients are informed of their legal rights with respect to the anticipated forensic service, of the purposes of any evaluation, of the nature of procedures to be employed, of the intended uses of any product of their services, and of the party who has employed the forensic psychologist.

1. Unless court ordered, forensic psychologists obtain the informed consent of the client or party, or their legal representative, before proceeding with such evaluations and procedures. If the client appears unwilling to proceed after receiving a thorough notification of the purposes, methods, and intended uses of the forensic evaluation, the evaluation should be postponed and the psychologist should take steps to place the client in contact with his/her attorney for the purpose of legal advice on the issue of participation.

2. In situations where the client or party may not have the capacity to provide informed consent to services or the evaluation is pursuant to court order, the forensic psychologist provides reasonable notice to the client's legal representative of the nature of the anticipated forensic service before proceeding. If the client's legal representative objects to the evaluation, the forensic psychologist notifies the court issuing the order and responds as directed.

3. After a psychologist has advised the subject of a clinical forensic evaluation of the intended uses of the evaluation and its work product, the psychologist may not use the evaluation work product for other purposes without explicit waiver to do so by the client or the client's legal representative.

F. When forensic psychologists engage in research or scholarly activities that are compensated financially by a client or party to a legal proceeding, or when the psychologist provides those services on a pro *bono* basis, the psychologist clarifies any anticipated further use of such research or scholarly product, discloses the psychologist's role in the resulting research or scholarly products, and obtains whatever consent or agreement is required by law or professional standards.

G. When conflicts arise between the forensic psychologist's professional standards and the requirements of legal standards, a particular court, or a directive by an officer of the court or legal authorities, the forensic psychologist has an obligation to make those legal authorities aware of the source of the conflict and to take reasonable steps to resolve it. Such steps may include, but are not limited to, obtaining the consultation of fellow forensic professionals, obtaining the advice of independent counsel, and conferring directly with the legal representatives involved.

Confidentiality and Privilege

A. Forensic psychologists have an obligation to be aware of the legal standards that may affect or limit the confidentiality or privilege that may attach to their services or their products, and they conduct their professional activities in a manner that respects those known rights and privileges.
   1. Forensic psychologists establish and maintain a system of record keeping and professional communication that safeguards a client's privilege.
   2. Forensic psychologists maintain active control over records and information. They only release information pursuant to statutory requirements, court order, or the consent of the client.
B. Forensic psychologists inform their clients of the limitations to the confidentiality of their services and their products (see also Guideline IV E) by providing them with an understandable statement of their rights, privileges, and the limitations of confidentiality.
C. In situations where the right of the client or party to confidentiality is limited, the forensic psychologist makes every effort to maintain confidentiality with regard to any information that does not bear directly upon the legal purpose of the evaluation.
D. Forensic psychologists provide clients or their authorized legal representatives with access to the information in their records and a meaningful explanation of that information, consistent with existing Federal and state statutes, the *Ethical Principles of Psychologists*, the *Standards for Educational and Psychological Testing*, and institutional rules and regulations.

Methods and Procedures

A. Because of their special status as persons qualified as experts to the court, forensic psychologists have an obligation to maintain current knowledge of scientific, professional and legal developments within their area of claimed competence. They are obligated also to use that knowledge, consistent with accepted clinical and scientific standards, in selecting data collection methods and procedures for an evaluation, treatment, consultation or scholarly/empirical investigation.
B. Forensic psychologists have an obligation to document and be prepared to make available, subject to court order or the rules of evidence, all data that form the basis for their evidence or services. The standard to be applied to such documentation or recording *anticipates* that the detail and quality of such documentation will be subject to reasonable judicial scrutiny; this standard is higher than the normative standard for general clinical practice. When forensic psychologists conduct an examination or engage in the treatment of a party to a legal proceeding, with foreknowledge that their professional services will be used in an adjudicative forum, they incur a special responsibility to provide the best documentation possible under the circumstances.
   1. Documentation of the data upon which one's evidence is based is subject to the normal rules of discovery, disclosure, confidentiality, and privilege that operate in the jurisdiction in which the data were obtained. Forensic psychologists have an obligation to be aware of those rules and to regulate their conduct in accordance with them.
   2. The duties and obligations of forensic psychologists with respect to documentation of data that form the basis for their evidence apply from the moment they know or have a reasonable basis for knowing that their data and evidence derived from it are likely to enter into legally relevant decisions.

C. In providing forensic psychological services, forensic psychologists take special care to avoid undue influence upon their methods, procedures, and products, such as might emanate from the party to a legal proceeding by financial compensation or other gains. As an expert conducting an evaluation, treatment, consultation, or scholarly/empirical investigation, the forensic psychologist maintains professional integrity by examining the issue at hand from all reasonable perspectives, actively seeking information that will differentially test plausible rival hypotheses.

D. Forensic psychologists do not provide professional forensic services to a defendant or to any party in, or in contemplation of, a legal proceeding prior to that individual's representation by counsel, except for persons judicially determined, where appropriate, to be handling their representation pro se. When the forensic services are pursuant to court order and the client is not represented by counsel, the forensic psychologist makes reasonable efforts to inform the court prior to providing the services.

  1. A forensic psychologist may provide emergency mental health services to a pretrial defendant prior to court order or the appointment of counsel where there are reasonable grounds to believe that such emergency services are needed for the protection and improvement of the defendant's mental health and where failure to provide such mental health services would constitute a substantial risk of imminent harm to the defendant or to others. In providing such services the forensic psychologist nevertheless seeks to inform the defendant's counsel in a manner consistent with the requirements of the emergency situation.

  2. Forensic psychologists who provide such emergency mental health services should attempt to avoid providing further professional forensic services to that defendant unless that relationship is reasonably unavoidable [see N(D)(2)].

E. When forensic psychologists seek data from third parties, prior records, or other sources, they do so only with the prior approval of the relevant legal party or as a consequence of an order of a court to conduct the forensic evaluation.

F. Forensic psychologists are aware that hearsay exceptions and other rules governing expert testimony place a special ethical burden upon them. When hearsay or otherwise inadmissible evidence forms the basis of their opinion, evidence, or professional product, they seek to minimize sole reliance upon such evidence. Where circumstances reasonably permit, forensic psychologists seek to obtain independent and personal verification of data relied upon as part of their professional services to the court or to a party to a legal proceeding.

  1. While many forms of data used by forensic psychologists are hearsay, forensic psychologists attempt to corroborate critical data that form the basis for their professional product. When using hearsay data that have not been corroborated, but are nevertheless utilized, forensic psychologists have an affirmative responsibility to acknowledge the uncorroborated status of those data and the reasons for relying upon such data.

  2. With respect to evidence of any type, forensic psychologists avoid offering information from their investigations or evaluations that does not bear directly upon the legal purpose of their professional services and that is not critical as support for their product, evidence or testimony, except where such disclosure is required by law.

  3. When a forensic psychologist relies upon data or information gathered by others, the origins of those data are clarified in any professional product. In addition, the forensic psychologist bears a special responsibility to ensure that such data, if relied upon,

were gathered in a manner standard for the profession.

G. Unless otherwise stipulated by the parties, forensic psychologists are aware that no statements made by a defendant, in the course of any (forensic) examination, no testimony by the expert based upon such statements, nor any other fruits of the statements can be admitted into evidence against the defendant in any criminal proceeding, except on an issue respecting mental condition on which the defendant has introduced testimony. Forensic psychologists have an affirmative duty to ensure that their written products and oral testimony conform to this Federal Rule of Procedure (12.2[c]), or its state equivalent.

1. Because forensic psychologists are often not in a position to know what evidence, documentation, or element of a written product may be or may lend to a "fruit of the statement," they exercise extreme caution in preparing reports or offering testimony prior to the defendant's assertion of a mental state claim or the defendant's introduction of testimony regarding a mental condition. Consistent with the reporting requirements of state or federal law, forensic psychologists avoid including statements from the defendant relating to the time period of the alleged offense.

2. Once a defendant has proceeded to the trial stage, and all pretrial mental health issues such as competency have been resolved, forensic psychologists may include in their reports or testimony any statements made by the defendant that are directly relevant to supporting their expert evidence, providing that the defendant has "introduced" mental state evidence or testimony within the meaning of Federal Rule of Procedure 12.2(c), or its state equivalent.

H. Forensic psychologists avoid giving written or oral evidence about the psychological characteristics of particular individuals when they have not had an opportunity to conduct an examination of the individual adequate to the scope of the statements, opinions, or conclusions to be issued. Forensic psychologists make every reasonable effort to conduct such examinations. When it is not possible or feasible to do so, they make clear the impact of such limitations on the reliability and validity of their professional products, evidence, or testimony.

Public and Professional Communications

A. Forensic psychologists make reasonable efforts to ensure that the products of their services, as well as their own public statements and professional testimony, are communicated in ways that will promote understanding and avoid deception, given the particular characteristics, roles, and abilities of various recipients of the communications.

1. Forensic psychologists take reasonable steps to correct misuse or misrepresentation of their professional products, evidence, and testimony.

2. Forensic psychologists provide information about professional work to clients in a manner consistent with professional and legal standards for the disclosure of test results, interpretations of data, and the factual bases for conclusions. A full explanation of the results of tests and the bases for conclusions should be given in language that the client can understand.

a. When disclosing information about a client to third parties who are not qualified to interpret test results and data, the forensic psychologist complies with Principle 16 of the *Standards for Educational and Psychological Testing*. When required to disclose results to a nonpsychologist, every attempt is made to ensure that test security is maintained and access to information is restricted to individuals with a legitimate and professional interest in the data. Other qualified mental health professionals who make a request for information pursuant to a lawful order are, by definition, "individuals with a legitimate and professional interest."

    b. In providing records and raw data, the forensic psychologist takes reasonable steps to ensure that the receiving party is informed that raw scores must be interpreted by a qualified professional in order to provide reliable and valid information.

B. Forensic psychologists realize that their public role as "expert to the court" or as "expert representing the profession" confers upon them a special responsibility for fairness and accuracy in their public statements. When evaluating or commenting upon the professional work product or qualifications of another expert or party to a legal proceeding, forensic psychologists represent their professional disagreements with reference to a fair and accurate evaluation of the data, theories, standards, and opinions of the other expert or party.

C. Ordinarily, forensic psychologists avoid making detailed public (out-of-court) statements about particular legal proceedings in which they have been involved. When there is a strong justification to do so, such public statements are designed to assure accurate representation of their role or their evidence, not to advocate the positions of parties in the legal proceeding. Forensic psychologists address particular legal proceedings in publications or communications only to the extent that the information relied upon is part of a public record, or consent for that use has been properly obtained from the party holding any privilege.

D. When testifying, forensic psychologists have an obligation to all parties to a legal proceeding to present their findings, conclusions, evidence, or other professional products in a fair manner. This principle does not preclude forceful representation of the data and reasoning upon which a conclusion or professional product is based. It does, however, preclude an attempt, whether active or passive, to engage in partisan distortion or misrepresentation. Forensic psychologists do not, by either commission or omission, participate in a misrepresentation of their evidence, nor do they participate in partisan attempts to avoid, deny, or subvert the presentation of evidence contrary to their own position.

E. Forensic psychologists, by virtue of their competence and rules of discovery, actively disclose all sources of information obtained in the course of their professional services; they actively disclose which information from which source was used in formulating a particular written product or oral testimony.

F. Forensic psychologists are aware that their essential role as expert to the court is to assist the trier of fact to understand the evidence or to determine a fact in issue. In offering expert evidence, they are aware that their own professional observations, inferences, and conclusions must be distinguished from legal facts, opinions, and conclusions. Forensic psychologists are prepared to explain the relationship between their expert testimony and the legal issues and facts of an instant case.

ABOUT THE EDITOR AND CONTRIBUTORS

Shane S. Bush, Ph.D., ABPP, ABPN is in independent practice in Smithtown N.Y. and is the Chief Science Officer for MemoryConcepts, LLC. He is board certified in Neuropsychology by the American Board of Professional Neuropsychology and board certified in Rehabilitation Psychology by the American Board of Professional Psychology. He is a member of the Ethics Committee of the Division of Neuropsychology and is Chair of the Social and Ethical Responsibility Committee of the Division of Rehabilitation Psychology of the American Psychological Association. He is a member of the New York State Psychological Association (NYSPA) Committee on Ethical Practice and is president-elect of NYSPA's Division of Neuropsychology. He is Chair of the Education Committee of the National Academy of Neuropsychology (NAN), is a member of the NAN Policy and Planning Committee, and is the coordinator of the Grand Rounds section of the *NAN Bulletin*. He is an editorial board member of *The Clinical Neuropsychologist*, co-editing the Ethical and Professional Issues section, and is an editorial board member of the Journal of Forensic Neuropsychology. He is co-editor of the textbook *Ethical Issues in Clinical Neuropsychology* and co-author of the textbook *Health Care Ethics for Psychologists: A Casebook*. He has presented on ethical issues in neuropsychology and rehabilitation psychology at national conferences. He is a veteran of both the U.S. Marine Corps and Navy.

Jeffrey N. Browndyke, Ph.D. is an assistant professor in the Department of Psychiatry and Behavioral Sciences and faculty member of the Joseph and Kathleen Bryan Alzheimer's Disease Research Center at Duke University Medical Center. Dr. Browndyke specializes in geriatric neuropsychology, geriatric neuroimaging, and computerized cognitive assessment. He has been actively involved in the development and use of Internet-based technologies for neuropsychological research and clinical application since the mid-1990s. He is the founder and editor-in-chief of Neuropsychology Central website; co-founder of the National Academy of Neuropsychology website; a member of the Society for Computers in Psychology; a member of the Information Technology Committee of the National Academy of Neuropsychology; and recipient of the Laird Cermak Award for Early Contributions to Memory Research from the International Neuropsychological Society. He has published research investigating the interaction between patient variables and computerized assessment performance; the development of Internet-based cognitive assessment measures; the cognitive consequences and structural neuroimaging markers of vascular dementia, ischemic cerebrovascular disease, and post-cardiosurgical intervention; and the functional neuroimaging of episodic memory deficits in Alzheimer's disease.

David R. Cox, PhD, ABPP is a licensed psychologist who is board certified in Rehabilitation Psychology. He is the Vice President of the American Board of Rehabilitation Psychology. His work focuses on patients with psychological and/or physiological injury, most often with patients who have primary brain injury or other medical illness. He is President of Neuropsychology & Behavioral Health Consultants, Inc. with offices in Winter Park, Florida and Chapel Hill, North Carolina. He maintains a private practice and holds an academic appointment as Courtesy Professor of Clinical and Health Psychology at the University of Florida. He is a Past-President of the Florida Psychological Association, and has served on the board of directors of the Brain Injury Association of Florida as well as the Orlando Metro Unit of the American Cancer Society. He is frequently called on to provide evaluations and impairment or disability ratings as part of his clinical work, including worker's compensation ratings for insurance carriers, attorneys and the courts. He is one of the original authors of the Computerized Assessment of Response Bias, a widely used measure in evaluation of response bias in neuropsychological assessment. His work has been presented at state, national and international conferences.

John A. Crouch, Ph.D., ABPP has worked in the field of clinical neuropsychology since 1981. He obtained his doctorate in clinical psychology (rehabilitation subspecialty) at the University of Kansas. He completed specialty training in clinical neuropsychology via an internship at the University of Florida (Shand's Hospital) and through a postdoctoral fellowship at the University of California, San Diego. Dr. Crouch is board certified in Clinical Neuropsychology through the American Board of Professional Psychology (ABPP) and the American Academy of Clinical Neuropsychology (AACN). Since becoming licensed as a psychologist in 1990, Dr. Crouch has worked in general medical, rehabilitation, university-based programs, and private practice settings. Dr. Crouch has worked with individuals from diverse clinical backgrounds including TBI, stroke, movement disorders, dementia, substance usage, and neuropsychiatric conditions. His numerous publications and presentations include work on ethical issues in clinical Neuropsychology. Dr. Crouch is currently in independent practice with offices in New Canaan and Glastonbury, CT. Current work involves assessment of brain functioning, formulating diagnoses, and treatment planning. Dr. Crouch's work involves assessment within the context of disability determination or litigation matters.

Duane E. Dede, Ph.D. is a Clinical Associate Professor in the Department of Clinical & Health Psychology at the University of Florida. He is also co-director of the University of Florida Mild Traumatic Brain Injury Clinic. He is a member of the Board of Directors of the Brain Injury Association of Florida. He served as the Program Chair of the International Neuropsychology Society's 22nd Neuropsychology Conference in South Africa in 1999. From 1997-2000 he served as Chairman, Division 40 (Neuropsychology) Committee on Minority Affairs, American Psychological Association. He has

twice been awarded the Hugh Davis Award for excellence in Clinical Teaching. He received his Ph.D. from the University of Louisville and completed postdoctoral training in clinical neuropsychology in the University of Michigan Neuropsychology Program. He conducts research on demographic variables (e.g., ethnicity, age) in neuropsychological functioning.

John DeLuca, Ph.D., ABPP is the Director of Neuroscience Research at the Kessler Medical Rehabilitation Research and Education Corporation (KMRREC), and a Professor in the Departments of Physical Medicine & Rehabilitation (PM&R), and Neurosciences at University of Medicine and Dentistry of New Jersey – New Jersey Medical School (UMDNJ-NJMS). He is a licensed Psychologist in the states of New Jersey and New York. Dr. DeLuca directs the Neuropsychology and Neuroscience Laboratory at KMRREC, and is director of the post-doctoral fellows program in Neuropsychology. He is currently studying disorders of memory and information processing in a variety of clinical populations, and has published over 180 articles, abstracts and chapters in these areas. He is the editor of an upcoming book entitled "Fatigue as a Window to the Brain". Dr. DeLuca is the recipient of early career awards for his research from both the American Psychological Association and the National Academy of Neuropsychology. Dr. DeLuca is Board Certified by the American Board of Professional Psychology in Rehabilitation Psychology. He is also a Fellow of the American Psychological Association and the National Academy of Neuropsychology.

Robert L. Denney, Psy.D., ABPP, ABPN received a doctor of psychology degree in clinical psychology from the Forest Institute of Professional Psychology in 1991. He has worked as a forensic psychologist and neuropsychologist at the U.S. Medical Center for Federal Prisoners in Springfield, Missouri, for over 12 Years. He is also an associate professor and director of neuropsychology at the Forest

Institute of Professional Psychology in Springfield. He is board certified in forensic psychology and clinical neuropsychology by the American Board of Professional Psychology and in neuropsychology by the American Board of Professional Neuropsychology. He has published in the scientific literature on such subjects as neuropsychological evaluation of criminal defendants, malingering, and professional licensure. He has also presented throughout the U.S. on neurolitigation, brain injury, malingering, and admissibility of scientific evidence. Opinions expressed here are those of the author and do not necessarily represent opinions of the Federal Bureau of Prisons or Department of Justice.

Eileen B. Fennell, Ph.D., ABPP is a Professor in the Departments of Clinical and Health Psychology and Neurology of the University of Florida, Gainesville. She also serves as the Co-Director of the University of Florida Center for Neuropsychological Studies and is a faculty member of the University of Florida Brain Institute. She has authored or co-authored over 50 refereed articles, 10 book chapters and one book, "Pediatric Neuropsychology in a Medical Setting". Dr. Fennell has served on a number of Boards and Committees of professional organizations in the field of clinical neuropsychology including Division 40 of APA, the National Academy of Neuropsychology, the American Board of Clinical Neuropsychology, and the Board of Trustees of the American Board of Professional Psychology. She was elected President of Division 40 for 1996-1997. She is Board Certified in Clinical Neuropsychology by the American Board of Professional Psychology and continues to teach, see patients, and supervise graduate students at the University of Florida, where she is Director of the Specialty Track in Clinical Neuropsychology.

Alan L. Goldberg, Psy.D., ABPP; J.D. has been a licensed psychologist for over 20 years (Psy.D., 1983 – Wright State University), and has been a member of the Tucson, Arizona legal community for 7 years (J.D., 1997 – The University of Arizona). He has 20 years of experience providing services to rehabilitation clients in hospital and outpatient settings. His current professional activities involve a blending of psychology and law. He conducts traditional and forensic neuropsychological evaluations, continues to provide psychotherapy to select clients, has served as a hearing officer for the Arizona Department of Education, is a provider for the State Bar of Arizona Member Assistance Plan, consults with businesses and schools concerning compliance with the Americans with Disabilities Act and the Individuals with Disabilities Education Act, and assists attorneys with medical record review & examination of expert witnesses. He is immediate past president of the Southern Arizona Psychological Association, where he also serves on the Social Policy, Psychology-Law, and Program Committees. Dr. Goldberg has served two terms as a Member at Large of the Executive Board of the American Psychological Association's Division of Rehabilitation Psychology. He also serves on that division's Pediatric, Program, Continuing Education, and Social and Ethical Responsibility Committees. He is the liaison between the Division of Rehabilitation Psychology and the American Psychological Association's Committee on disability Issues in Psychology. He is a Diplomate in Rehabilitation Psychology, American Board of Professional Psychology. Dr. Goldberg has published more than 20 book chapters, articles, and abstracts, and he has presented more than 50 papers and symposia at state, national, and international conferences.

Charles J. Golden, Ph.D., ABPP is currently Professor of Psychology and Director of the Neuropsychology Assessment Center at Nova Southeastern University in Fort Lauderdale, Florida. Dr. Golden is a 1975 graduate of the University of Hawaii who is board certified in clinical psychology, clinical neuropsychology, and assessment psychology. He has over 300 publications primarily in the area of neuropsychology. He is a past-president of the National Academy of Neuropsychologists as well as current past president of the Assessment Section (Section 9) of Division 12 of APA. He has worked in both clinical and professional settings throughout his career and is best known for the development of the Luria-Nebraska Neuropsychological Battery as well as the popularization the Stroop Color and Word Test.

Christopher L. Grote, Ph.D, ABPP is an Associate Professor and co-director of the neuropsychology program in the Department of Psychology at Rush-Presbyterian-St. Luke's Medical Center in Chicago. He is board certified in Clinical Neuropsychology by the American Board of Professional Psychology, and is a member of the Board of Directors of the American Academy of Clinical Neuropsychology. He also serves as Local Arrangements Coordinator for the oral exams for the American Board of Clinical Neuropsychology. He previously served as director of the Midwest Neuropsychology Group and as chair of the Division 40 Practice Advisory Committee. He has published primarily in the areas of epilepsy and ethics in neuropsychology.

Stephen Honor, Ph.D., ABPP obtained his doctoral degree at Hofstra University in New York. He is in the full time practice of forensic and clinical neuropsychology in Smithtown, NY. He is board certified in clinical psychology, clinical neuropsychology, and forensic psychology by the American Board of Professional Psychology. Dr. Honor is a Medical Advisor to the U.S. Department of Health and Human Services and a member of the New York State Department of Health Medical Records Access Review Committee. He has testified locally and nationally in a number of legal cases, including murder, personal injury and custody evaluation. He lectures to professional groups including physicians, psychologists, attorneys and mental health specialists. Dr. Honor is on the faculty of Touro College,

School of Health Sciences, where he teaches in the graduate program in Forensic Examination.

Doug Johnson-Greene, Ph.D., ABPP is an Associate Professor and Director of the postdoctoral fellows program in Neuropsychology in the Department of Physical Medicine and Rehabilitation at the Johns Hopkins University School of Medicine where he maintains a clinical practice, teaching, and active research program. A 1993 graduate of the University of Mississippi, Dr. Johnson-Greene completed his internship at the Portland VA and Oregon Health Sciences University, and residency at the University of Michigan Medical Center. He is currently studying neuropsychological aspects of alcohol abuse, premorbid ability estimation, ecological validity, and cerebrovascular disorders. An NIH-funded researcher, Dr. Johnson-Greene has published more than 80 articles, chapters, and abstracts. He has been a member of numerous professional committees and currently serves on the APA Division 40 Ethics Committee and has held an appointment with the Maryland Board of Examiners of Psychologists since 2000. He is the recipient of the Early Career Award in Research by APA Division 22, Dr. Johnson-Greene is Board Certified by the American Board of Professional Psychology in Clinical Psychology, Rehabilitation Psychology, and Clinical Neuropsychology and is a Fellow of the National Academy of Neuropsychology.

Michael F. Martelli, Ph.D. directs Rehabilitation Neuropsychology at Concussion Care Centre of Virginia and Tree of Life. He has 16 years of experience in rehabilitation psychology and neuropsychology with specialization in practical, holistic assessment and treatment services primarily in the areas of rehabilitation of neurologic and chronic pain disorders. He has produced a Habit Retraining Model and Methodology for Neurologic Rehabilitation. He is the commissioner of psychology for the Commission on Disability Examiner Certification, has academic appointments in three departments at VCU and one at University of Virginia, serves on several editorial review boards and brain injury related boards, and is the current President of the Brain Injury Association of Virginia, and High Hopes, Inc, a non-profit organization dedicated to providing affordable housing opportunities for persons with disabilities. He frequently lectures and publishes, with over 300 papers, abstracts, articles, chapters and talks in numerous areas relating to disability, rehabilitation, neuropsychology and chronic pain.

Thomas A. Martin, Psy.D., ABPP is Chief of Psychology Services at Missouri Rehabilitation Center and a Clinical Assistant Professor in the Department of Health Psychology at University of Missouri–Columbia. He earned his doctoral degree from the Adler School of Professional Psychology and completed a post-doctoral fellowship in Clinical Neuropsychology and Rehabilitation Psychology at the University of Missouri–Columbia. He currently serves on the Board of Directors of the Brain Injury Association of Missouri, is a member of the Social and Ethical Responsibility Committee of APA's Division of Rehabilitation Psychology, and is a member of the Education Committee of the National Academy of Neuropsychology. He has published in the areas of clinical neuropsychology and rehabilitation psychology, and he is currently conducting research in the area of traumatic brain injury and treatment outcomes. Dr. Martin is board certified in Rehabilitation Psychology by the American Board of Professional Psychology.

A. John McSweeny, Ph.D., ABPP is Professor of Psychiatry and Neurology, and Director of the Neuropsychology Laboratory, at the Medical College of Ohio (MCO). He received his Ph.D. in clinical psychology from Northern Illinois University in 1975. He completed his clinical psychology internship at Baylor College of Medicine in Houston, Texas and a post-doctoral fellowship in methodology and evaluation research at

Northwestern University in Evanston, Illinois. He was a member of the faculties at Northwestern University and West Virginia University before coming to MCO. Dr. McSweeny is a Diplomate in Clinical Neuropsychology of the American Board of Professional Psychology and a Fellow of the American Psychological Association and the National Academy of Neuropsychology. He served on the APA Division 40 Ethics Committee from 1992 to 2000 and chaired the Committee from 1993-1996. Dr. McSweeny has conducted research on several topics in neuropsychology for 25 years and is the author of multiple research articles and the co-editor of two books.

Paul J. Moberg, Ph.D., ABPP is an Associate Professor of Neuropsychology in the Departments of Psychiatry, Neurology and Otorhinolaryngology: Head and Neck Surgery at the University of Pennsylvania School of Medicine. He is the Director of Clinical Services for the Brain-Behavior Laboratory. He received his B.A. in Psychology from Augsburg College in Minneapolis, Minnesota in 1982 and his M.A. in Clinical Psychology from Loyola College in Baltimore, Maryland in 1985. He received his initial training in Neuropsychology at the Johns Hopkins University School of Medicine in Baltimore and subsequently obtained his Ph.D. in Clinical Psychology (1990) from the University of Health Sciences/The Chicago Medical School in North Chicago, Illinois. Dr. Moberg completed his Predoctoral internship at the University of Florida in Gainesville with an emphasis in Neuropsychology. He subsequently completed Postdoctoral training in Neuropsychology at the same institution. Dr. Moberg is board certified in Clinical Neuropsychology by the American Board of Professional Psychology.

Joel E. Morgan, Ph.D., ABPP practices clinical neuropsychology in New Jersey and is an Assistant Professor in the Department of Neurology and Neuroscience at UMDNJ-New Jersey

Medical School. For nearly 20 years he was Director of Neuropsychology and Director of Training at the Department of Veterans Affairs in New Jersey. Dr. Morgan is now in full time private practice where he is active in many professional organizations in neuropsychology. He is board certified in clinical neuropsychology by the American Board of Clinical Neuropsychology/American Board of Professional Psychology. He is a Fellow of the National Academy of Neuropsychology (NAN) and an Accreditation Site Visitor for the Committee on Accreditation of the American Psychological Association (APA). Dr. Morgan devotes a good deal of time to professional activities, and serves as the Editor of Division 40's Newsletter, Newsletter40, is on the board of the American Academy of Clinical Neuropsychology, and the editorial board of a leading neuropsychology journal, as well as an external reviewer for many neuropsychology journals. He is also a Past-President of the Association for Internship Training in Clinical Neuropsychology, which represents neuropsychology specialty track internships at the division level of APA. Dr. Morgan developed NAN's DistanCE Program on Ethics in Neuropsychology, which will be presented as a web-based CE program in 2003-4. Dr. Morgan maintains an active clinical and forensic neuropsychology practice.

Richard I. Naugle, Ph.D., ABPP is Head of the Section of Neuropsychology at the Cleveland Clinic Foundation in Cleveland, Ohio, where he maintains an active clinical practice, teaches, and is involved in research. Dr. Naugle is an active member of the Division 40 of the American Psychological Association, the International Neuropsychological Society, and the National Academy of Neuropsychology and has served on a number of executive boards and committees, including the Ethics Subcommittee of Division 40, which he chaired from 1999 through 2002. He is currently serving in an elected capacity on the Executive boards of the Association of

Postdoctoral Programs in Clinical Neuropsychology and the American Board of Clinical Neuropsychology. He was board certified in clinical neuropsychology in 1993 and is a fellow in the National Academy of Neuropsychology and the American Psychological Association through Division 40. He has authored or co-authored a number of refereed articles, book chapters, and one book. His current research interests include the use of neuropsychological data to inform medical and surgical decisions. He has written on a number of ethical issues and currently co-edits the Ethical and Professional Issues Section of *The Clinical Neuropsychologist*.

Keith Nicholson, Ph.D., is a psychologist currently working with the Comprehensive Pain Program at Toronto Western Hospital and as a consulting psychologist with several community clinics. He also maintains an independent private practice with a focus on clinical neuropsychology and chronic pain. He has particular interest in the confounding effects of pain and related problems on neuropsychological test performance and what may be the psychoneurobiological interface in chronic pain.

James B. Pinkston, Ph.D. earned his BS in Psychology from Brigham Young University and his doctorate in Clinical Psychology with an emphasis in neuropsychology from Louisiana State University. He completed his pre-doctoral internship in Clinical Psychology with an emphasis in neuropsychology at the University of Oklahoma Health Sciences Center and a post-doctoral fellowship in neuropsychology at The Cleveland Clinic Foundation. He is currently employed as a staff neuropsychologist within the department of neurology at the LSU Health Sciences Center and School of Medicine in Shreveport, Louisiana.

Brad L. Roper, Ph.D., ABPP, is Director of Neuropsychology and Associate Training Director at the Department of Veterans Affairs Medical Center in Memphis, TN. He is also

Associate Professor in the Department of Psychiatry at the University of Tennessee, Memphis, and holds joint appointments in the Department of Neurology and the College of Nursing. He holds adjunct appointments in the Departments of Psychology at the University of Memphis and the University of Mississippi. He is board certified in Clinical Neuropsychology by the American Board of Professional Psychology. He currently serves as Past President of the Association for Internship Training in Clinical Neuropsychology. He is Director of Neuropsychology Residency Training at the Memphis VAMC, LeBonheur Children's Medical Center, and St. Jude Children's Research Hospital, and he serves on the Board of Directors of the Association of Postdoctoral Programs in Clinical Neuropsychology. He is Associate Editor for Neuropsychology for the newsletter of the Association of Psychology Postdoctoral and Internship Centers. He received his B.S. in Industrial Engineering at Texas A&M University and his Ph.D. in Clinical Psychology at the University of Minnesota.

Philip Schatz, Ph.D. is an Assistant Professor of Psychology at Saint Joseph's University in Philadelphia, PA. He is a Neuropsychology Consultant to the Department of Health's Pennsylvania Head Injury program, the President of the Philadelphia Neuropsychology Society, and a site coordinator and member of the executive committee of the Philadelphia Sports Concussion Research program. A self-professed technophile, he is a co-founder of the National Academy of Neuropsychology distance program, and the current web coordinator and Chair of the Information Technology Committee of the National Academy of Neuropsychology. He is an active researcher in the areas of assessment and prediction of outcome following moderate and severe traumatic brain injury, assessment and diagnosis of sports-related concussion, and computer-based neuropsychological assessment.

Abigail B. Sivan, Ph.D. received her AB degree from Oberlin College, and her MA and PhD from New York University where she specialized in Educational Research and worked with L. Diller at Rusk Rehabilitation Institute on her dissertation research. While teaching at Michigan State University, she continued her education in Clinical Psychology. From 1975-1981, Dr. Sivan lived in Israel where she worked with Y. Ben-Yishay at the Rehabilitation Division of the IDF, directed the Kibbutz Child Development Center, taught at several medical schools, and did research with A. Carmon at the Brain Behavior Research Unit at Hadassah/Hebrew University Hospital. After returning to the U.S. in 1981, Dr. Sivan completed her internship with Dr. Nils Varney at the VAMC in Iowa City where she also researched the applicability of adult neuropsychological measures to normal and special children. Between 1983 and 1987, Dr. Sivan was the staff psychologist on a multidisciplinary team at the Child Development Clinic at the Division of Developmental Disabilities at the University of Iowa. Between 1988-1999, Dr. Sivan worked as a pediatric neuropsychologist in the Section of Child Psychiatry at Rush Presbyterian St. Luke's Medical Center, Chicago. After two years at Evanston Northwestern Healthcare, in January, 2001, she entered private practice; she also maintains an appointment as a Clinical Associate Professor at Feinberg School of Medicine, Northwestern University, in the Department of Psychiatry and Behavioral Sciences. Her research has focused on neuropsychological test development for children and adults. Dr. Sivan served on the Iowa Board of Psychology Examiners (1985-1987) and most recently on the APA Ethics Committee (1999-2001) and the APA Ethics Code Task Force (2000-2001). In 1994, Dr. Sivan consulted with the UN Commission on War Crimes in the former Yugoslavia.

Jerry J. Sweet, Ph.D., ABPP is Director of the Neuropsychology Service and Vice Chairman of the Psychiatry & Behavioral Sciences Department at Evanston Northwestern Healthcare, Evanston,

IL. He holds an academic rank of Professor of Psychiatry and Behavioral Sciences in the Feinberg School of Medicine of Northwestern University, and is board certified in clinical neuropsychology and clinical psychology by the American Board of Professional Psychology. He is presently on the Board of Directors of the American Academy of Clinical Neuropsychology. He is a Fellow of the Division of Clinical Neuropsychology (Division 40) and the Division of Clinical Psychology (Division 12) of the American Psychological Association. He served on the Ethics Committee of the Illinois Psychological Association for four years. Dr. Sweet edited the textbook *Forensic Neuropsychology: Fundamentals and Practice*, co-authored *Psychological Assessment in Medical Settings* and co-edited *Handbook of Clinical Psychology in Medical Settings*. He has authored and co-authored numerous book chapters and peer-reviewed research studies. He presently serves as Co-Editor of *The Clinical Neuropsychologist*, Associate Editor of *Journal of Clinical Psychology in Medical Settings*, and is on the editorial boards of *Archives of Clinical Neuropsychology*, *Journal of Forensic Neuropsychology*, *Neuropsychology Review*, and *International Journal of Forensic Psychology*.

Laetitia L. Thompson, Ph.D., ABPP is an associate professor in the departments of psychiatry and neurology and she is the Director of the UCHSC Neuropsychology Laboratory. She obtained her Ph.D. in clinical psychology from the University of Kansas in 1980. Her postdoctoral fellowship in clinical neuropsychology was completed at the University of Oklahoma Health Sciences Center in 1983. She then joined the faculty at the University of Colorado School of Medicine and has remained there since. She is board certified in Clinical Neuropsychology by the American Board of Professional Psychology. She is a Fellow of the National Academy of Neuropsychology and was Treasurer of NAN from 1998-2000. She has had an interest in ethical issues for a number of years. She co-authored with Dr. Laurence Binder one of the first articles relating the 1992 APA Ethics Code to neuropsychological assessment, published in the *Archives of Clinical Neuropsychology* in 1995. She also served on the APA Division 40 Ethics Committee from 1995 to 1999.

Wilfred G. van Gorp, Ph.D., ABPP is Professor of Clinical Psychology in the Department of Psychiatry of Columbia University College of Physicians and Surgeons and is the Director of the Neuropsychology Program there. Dr. van Gorp is a Fellow of the American Psychological Association (Division 40) and a Diplomate in Clinical Neuropsychology from the American Board of Professional Psychology. He is on the Executive Committee of Division 40 of the American Psychological Association and is a past President of the American Academy of Clinical Neuropsychology. Dr. van Gorp is Editor of the *Journal of Clinical and Experimental Neuropsychology*, and is on the editorial boards of the *Journal of the International Neuropsychological Society* and *The Clinical Neuropsychologist*. He has authored over 120 peer reviewed research papers, book chapters, and books.

Elisabeth A. Wilde, Ph.D. is a faculty member in the Department of Physical Medicine and Rehabilitation and the Cognitive Neuroscience Laboratory at Baylor College of Medicine. She received her Ph.D. from Brigham Young University and completed a post-doctoral fellowship in neuropsychology at the University of Michigan. She has published reviews on competency issues in older, cognitively-impaired patients and on the application of ethics for neuropsychologists in medical settings. Other research interests include clinical interventions in traumatic brain injury patients, age-related cognitive changes, and structural and functional neuroimaging.

Allan Yozawitz, Ph.D., ABPP is board certified in Clinical Neuropsychology by the American

Board of Professional Psychology and the American Board of Clinical Neuropsychology. He maintains a private practice in Syracuse, N.Y. and a faculty appointment as an Associate Professor in the Department of Psychiatry at Upstate Medical University. He also holds a faculty appointment as an Adjunct Associate Professor in the Department of Psychology at Syracuse University. Until his recent retirement from public service, Dr. Yozawitz was Director of Neuropsychology at Hutchings Psychiatric Center for 26 years. In that role, he was a pioneer for the practice of clinical neuropsychology in a psychiatric setting and for the application of neuropsychological rehabilitation strategies to a psychiatric population. Additionally, through task force memberships and leadership appointments in professional societies, he participated in developing guidelines for education, accreditation, and credentialing in neuropsychology. As a two-term member and former chairperson of the New York State Board for Psychology, Dr. Yozawitz also participated in developing licensure standards and professional practice guidelines for the field of psychology. He continues to serve on the New York State Board for Psychology's Licensure/Disciplinary Panel to assist in adjudicating charges of unprofessional conduct filed against psychologists. Dr. Yozawitz was Director of Continuing Education for the International Neuropsychological Society for nine years, served on the editorial board of three neuropsychology journals, functioned as a reviewer for six other psychology journals, contributed to two sections of the DSM-IV as a work group advisor, and authored book chapters and research papers on a variety of topics.

CONTACT INFORMATION

Editor

Shane S. Bush, Ph.D., ABPP, ABPN
26 Pembrook Dr., Stony Brook, NY 11790
USA
(631) 334-7884
sbushphdnp@medscape.com

Contributors

Jeffrey N. Browndyke, Ph.D.
Assistant Professor, Dept. of Psychiatry &
Behavioral Sciences
Duke University Medical Center
Bryan Alzheimer's Disease Research Center
2200 W. Main St., Suite A-230
Durham, NC 27705, USA
(919) 416-5383
j.browndyke@duke.edu

David R. Cox, Ph.D., ABPP
Neuropsychology & Behavioral Health
Consultants, Inc.
1555 Howell Branch Road
Suite C-210
Winter Park, FL 32789, USA
(407) 740-0007
drcox@iag.net

John A. Crouch, Ph.D., ABPP
21 Locust Avenue, Suite 1-D
New Canaan, CT 06840, USA
(203) 972-1177
johncrouchphd@hotmail.com

Duane E. Dede, Ph.D.
PO Box 100165
Gainesville, FL, USA
32610-0165
(352) 265-0680 x46890
DDede@hp.ufl.edu

John DeLuca, Ph.D., ABPP
Professor of Physical Medicine and
Rehabilitation
UMD-New Jersey Medical School, Newark,
New Jersey, USA
and
Director of Neuroscience Research
Neuropsychology and Neuroscience
Laboratory
Kessler Medical Rehabilitation Research and
Education Corporation
1199 Pleasant Valley Way
West Orange, New Jersey, 07052, USA
jdeluca@kmrrec.org
(973) 243-6974 (office)
(973) 243-6984 (fax)

Robert L. Denney, Psy.D., ABPP, ABPN
U.S. Medical Center for Federal
Prisoners
PO Box 4000
Springfield, MO 65801-4000, USA
rdenney@bop.gov

Eileen B. Fennell, Ph.D., ABPP
Professor, Department of Clinical and Health
Psychology
University of Florida
PO Box 100165 HSC
Gainesville, FL 32610-0165, USA
352-273-6151
EFennell@phhp.ufl.edu

Alan L. Goldberg, Psy.D., ABPP; J.D.
4641 E. Coronado Dr.
Tucson, AZ 85718-1643, USA
(520) 529-0878
ALG2000@aol.com

Charles J. Golden, Ph.D., ABPP
Professor of Psychology
Center for Psychological Studies
Nova Southeastern University
3301 College Avenue
Fort Lauderdale, Fl 33314, USA
954-262-5715
goldench@nova.edu

Christopher L. Grote, Ph.D., ABPP
Rush Presbyterian – St. Luke's Medical
Center
Department of Psychology
1653 W. Congress Parkway
Chicago, IL 60612, USA
(312) 942-5932
cgrote@rush.edu

Stephen Honor, Ph.D., ABPP
222 Middle Country Rd., Suite 215
Smithtown, NY 11787, USA
(631) 979-6226
shonorphd@juno.com

Doug Johnson-Greene, Ph.D., ABPP
Assistant Professor of Physical Medicine and
Rehabilitation
Johns Hopkins University School of
Medicine
Good Samaritan POB Suite 406,
5601 Lock raven Blvd.
Baltimore, MD 21239, USA
Phone: (410) 532-4700
johnsong@jhmi.edu

Michael F. Martelli, Ph.D., ABPP
Director, Medical Psychology and
Rehabilitation Neuropsychology
Concussion Care Centre, and Tree of Life
10120 West Broad Street, Suites G-H
Glen Allen, Virginia 23060, USA
(804) 747-8429
MFMartelli@ccc-ltd.com

Thomas A. Martin, Psy.D., ABPP
Missouri Rehabilitation Center
600 N. Main Street
Mt. Vernon, MO 65712, USA
(417) 461-5238
martinta@health.missouri.edu

A. John McSweeny, Ph.D. ABPP
Medical College of Ohio
Department of Psychiatry
3120 Glendale Avenue
Toledo, OH 43614-5809, USA
(419) 383-5665
jmcsweeny@mco.edu

Paul J. Moberg, Ph.D., ABPP
Hospital of the University of Pennsylvania
Brain Behavior Lab., Dept. of Psychiatry
10th Floor Gates Bldg.
3400 Spruce St.
Philadelphia, PA 19104, USA
(215) 662-2826
moberg@bbl.med.upenn.edu

Joel E. Morgan, Ph.D., ABPP
Assistant Professor of Neurosciences,
UMDNJ-New Jersey Medical School
49 Greenwood Drive
Millburn, NJ 07041, USA
973-921-2889
joelmor@comcast.net

Richard I. Naugle, Ph.D., ABPP
Cleveland Clinic Foundation
9500 Euclid Avenue (P57)
Cleveland, OH 44195-0001, USA
(216) 444-7748
naugler@ccf.org

Keith Nicholson, Ph.D.
Psychologist
Comprehensive Pain Program
Toronto Western Hospital
4th Floor, Fell Pavillion, Room 4F-811
399 Bathurst St.
Toronto, Ontario M5T 2S8
Canada

keith@uhnres.utoronto.ca
(416) 603-5800 x. 2969

James B. Pinkston, Ph.D.
LSU Health Sciences Center
Department of Neurology
1501 Kings Highway
PO Box 33932
Shreveport, LA 71103-3932, USA
(318) 675-4679
ipinks@lsuhsc.edu

Brad L. Roper, Ph.D., ABPP
Mental Health Service (116A4)
Memphis VAMC
1030 Jefferson Ave.
Memphis, TN 38104
(901) 523-8990 ext. 5783
Brad.Roper@med.va.gov

Philip Schatz, Ph.D.
Assistant Professor of Psychology
Saint Joseph's University
Philadelphia, PA 19131, USA
pschatz@sju.edu

Abigail B. Sivan, Ph.D.
2000 Dewes St.
Glenview, IL 60025-4239, USA
(847) 730-3100
a-sivan@northwestern.edu

Jerry J. Sweet, Ph.D., ABPP
Evanston Northwestern Healthcare
909 Davis St., Suite 160
Evanston, IL 60201, USA
(847) 425-6407
j-sweet@northwestern.edu

Laetitia L. Thompson, Ph.D., ABPP
University of Colorado Health Sciences Center
Neuropsychology Lab
4200 E. 9th Avenue, #C268-29
Denver, CO 80220, USA
(303) 315-2511
laetitia.thompson@uchsc.edu

Wilfred G. van Gorp, Ph.D., ABPP
Professor of Clinical Psychology and
Director, Neuropsychology
Columbia University
College of Physicians and Surgeons
Department of Psychiatry
16 E. 60th St., Suite 400
New York, NY 10022, USA
(212) 543-6940
vangorp@pi.cpmc.columbia.edu

Elisabeth A. Wilde, Ph.D.
Cognitive Neuroscience Laboratory
Baylor College of Medicine
6560 Fannin St., Suite 1144, Box 67
Houston, TX 77030, USA
(713) 798-7331 office
ewilde@bcm.tmc.edu

Allan Yozawitz, Ph.D., ABPP
1101 Erie Blvd. E., Suite 207
Syracuse, New York 13210, USA
(315) 472-7947
yozawitza@aol.com

AUTHOR INDEX

SUBJECT INDEX